Ball and Moore's
Essential Physics for Radiographers

Other titles of interest

Imaging Science
P. Carter
978-0-632-05656-9

MRI in Practice
Third Edition
C. Westbrook, C. Kaut, J. Talbot
978-1-4051-2787-5

Handbook of MRI Technique
Third Edition
C. Westbrook
978-1-4051-6085-8

Review Questions for MRI
C. Kaut and W. Faulkener
978-0-632-03905-0

Chesneys' Radiographic Imaging
Sixth Edition
J. Ball and T. Price
978-0-632-03901-2

Ball and Moore's
Essential Physics for Radiographers

John Ball
TDCR FBIS
Formerly Principal
South West Wales
School of Radiography
Swansea

Adrian D. Moore
MA TDCR FCR
Professor of Health Sciences
Dean of Faculty of Science and Technology
Pro Vice-Chancellor
Anglia Ruskin University
Cambridge

Steve Turner
MSc TDCR DRI
Head of Division of Radiography
Birmingham City University
Birmingham

Fourth Edition

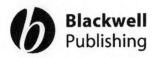
Blackwell
Publishing

This edition first published 2008
© 2008, 1986, 1979 by Blackwell Science Ltd, a Blackwell Publishing company
© 2008 by John Ball, Adrian Moore and Steve Turner

Blackwell Publishing was acquired by John Wiley & Sons in February 2007. Blackwell's publishing programme has been merged with Wiley's global Scientific, Technical, and Medical business to form Wiley-Blackwell.

Registered office
John Wiley & Sons Ltd, The Atrium, Southern Gate, Chichester, West Sussex, PO19 8SQ, United Kingdom

Editorial office
9600 Garsington Road, Oxford, OX4 2DQ, United Kingdom

For details of our global editorial offices, for customer services and for information about how to apply for permission to reuse the copyright material in this book please see our website at www.wiley.com/wiley-blackwell.

Library of Congress Cataloging-in-Publication Data

Ball, John, TDCR.
Ball and Moore's essential physics for radiographers / John Ball, Adrian D. Moore, Steve Turner. – 4th ed.
   p. ; cm.
  Rev. ed. of: Essential physics for radiographers / John Ball, Adrian D. Moore. 3rd ed. 1997.
  Includes bibliographical references and index.
  ISBN-13: 978-1-4051-6101-5 (pbk. : alk. paper)
  ISBN-10: 1-4051-6101-9 (pbk : alk. paper)
  1. Medical physics.   2. Radiography.   I. Moore, Adrian D. II. Turner, Steve, 1950–   III. Ball, John.
Essential physics for radiographers.   IV. Title.   V. Title: Essential physics for radiographers.
  [DNLM: 1. Health Physics.   2. Radiography. WN 110 B187b 2008]

  R895.B28 2008
  610.1'53–dc22

                                             2007044467

A catalogue record for this book is available from the British Library.

Set in 10/12 Palatino by Aptara Inc., New Delhi, India
Printed in Singapore by C.O.S. Printers Pte Ltd

9 2015

Contents

Preface

The decade leading up to the publication of the third edition of *Essential Physics for Radiographers* in 1997 saw a revolution in the education and training of radiographers in the UK. By contrast, the 10 years which have elapsed since then have been a period of consolidation. Although in most 'schools of radiography' traditional physics and equipment are no longer taught as separate subjects, we have remained faithful to our original concept of focusing on the physical principles underpinning radiography and have resisted the temptation to write an integrated physics and equipment book. Our aim remains to ensure the 'essential physics' on which the integrated approach is based is made clear and readily understandable to students. Consequently, some sections remain largely unchanged except for the updating of references to the applications of physical principles.

However, the introduction of new radiation safety legislation in the past decade demanded that we employ a more drastic approach to the revision of the chapter on radiation safety. With this in mind, and with an eye on the future of 'Ball and Moore', we took the opportunity to invite long-time friend and colleague Steve Turner onto our writing team. Steve has brought a fresh mind and valuable expertise to the project. He has contributed the whole of Chapter 21 as well as influencing the revision of other chapters.

We have retained the extremely successful and popular innovations introduced in the last edition: the *Maths Help File*, decimal numbering of paragraphs and sections, and reference citations, updated to include Internet sources. The physical principles of magnetic resonance imaging form the basis of a new chapter, Chapter 23.

We are happy to acknowledge the help we have received from many sources during the 2-year revision period. As always, we have been sustained in our efforts by the support and encouragement offered by our professional colleagues and by our friends and families. We also thank the editorial staff of Blackwell Publishing for their continuing commitment to our work.

John Ball
Adrian D. Moore
Steve Turner
2007

How to use the Maths Help File

A note to the reader

It has been our experience as teachers that students of radiological physics are frequently confused by some of its mathematical aspects. Often, the student may merely need to be reminded of the mathematical procedures involved. In other cases, the student may be totally unfamiliar with a particular procedure or concept and will benefit from a fuller explanation.

To overcome these difficulties, we have provided an appendix called the *Maths Help File*, following Chapter 23, which offers extra help on some of the mathematical methods and concepts found in the main text.

As you work through the book, you will encounter the *Maths Help File* icon in the left-hand margin, particularly alongside many of the mathematical worked examples, e.g.

The icon indicates that extra help is available, if you require it, in the *Maths Help File*. The number on the calculator (e.g. 12) tells you in which section of the *Maths Help File* you will find guidance and explanation relevant to the specific mathematical problem involved.

We hope that you will find the *Maths Help File* both easy to use and a valuable resource.

Chapter 1
General Physics

1.1   Energy and matter

Physics is concerned with the study of two concepts: energy and matter, and the relationships between them.

1.1.1   Energy

Energy is described as the ability to do work. Consider what would happen if there were no energy available. Without energy nothing would happen, nothing would ever change and nothing would ever get done. Energy is needed to make things happen. It exists in many forms and can be converted from one form to another, e.g.

- The human body converts chemical energy (obtained from the food we eat and the oxygen we breathe) into energy of movement (kinetic energy) when we walk or run.
- Light energy is converted into electrical energy in a solar-powered electronic calculator.

1.1.1.1   Conservation of energy

As well as being converted from one form to another, energy can also be stored, but it is not possible to create or destroy energy. In other words, in a self-contained or closed system (i.e. one with no 'leaks') the total amount of energy does not change. This concept is embodied in the **law of conservation of energy**, which states that the total energy in the universe is constant. This concept is fundamental to our understanding of physics.

1.1.2   *Matter*

Matter is the name given to the material of which all things, including us, are made. It normally exists in one or more of the three main physical states of matter **solid**, **liquid** and **gas**, but it may also exist in **liquid crystal** and **plasma** states.

Matter can be converted from one form to another by physical or chemical means, e.g.

- Ice can be melted and turned from a solid into a liquid. This is a *physical* change because both the solid and the liquid are made of the same substance (water). The process is reversible: liquid water can be frozen back into ice.
- Wood can be burned and changed into ash. This is a *chemical* change because wood and ash are fundamentally different materials. Although it is not possible to reverse this process by converting ash back into wood, some chemical changes *are* reversible; e.g. the chemical combination of oxygen with the haemoglobin of red blood cells, which takes place in the lungs, is reversed when oxygen is released from haemoglobin in the tissues.

1.1.2.1   Is matter conserved?

In most everyday situations, when a physical or chemical change occurs matter is neither created nor destroyed: the total amount of matter involved remains constant. For example, when melted, a 1-kilogram block of ice forms 1 kilogram of liquid water: there is no net gain or loss of matter. In the case of the burning of wood, however, matter does not at first sight appear to have been conserved: 1 kilogram of wood produces less than 1 kilogram of ash. Nevertheless, if all the matter involved in the process is taken into account (i.e. the oxygen gas consumed and the smoke particles, gases and water vapours produced during combustion), a balance *can* be demonstrated and it is found that matter *has* been conserved.

For many years, the conservation of matter was believed to be as fundamental a concept as the conservation of energy. All the experiments and observations seemed to confirm that matter was indeed conserved. Since the beginning of the twentieth century, however, it has been known that there are processes in which matter is *not* conserved; e.g. the nuclear fusion process which generates the energy output of the sun involves a net loss of matter and a net gain of energy. Consequently, although the conservation of matter remains a useful concept, it no longer warrants the status of a physical law because it is not universally true.

1.1.3   *The relationship between energy and matter*

Albert Einstein showed that energy and matter are not two entirely different concepts and that it is possible to convert one into the other. It seems that matter is a special form of stored energy and, in certain circumstances, its energy can be released and used.

Einstein's famous equation $E = mc^2$ (see Section 17.2.4) quantifies the relationship between matter and energy. It shows us that the conversion of only a minute amount of matter releases an enormous quantity of energy (as in a nuclear explosion). Conversely, a massive amount of energy must be converted to produce even a small quantity of matter.

In some respects, energy is rather like money:

- You can do lots of things with it, but you cannot do an awful lot without it!
- Energy can be converted from one form to another (just as currency can be converted, e.g. from US dollars to pounds sterling).
- Energy can be stored, e.g. in an electrical battery, and released on demand (rather like keeping cash in a purse or trouser pocket).
- Energy can be converted into matter (and money can be converted into assets, e.g. by buying antiques) and can be released when required. (The assets can be realised by selling the antiques!)

However, it is wise not to take this analogy too far. For example, one would hope to make a profit when selling an antique, but energy stored as matter neither appreciates nor depreciates over a period of time. Moreover, when energy is obtained from its conversion from matter, it may not necessarily appear in the most desirable form; e.g. it often appears as **internal energy** (Section 2.1) rather than as the more versatile electrical energy.

1.2   Measurement and units

Physics is concerned with quantities. As well as knowing what and why things happen, physicists also like to know *how much*; i.e. measurements are essential in physics.

In order for measurements to have meaning, units of measurement have to be created and be widely accepted among those who are going to make and use the measurements.

In science, there is a vast range of different quantities that may require measurement, each of these quantities requiring its own properly defined unit of measurement (Darton & Clark, 1994). Furthermore, relationships often exist between different quantities. For example, relationships exist between the quantities *speed*, *distance* and *time*:

$$\text{Speed} = \frac{\text{distance}}{\text{time}} \qquad \text{Distance} = \text{speed} \times \text{time} \qquad \text{Time} = \frac{\text{distance}}{\text{speed}}$$

The same relationships must apply between the *units* of speed, distance and time; i.e. the units must be mutually compatible.

1.2.1   Systems of units

A comprehensive set of properly defined and mutually compatible units of measurement is termed a *system* of units. A number of such systems have evolved or been devised and are discussed in the following sections.

1.2.1.1 British imperial system

This system evolved over hundreds of years and was in common use in the United Kingdom until recently, both in everyday life and in engineering. Imperial units include the *foot* (length), the *pound* (mass) and the *second* (time). Interestingly, in the year 1305, the yard (=3 feet) was defined as the length of the arm of King Edward I, while the inch (=one-twelfth of a foot) was the width of a thumb (Ramsey, 1970). Although more precise definitions were to follow, the imperial system has largely been abandoned in science and engineering, but it is still widely used in everyday life despite attempts to phase it out.

1.2.1.2 Continental or metric system

This is a system for which Napoleon Bonaparte was partly responsible. Its units include the *centimetre* (length), the *gram* (mass) and the *second* (time). The metre (=100 centimetres) was originally defined as one ten-millionth part of a quadrant of the earth's circumference, while the gram was the mass of one cubic centimetre of water. Again, these early definitions were later refined or replaced by more constant standards. This metric *centimetre–gram–second*, or 'cgs', system has a long tradition of application in science, and examples may still be seen in many scientific texts written before the mid-1960s.

1.2.1.3 International System of Units (in French, Le Système International d'Unités)

This is the name adopted by the *Eleventh General Conference on Weights and Measures*, held in Paris in 1960, for a universal, unified, self-consistent system of measurement units. The international system is commonly referred to as *SI*, after the initials of Système International. Its units include the *metre* (length), the *kilogram* (mass) and the *second* (time). This system is now used throughout the world in science and engineering and is gradually gaining more general everyday use in Europe and, to a lesser extent, in the USA. However, it is not uncommon for UK radiographers to quote X-ray film and cassette sizes in inches (e.g. 17″ × 14″, 12″ × 10″, etc.), even though for over 30 years manufacturers' catalogues have specified these dimensions in centimetres (e.g. 35 × 43 cm, 24 × 30 cm, etc.).

We shall use SI as our basic measuring system throughout this book, although other units will be included where appropriate.

1.2.2 Base units and derived units

When devising a coherent system of units it is not necessary to create completely new units for each different physical quantity to be measured. Instead, it may be possible to express one quantity by combining previously established units; e.g. the quantity speed may be expressed by combining a unit of length (the metre) and a unit of time (the second) (i.e. speed may be quoted in metres per second). However, a minimum number of **base units** must be established, from which the combination or **derived units** can be constructed. In our example, the *metre* and the *second* are base units, while the *metre per second* is a derived unit.

Table 1.1   SI base units

Quantity	Unit	Symbol
Length	metre	m
Mass	kilogram	kg
Time	second	s
Electric current	ampere	A
Thermodynamic temperature	kelvin	K
Amount of substance	mole	mol
Luminous intensity	candela	cd

1.2.3   SI units

Standards have been defined for the seven base units listed in Table 1.1. The aim is to define each of the base units in terms of a laboratory procedure which can be reproduced under identical conditions throughout the world. Only the definition of the kilogram (see Section 1.3.1) fails in this respect but a new approach to defining and realising the kilogram is being explored by the **Avogadro Project** (NPL, 2007). The definitions themselves are revised periodically as the technology of measurement improves; e.g. the metre was redefined in 1983 as the length of the path travelled by light in a vacuum during a time interval of $1/299\,792\,458$ of a second. The symbols (m, kg, s, etc.) given in the right-hand column of Table 1.1 are the authorised abbreviations and are the same in all languages.

The SI units for all other quantities are derived from the seven base units. Examples of some SI-derived units, expressed in terms of base units, are shown in Table 1.2. Some derived units are used so often that they have been assigned special names, usually those of scientists or engineers, as shown in Table 1.3. In addition to the seven base units described above, there are two **supplementary units** used to express angular measurements. The **radian** (rad) is the unit for two-dimensional or *plane* angles, while the **steradian** (sr) is the unit for three-dimensional or *solid* angles. Some derived units may incorporate supplementary as well as base units; e.g. angular velocity is expressed in radians per second (rad s^{-1}).

Table 1.2   Some examples of SI-derived units, expressed in terms of base units

Quantity	Derived SI unit	Symbol
Acceleration	Metres per second squared	m s^{-2}
Area	Square metres	m^2
Density	Kilogram per cubic metre	kg m^{-3}
Luminance	Candela per square metre	cd m^{-2}
Magnetic field strength	Ampere per metre	A m^{-1}
Velocity	Metres per second	m s^{-1}
Volume	Cubic metres	m^3

Table 1.3   Some examples of SI-derived units named after scientists and engineers

Quantity	Name of unit	Symbol	Equivalent in other SI units
Absorbed dose (radiation)	gray	Gy	$J\ kg^{-1}$
Energy, work	joule	J	N m
Electrical capacitance	farad	F	$C\ V^{-1}$
Electric charge	coulomb	C	A s
Electrical potential	volt	V	$J\ C^{-1}$
Electrical resistance	ohm	Ω	$V\ A^{-1}$
Force	newton	N	$kg\ m\ s^{-2}$
Frequency	hertz	Hz	s^{-1}
Magnetic flux	weber	Wb	V s
Magnetic flux density	tesla	T	$Wb\ m^{-2}$
Power	watt	W	$J\ s^{-1}$
Pressure	pascal	Pa	$N\ m^{-2}$
Radioactivity	becquerel	Bq	s^{-1}

1.2.3.1   Conventions for writing SI units

To avoid ambiguity, there are strict conventions for the way SI units are written down:

- When abbreviated, no punctuation marks are used; e.g. 1 kilogram is written as '1 kg', *not* '1 Kg.'.
- The abbreviations have no plural form; e.g. 500 metres is written as 500 m, *not* 500 ms.
- When written in full, the names of units never commence with a capital (uppercase) letter, e.g. 310 kelvin, *not* 310 Kelvin. (Note also that no 'degree' symbol (°) is used when expressing temperature in kelvin units; write 310 K, *not* 310° K.)
- Mathematical indices notation should be used rather than the slash sign (/) when dividing units; e.g. metres per second should be abbreviated to m s^{-1}, *not* m/s.

- Abbreviation symbols employ an uppercase letter only if the unit is named after a person; e.g. 1.5 ampere is written as 1.5 A. (The ampere is named after André Marie Ampère, a nineteenth-century French scientist.) Note, however, that some prefixes employ uppercase letters in their abbreviated form (see Table 1.4).

1.2.3.2   The use of prefixes

One advantage of SI over other systems of measurement is that it is a *coherent* system; i.e. its derived units are expressed as products and ratios of the base and derived units, *without the need for numerical conversion factors*. Unfortunately, this results in some units being far too large for practical purposes and others far too small. For example, the SI unit of radioactivity (the becquerel) is so miniscule that even the very low activities of the radiopharmaceuticals used for radionuclide

Table 1.4 Some of the prefixes used with SI base and derived units[a]

Multiplication factor	Prefix	Symbol
10^9	Giga	G
10^6	Mega	M
10^3	Kilo	k
10^{-1}	Deci	d
10^{-2}	Centi	c
10^{-3}	Milli	m
10^{-6}	Micro	μ
10^{-9}	Nano	n
10^{-12}	Pico	p

[a] Only those most commonly encountered in radiographic science are included.

imaging have to be measured in millions or even billions of becquerels (see Chapter 20). To overcome this difficulty, prefixes such as those given in Table 1.4 are used with base and derived units. Examples relevant to radiography include the *gigabecquerel* (GBq), *megajoule* (MJ), *kilovolt* (kV), *centigray* (cGy), *milliampere* (mA), *microfarad* (μF) and *nanometre* (nm). Because double prefixes are not used, and because the base unit name *kilogram* already contains a prefix, prefixes are used with the gram rather than the kilogram, so a gram (equal to one-thousandth of a kilogram) is never called a millikilogram!

1.3 Physical quantities

In physics many commonplace terms have very specialised meanings. We shall consider five of the most important quantities: mass, force, work, energy and power.

1.3.1 Mass

Matter, the material of which everything is made, can be quantified in a number of ways. For example, we could express the amount of matter in a body by:

- Stating the number of *elementary particles* (e.g. atoms or molecules) it contains. The SI unit known as the **mole** is based on this approach. One mole of matter contains 6×10^{23} elementary particles. (6×10^{23} is a fundamental physical constant known as **Avogadro's number**.)
- Judging how successfully the body resists an attempt to change its state of rest or its state of movement. In other words, we can measure a quantity of matter by reference to its *inertia* (if it is at rest) or its *momentum* (if it is in motion).

Mass is a method of quantifying matter based on the latter approach. The kilogram is the SI unit of mass.

Definition. The kilogram is the mass of the *International Prototype Kilogram*, a platinum–iridium cylinder kept at Sèvres near Paris in France.

1.3.2   Force

Physical sciences are concerned with understanding why things happen. Every effect must have a cause. Consider two simple observations:

- If we release a pencil we are holding, it falls.
- If we are cycling along a level track and stop pedalling, we slow down and eventually come to a halt.

Why is this so? Although the two events described above at first seem quite different, there are similarities between them, which suggest a common cause. In both cases, a *change* in the motion has occurred. In general, a change in the motion of an object is said to be due to the presence of a force. In the case of the falling pencil, the force causing it to fall is called the force of gravity; in the case of the cycle, it is the forces of air resistance and friction which cause it to slow down and stop.

Force is thus a generalised concept, which encompasses all the various reasons why objects speed up, slow down or change their direction of travel. In 1687, Sir Isaac Newton encapsulated this idea in his first law of motion: *a body will continue in its state of rest or uniform motion in a straight line, unless it is acted upon by an external force.* In other words, force is the *agency* by which a body's state of motion is changed.

In physics, any change in the motion of a body is described as acceleration, so we can deduce that acceleration is *always* caused by the action of one or more forces. There are many different kinds of forces: electric forces, magnetic forces, mechanical forces, as well as the gravitational and resistance forces mentioned above, but each of these forces satisfies the general description set out in the definition of a force.

Definition. Force is that which disturbs the state of rest or uniform motion of a body.

The unit of force is obtained by specifying the amount of acceleration achieved when a force is applied to a body of known mass. A simple relationship exists between a force (F), the mass (m) and the acceleration (a), which results:

$$F = ma$$

In SI units, mass is expressed in kilograms and acceleration in metres per second squared ($m\ s^{-2}$) (Table 1.2), so force is expressed in kilogram metres per second squared ($kg\ m\ s^{-2}$). This derived unit is called the **newton** (N).

Definition. A force of 1 N will produce an acceleration of $1\ m\ s^{-2}$ in a body whose mass is 1 kg, if it is free to move and not acted upon by any other forces.

1.3.2.1   Scalar and vector quantities

When describing a force it is not enough to quote the magnitude (i.e. strength) of the force, e.g. 6 N. It is also necessary to specify its direction, e.g. vertically downwards. Quantities such as this, having direction as well as magnitude, are known as *vector* quantities, or *vectors*. Quantities having only magnitude (e.g. mass) are known as *scalar* quantities.

1.3.2.2   Gravitational force

On the earth's surface, when a body is released it falls downwards, accelerating at a rate of 9.81 m s^{-2} (i.e. every second its downward speed increases by 9.81 m s^{-1}). This value of acceleration is often called *g*, the acceleration due to gravity. In 1589, Galileo is reported to have performed a famous experiment in which he dropped two cannonballs of different masses from the top of the Leaning Tower of Pisa in Italy. Because the two objects hit the ground at the same time, Galileo had confirmed that the value of *g* was the same for both masses. Further investigation led Galileo to conclude that the value of *g* was the same for *all* values of mass. In 1971, the astronaut Alan Shepard repeated Galileo's experiment on the surface of the Moon, using a feather and a hammer instead of cannonballs. It was an effective, if crude, confirmation of Galileo's findings.

The gravitational force acting on a body (commonly known as its weight) is the agency which causes it to accelerate downwards, so the relationship $F = ma$ applies. In this case the force is the weight of the body (*W*), the mass is *m* and the acceleration is *g*. Thus, $F = ma$ becomes

$$W = mg$$

This tells us, for example, that the weight of a 1-kg mass is 9.81 N. When we support a 1-kg bag of sugar on our hand, we are experiencing a force slightly less than 10 N. This gives us an idea of the size, in everyday terms, of the SI unit of force.

Force fields and field strength
It may be timely here to introduce the general concept of a **force field**, which is simply the name given to a region in which forces are acting. We can specify the magnitude of such a force field by quoting its **field strength**.

Gravitational field strength
The **gravitational field strength** at a particular location is the strength of gravitational force (i.e. weight) experienced by one unit of mass placed at that location. In SI units, gravitational field strength is expressed in newtons (of force) per kilogram (of mass), or N kg^{-1}. At the earth's surface, the gravitational field strength is therefore 9.81 N kg^{-1}. A similar concept can be applied to other types of force fields, e.g. an electric field (see Section 3.4.2).

The difference between mass and weight
No matter where we are on the earth's surface, the value of *g* is practically the same. In these circumstances, weight is *directly proportional* to mass and we are accustomed to using our weight (e.g. as measured on bathroom scales) to indicate how 'massive' we are.

For astronauts, the situation is more complex because they may experience gravitational forces very different from our own. On the moon's surface, the acceleration due to gravity is only 1.62 m s^{-2}, about one-sixth of that on the earth's surface (Moore & Hunt, 1997). An astronaut's weight measured on *lunar* bathroom scales would be only one-sixth of its terrestrial value. However, the astronaut's mass would *not* have changed because the mass of a body is independent of the value of gravitational field strength. A stretcher trolley bearing an obese patient would be just as difficult to manoeuvre around the tortuous corridors of a lunar hospital as it would here on earth because it is the *inertia* of the patient and trolley (which depends only on mass) rather than their weight (which depends on gravity and mass) that creates most of the problems. However, a moon-based radiographer would find it a lot easier to *lift* the obese patient if that proved necessary!

1.3.3 Work

If a force succeeds in changing the motion of a body we say that *work* has been done and we define the work done as the product of the magnitude of the force and the distance moved; i.e.

Work done = force × distance moved
(in the direction of the force)

The SI units in which work is measured are newton metres (i.e. newtons × metres) and are called *joules* (J) (1 joule = 1 newton metre).

The scientific meaning of the term 'work' can produce consequences which seem at odds with our everyday experiences. Suppose a patient has collapsed on the floor and we try to lift him onto a stretcher trolley. If we succeed in lifting him up we have done work (we have applied a force, the lift, and moved the patient through a certain distance upwards in the direction of the force).

So far, so good. But what if, despite our exertions, we were unable to lift the unfortunate patient because of his weight? The physicist would say we had done *no* work on the patient because we had not moved him. However, we may well feel that we tried very hard to achieve the lift and even though our efforts were in vain we had definitely been working!

Work can be thought of as being energy *usefully* expended, and since, in our example, we did not move the patient in the direction of our applied force, any energy we used was 'wasted'.

1.3.4 Energy

As we saw in Section 1.1.1, energy is defined as the ability to do work.

Its SI unit of measurement is the same as the unit of work, i.e. the joule. In fact, the joule is a rather small unit and we shall meet larger units of energy later.

Energy can appear in many forms, e.g. potential energy and kinetic energy.

1.3.4.1 Potential energy

This is the energy stored in a body due to its position or state; e.g. a compressed spring and a book on a shelf have potential energy (often abbreviated to PE).

The potential energy possessed by a body is equal to the amount of work required to 'raise' the body to its particular position or state.

Potential energy is a *relative* quantity; it has no absolute value. It is always quoted in relation to some chosen reference level or baseline, which may be stated explicitly, but is often merely implied. For a compressed spring, the baseline might be the relaxed state of the spring; for the book on the shelf, a sensible choice of baseline would be floor level. At floor level, the book would be said to have zero potential energy. Raising the book above floor level would increase its potential energy *above* zero (i.e. its potential energy would have a *positive* value). Taking the book downstairs to the floor below would reduce its potential energy *below* zero (i.e. its potential energy would take on a *negative* value).

Although bodies have a natural tendency to move from a high (positive) potential-energy state, or position, to one which is lower (i.e. less positive, or more negative), whether they actually achieve this reduction in potential energy depends on the presence or absence of factors preventing change. For example, a ball has a natural tendency to roll down a slope, but it cannot do so if we put an obstacle in its path.

Worked example

Let us consider a case involving gravitational potential energy. Suppose a 50-kg patient seated in a wheelchair has to be lifted onto an examination couch which is 25 cm higher than the wheelchair. How much work must be done to achieve such a task and how much potential energy will the patient acquire as a result?

From our discussion of work in Section 1.3.3, we know that:

Work done = force × distance

In our present example, the minimum force required is equal to the weight (W) of the patient since we need to apply an upward force of at least this magnitude in order to raise the patient. From Section 1.3.2.1:

$W = mg$

and because $m = 50$ kg, and $g = 9.81$ m s^{-2}, the weight of the patient must be:

$W = 50 \times 9.81$ N

The patient is raised through a distance of 25 cm, but we must convert this into metres in order to be consistent with the other units we are using (25 cm = 0.25 m).

We can now calculate the work done in raising the patient:

Work done = force × distance (which, in this case, is weight × height, or *mgh*)

$\quad\quad\quad\quad$ = $50 \times 9.81 \times 0.25$ N m

$\quad\quad\quad\quad$ = 120 N m (to two significant figures)

$\quad\quad\quad\quad$ = 120 J

So, 120 J of work has to be done to lift the patient.

How does this affect the potential energy possessed by the patient? Reference to the statements at the beginning of this section confirms that the patient's potential energy will have been increased by an amount equal to the work done in lifting him. In other words, his potential energy will be increased by 120 J.

1.3.4.2   Kinetic energy

This is the energy possessed by a body because of its movement; e.g. both a falling X-ray cassette and a moving stretcher trolley have kinetic energy (as we would no doubt appreciate if we happened to get in their way!).

The kinetic energy (KE) of a body depends on its mass (*m*) and its speed or velocity (*v*), linked by the relationship:

$$KE = \frac{1}{2}mv^2$$

Worked example

Suppose a 35 × 43-cm X-ray cassette is accidentally knocked off a shelf onto the floor. The shelf is 1.50 m high and the cassette has a mass of 2.00 kg. How much kinetic energy will the cassette possess at the instant it hits the floor, and how fast will it then be travelling? The best way of approaching the problem is to first find the kinetic energy and then from that compute the speed.

To determine the kinetic energy we must consider the *origin* of the cassette's kinetic energy. Its kinetic energy is the result of the conversion of the potential energy possessed by the cassette when it was resting on the shelf. As we saw in our earlier worked example:

$$PE = mgh(\text{i.e. weight} \times \text{height})$$

so

$$PE = 2 \times 9.81 \times 1.50$$
$$= 29.4 \text{ J}$$

That is, when the cassette was on the shelf its potential energy was 29.4 J greater than that when it was on the floor. Remembering the principle of conservation of energy (Section 1.1.1.1), it is reasonable to assume that as the cassette fell, it converted *all* 29.4 J of its potential energy into kinetic energy. So, at the moment it struck the floor, its kinetic energy was 29.4 J. How fast was it then travelling? We know that $KE = \frac{1}{2}mv^2$ and we know the values of KE and *m*, so we should now be able to find *v*.

It is helpful to rearrange the relationship into a form which puts all the known quantities on the right-hand side of the equation:

$$v^2 = \frac{2 \times KE}{m}$$
$$= \frac{2 \times 29.4}{2}$$
$$= 29.4 \text{ m}^2\text{s}^{-2}$$

So

$$v = \sqrt{29.4}$$
$$= 5.4 \text{ m s}^{-1}$$

The cassette was therefore travelling at nearly $5\frac{1}{2}$ m s^{-1} when it struck the ground (or struck our toes if we were slow in moving out of the way!).

There are many other forms of energy in addition to the two we have considered above, e.g. chemical energy, internal energy, electrical energy, nuclear energy, sound energy, X-ray energy, etc. We shall be looking at some of these in later chapters.

1.3.5 *Power*

It may be important, on many occasions, to know the *rate* at which we are expending energy in a particular process or action. We call the rate of using energy **power**. It can also be defined as the rate of doing work; i.e.

$$\text{Power} = \frac{\text{work done}}{\text{time taken}}$$

The unit of power is therefore the joule per second ($J\ s^{-1}$). This derived unit is also known as the watt (W); i.e. 1 watt = 1 joule per second. The watt is a relatively small unit, being hundreds of times smaller than the older, more well known unit, the horse power (1 horse power = 746 watts).

The ideas introduced in this chapter will be referred to many times in later chapters. If possible, talk over the work with your tutors and with your fellow students until you are confident that you understand it. Some simple problems follow which should help you achieve a proper understanding. The answers are given in brackets after each question.

1.4 Problems

(1) An 18-month-old baby has a mass of 10 kg (22 lb). What is its weight in newtons? (Assume 'g' is 9.81 m s^{-1}.) (98.1 *N*)

(2) A volume of 1 mL of water has a mass of 1 g. What is the weight of 1 L of water? (9.81 *N*)

(3) How fast will a body be travelling after it has fallen under gravity for 10 s? (Neglect air resistance.) (98.1 *ms^{-1}*)

(4) How much work is done in lifting a 100-kg patient from the floor onto a stretcher trolley 1 m high? (981 *J*)

(5) How much power would be required to achieve this lift in 1 s? (981 *W*)

(6) How much energy would be released if the same patient fell off the stretcher trolley onto the floor? (981 *J*)

(7) At what speed would he hit the floor? (*Hint*: Think about kinetic and potential energy.) (4.3 *m s^{-1}approx.*)

(8) What force would be required to accelerate a stretcher trolley at 1 m s^{-2} if its mass is 20 kg and it carries a patient of 80 kg? (100 *N*)

(9) How fast will it be travelling if this force is maintained for 5 s? (5 *m s^{-1}*)

(10) How much energy would be needed to bring the trolley to rest? (1250 *J*)

Chapter 2
Internal Energy, Temperature and Heat

2.1 Internal energy

All matter is made up of minute particles, too small to be seen even with a good microscope. The particles are called **atoms** and **molecules**, and we shall consider them in detail in Chapter 4. The important property of these particles that we are concerned with in this chapter is the fact that they are always in motion. The type of motion depends on whether the material is a solid, liquid or gas (see Fig. 2.1).

In solids, the molecules vibrate about fairly fixed positions. This is the reason why solids do not alter their shape easily. In liquids and gases, the molecules move randomly. Liquids and gases do not have fixed shapes for this reason.

Because these particles are in constant motion, they possess **kinetic energy**. The molecules, particularly in solids and liquids, also possess **potential energy** because of the forces of attraction between them. (These **intermolecular** forces are strongest in solids and weakest, or absent altogether, in gases.) We call the total kinetic and potential energy of the molecules in a system its **internal energy**.

2.2 Temperature

The concept of temperature arises from the idea of measuring the relative hotness and coldness of a body and from the observation that increasing the internal energy of a body leads to an increase in its temperature as long as no melting or boiling occurs.

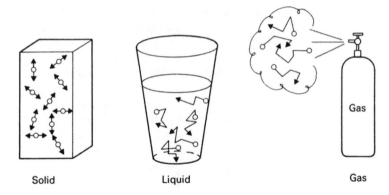

Fig. 2.1   Motion of particles in solids, liquids and gases.

The temperature of a body depends on the average kinetic energy of its particles (and hence their speed of movement). A high temperature means that the particles are in vigorous motion, while a low temperature indicates that they are moving more slowly.

Temperature is a property of a body, a material or a substance. Thus, a vacuum (or 'space') cannot have a temperature. Temperature changes in a substance are measured by observing changes taking place in its *other* properties, as discussed below.

2.2.1 *Expansion and contraction*

If the temperature of a substance is increased, it expands if free to do so; if its temperature falls, it contracts. This is because as the motion of its molecules becomes more violent they occupy more space. If the specimen is *prevented* from expanding or contracting, e.g. because it is sealed in a strong containing vessel, the changes in temperature will be associated with changes in the **pressure** the substance exerts on the walls of the vessel.

Mercury thermometers allow us to measure temperature by observing the expansion of a mercury column in a glass capillary. The change in length of the mercury column is related to the temperature change.

2.2.2 *Melting and boiling*

If the temperature of a solid is increased, it eventually melts, changing from the solid into the liquid state. If the temperature of a liquid is increased, it eventually boils and changes from a liquid into a gas.

2.2.3 *Other effects of temperature*

Changes of temperature may also be associated with numerous other effects on the property of materials; e.g. electrical resistance and conductivity may change (Section 7.4.4.3); fluids may become more or less viscous; the rate of chemical

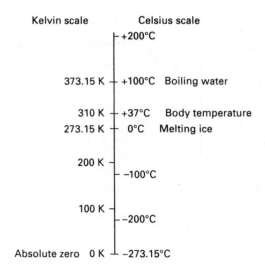

Fig. 2.2   The kelvin and Celsius scales compared.

reactions may alter (e.g. body metabolism is markedly affected by temperature, hence the need to maintain a constant body temperature).

2.2.4   Scales of temperature

The changes in the physical state of a substance from solid to liquid and from liquid to gas are easy to recognise. Furthermore, for water, these effects occur at temperature levels which are well within our everyday experience. For this reason, the melting point of ice and the boiling point of water have been used to define scales of measurement.

The **Celsius scale** divides the range between melting point and boiling point into 100 intervals called degrees (100°C). The temperature of melting ice is zero (0°C), while the temperature of boiling water is 100°C.

The **kelvin scale**, which provides the SI unit of temperature, employs intervals of the same size as Celsius degrees, but places melting ice at 273.15 K and boiling water at 373.15 K. The significance of this scale is that at zero (0 K) the atomic particles which are normally in motion are at rest. In other words, at 0 K, a body has no internal energy at all. This temperature, which has never been achieved except in the imagination, is known as **absolute zero**. Scientists have approached this temperature very closely but have not been able to bring those last few particles to rest.

The **Fahrenheit scale** divides the range between melting ice and boiling water into 180 degrees, melting ice being at 32°F and boiling water at 212°F. Body temperature is about 98.4°F, 37°C or 310 K (see Fig. 2.2).

2.3   Heat and temperature gradients

Heat is the *transfer* of internal energy from one part of a body of matter to another, or from one body to another, as a result of a difference in temperature known as a **temperature gradient**. Heat is energy in transit; its tendency is always to flow *down* a temperature gradient, i.e. from a substance at a higher temperature to a substance at a lower temperature, raising the temperature of the latter and lowering that of the former.

Consider two examples:

- A hot drink placed on a table gradually cools down because it is hotter than its surroundings. Energy is transferred down the temperature gradient from the drink to the surroundings. The surroundings get slightly warmer as a result of the energy they have gained.
- A cold drink placed on the same table gets warmer because it is colder than its surroundings. Energy is transferred down the temperature gradient from the surroundings to the drink. The surroundings get slightly cooler as a result of the energy they have lost.

In both these examples, energy is being transferred *down* a temperature gradient. If we want energy to flow *up* a temperature gradient, we have to force it to do so by doing work using a system known as a **heat pump**. For example, the environment inside a refrigerator is cooled below the temperature of its surroundings by extracting energy from inside the fridge and releasing it to its external surroundings, which become warmer as a result. An energy supply (usually electricity) is necessary to do this work.

A note about terminology. It is quite common for the terms *heat* and *heat energy* to be used when what is really meant is *internal energy*. This confusion is perhaps understandable: after all, all three are measured in the same units (joules) and many sources (including the early editions of this book!) have perpetuated the error. However, the three terms are *not* synonymous:

- *Heat* is energy transferred as a result of a temperature gradient.
- *Internal energy* is the sum of all the molecular kinetic and potential energies in an object.
- *Heat energy* is an in-between term and we should replace it either by the term *heat* or by the term *internal energy*, according to the exact meaning we wish to convey.

2.3.1   *Latent heat*

A solid at melting point or a liquid at boiling point can absorb energy without experiencing a rise of temperature. Similarly, a gas which condenses into a liquid, or a liquid which freezes into a solid, can release energy without suffering a fall in temperature. This is because rather than being used to change the kinetic energy of the particles (seen as a temperature change), the energy is used to achieve the rearrangement of particles, which characterises a change of physical state (from solid to liquid, or liquid to gas). This energy change, which is not accompanied by a change of temperature, is known as **latent heat** (i.e. 'hidden' heat). For example:

- To melt 1 kg of ice (at 0°C) into water (also at 0°C) requires about 330 kJ of energy.

- When 1 kg of liquid water (at 0°C) freezes (or 'fuses') to form ice (also at 0°C), about 330 kJ of energy is released.

We say that the **specific latent heat of fusion** for water is about 330 kJ kg^{-1}:

- To boil 1 kg of water (at 100°C) into water vapour (also at 100°C) requires about 2300 kJ of energy.
- When 1 kg of water vapour (at 100°C) is condensed into liquid water (also at 100°C), about 2300 kJ of energy is released.

We say that the **specific latent heat of vaporisation** for water is about 2300 kJ kg^{-1}. Other materials have different values of specific latent heat.

2.3.2   Heat capacity (thermal capacity)

Assuming a body does not undergo a change of state, the temperature change in a body associated with the addition or removal of internal energy depends on the amount of energy involved, the size of the body and the nature of the material of which it is made. For a particular object, the change in internal energy which accompanies a one-unit temperature change in the object is known as the **heat capacity** (or thermal capacity) of the object; i.e.

$$\text{Heat capacity} = \frac{\text{internal energy change}}{\text{temperature change}}$$

and

$$\text{Internal energy change} = \text{heat capacity} \times \text{temperature change}$$

or

$$Q = C\Delta\theta$$

where C is heat capacity, Q is internal energy change and $\Delta\theta$ is temperature change. The SI units of these quantities are as follows: internal energy change, joules (J); temperature change, kelvin (K); heat capacity, joules per kelvin (J K^{-1}).

2.3.3   Specific heat capacity

Specific heat capacity (c) is a property of a *material* or *substance* rather than a particular body or object. Like heat capacity, it expresses the change in internal energy associated with a unit change in temperature but for a *unit mass* of substance; i.e.

$$\text{Specific heat capacity} = \frac{\text{internal energy change}}{\text{temperature change} \times \text{mass}}$$

or

$$\text{Internal energy change} = \text{mass} \times \text{specific heat capacity} \times \text{temperature change}$$

and

$$Q = mc\Delta\theta$$

Table 2.1 Examples of specific heat capacity (c)

Material	Specific heat capacity (c) ($J kg^{-1} K^{-1}$)
Tungsten	130
Rhenium	130
Lead	130
Molybdenum	250
Copper	380
Steel	500
Glass	700
Carbon (graphite)	710
Aluminium	910
Water	4200

where m represents mass. The SI unit of specific heat capacity is the joule per kilogram kelvin ($J kg^{-1}K^{-1}$). Table 2.1 shows examples of the values of specific heat capacity for different materials.

2.3.4 Heat sinks

A component designed with a large heat capacity is able to absorb vast quantities of heat, with only a small change in temperature. Such a component, known as a **heat sink**, is extremely useful because it can store a potentially dangerous amount of energy, without reaching excessively high temperatures. In a modern X-ray tube, the component known as the **anode disc** is designed to act as a heat sink, absorbing the energy placed on it by a heavy radiography workload, yet remaining well below its melting point (see Section 12.5.2).

Examination of Table 2.1 enables us to identify which materials are likely to make good heat sinks. Those with high specific heat capacity will resist temperature changes better than those with low values, so water seems outstanding in this respect. Indeed, for some purposes water makes an excellent temperature stabiliser; e.g. because the human body consists largely of water, it has a natural resistance to temperature change, increasing the effectiveness of its sophisticated physiological temperature-regulating systems. The presence of vast quantities of water in the earth's oceans plays a large part in maintaining the planet at an equable temperature. However, for some applications, e.g. for the anode of an X-ray tube, water is totally unsuitable as a heat sink material, not least because it would vaporise at the temperatures encountered inside an X-ray tube!

Worked example
The anode disc of an X-ray tube is made largely of molybdenum and has a mass of 0.7 kg. During a very rapid angiographic exposure series, 75 kJ of energy is deposited on the anode disc. Ignoring any energy lost *during* the exposure series, estimate the approximate temperature rise experienced by the anode disc. (Specific heat capacity of molybdenum is approximately 250 $J kg^{-1} K^{-1}$.)

Remember the relationship given in Section 2.3.3:

Internal energy change = mass × specific heat capacity × temperature change

which we expressed symbolically as:

$$Q = mc\,\Delta\theta$$

which can also be written as:

$$\Delta\theta = \frac{Q}{mc}$$

In our problem, we know the values of:

Internal energy change, $Q = 75\text{ kJ} = 75 \times 10^3 \text{ J}$
Mass, $m = 0.70\text{ kg}$
Specific heat capacity, $c = 250\text{ J kg}^{-1}\text{ K}^{-1}$

So, we should be able to calculate the value of the temperature rise, $\Delta\theta$:

$$\begin{aligned}
\Delta\theta &= \frac{Q}{mc} \\
&= \frac{75 \times 10^3}{0.7 \times 250} \\
&= 430\text{ K (corrected to two significant figures)}
\end{aligned}$$

Discussion. Our calculations show that the anode disc would experience a rise in temperature of around 430 K. If we assume the anode was at room temperature (say, 20°C or 293 K) before the angiographic exposure, then its temperature would rise by 430 K to about 720 K. This is well below the melting point of molybdenum (approximately 2900 K).

Note that to simplify our calculation, we chose to ignore the fact that some of the energy deposited on the anode would, in reality, have been dissipated during the exposure series. This suggests that our answer is an overestimate of the actual temperature rise but, even so, it is probably not too far from the truth. Certainly, one can infer that repeating the exposure series a number of times, without allowing time for the anode to cool down, could eventually cause overheating and endanger the integrity of the anode disc. To avoid this problem, the anodes of some modern heavy-duty X-ray tubes are designed to hold several megajoules of energy without damage.

2.4   Conduction, convection and radiation

There are three mechanisms through which energy is transferred by heat: **conduction**, **convection** and **radiation**. Although these processes can occur simultaneously, it is not uncommon for one process to predominate over the other two. For example, conduction is the dominant process in solids, convection in fluids (liquids and gases), and radiation in a vacuum.

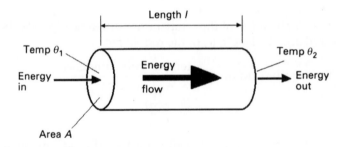

Fig. 2.3   Energy being conducted through a solid rod.

2.4.1   *Conduction*

In solids, heat transfers energy by conduction. This is the transfer of internal energy through the material by collisions between neighbouring atoms. In this way the vibrational energy of the molecules is able to spread throughout the entire solid.

Figure 2.3 shows a solid rod of length l and uniform cross-sectional area A. One end of the rod is maintained at temperature θ_1 and the other end at a lower temperature θ_2. Thus, a **temperature gradient** is established across the ends of the rod. In these circumstances, as we saw in Section 2.3, energy will flow down the temperature gradient. Energy injected at the high-temperature end will flow (by conduction) along the rod and leave at the low-temperature end. For the purposes of this discussion we will assume that the rod is surrounded by thermal insulation such that no energy is lost or gained through its sides; i.e. there is no 'leakage' of energy. Scientists performed experiments under the above conditions to investigate the factors on which the rate of flow of energy through a solid depends. Rate of flow of energy, which means the quantity of energy (Q) entering (or leaving) one end of the rod in one unit of time, is represented by the term dQ/dt, which in SI units would be expressed in joules per second.

2.4.1.1   Factors affecting conduction

Cross-sectional area (A)
The greater the value of A, the greater the rate of energy flow. In fact, the rate of flow is *directly proportional* to cross-sectional area:

$$\frac{dQ}{dt} \propto A$$

An engineer designing a rod-shaped component to encourage rapid heat flow would bear this in mind. The anode stem of a stationary-anode X-ray tube employs this principle (Section 12.8.2). Conversely, if the purpose of a rod-shaped component was to inhibit heat flow, a narrow rod, with a small cross-sectional area, would be more suitable. The anode stem in a rotating-anode X-ray tube follows this pattern (see Section 12.8.1 and the worked example at the end of this section).

Temperature gradient

This is a combination of the temperature difference $(\theta_1 - \theta_2)$ between the ends of the rod and the length (l) of the rod. In fact:

$$\text{Temperature gradient} = \frac{\text{temperature difference}}{\text{length}}$$

$$= \frac{(\theta_1 - \theta_2)}{l}$$

In SI units, temperature gradient is measured in kelvin per metre (K m^{-1}). It represents the suddenness with which temperature changes with distance. Rate of heat flow is *directly proportional* to temperature gradient:

$$\frac{dQ}{dt} \propto \frac{(\theta_1 - \theta_2)}{l}$$

Thermal conductivity (k)

Some materials are inherently better conductors of internal energy than are others. In particular, *metals* (iron, copper, aluminium, etc.) are better thermal conductors than are *non-metals* (carbon, wood, brick, plastics, etc.). The property of a material which affects its inherent ability to conduct thermal energy is called its **thermal conductivity** (k). In SI units, thermal conductivity is measured in joules per second metre kelvin $(\text{J s}^{-1}\,\text{m}^{-1}\,\text{K}^{-1})$, but because the joule per second is known as a watt (Section 1.3.5), the unit of thermal conductivity is often quoted as the watt per metre kelvin $(\text{W m}^{-1}\,\text{K}^{-1})$. For the experimental set-up illustrated in Fig. 2.3, the rate of heat flow is *directly proportional* to thermal conductivity:

$$\frac{dQ}{dt} \propto k$$

Examples of the values of thermal conductivity for various materials are listed in Table 2.2. Note, however, that the thermal conductivity of a substance is not necessarily constant; e.g. for metals, its value tends to decrease as temperature increases.

The three factors affecting the rate of conduction of energy can be combined into one expression:

$$\frac{dQ}{dt} = kA\frac{(\theta_1 - \theta_2)}{l}$$

But strictly, this formula can only be applied to conditions similar to those illustrated in Fig. 2.3, where no leakage of energy takes place, i.e. where the energy flow is parallel to the long axis of the conductor.

Worked example

A component consists of a solid molybdenum cylinder, with length 30 mm and diameter 5.0 mm. One end of the cylinder is at a temperature of 2000 K, while the temperature of the other end is kept below 600 K. Estimate the maximum rate at which thermal energy is being conducted through the component, assuming no leakage of energy occurs along its length. The thermal conductivity of molybdenum is approximately 100 $\text{W m}^{-1}\,\text{K}^{-1}$ under these conditions.

Table 2.2 Examples of approximate values of thermal conductivity (*k*) at room temperature (20°C) and at 500°C

Material	Thermal conductivity (k) (W m^{-1} K^{-1})	
	At 20°C	At 500°C
Silver	420	380
Copper	400	350
Aluminium	240	90 (liquid Al)[a]
Tungsten	170	120
Molybdenum	140	110
Carbon (graphite)	80–200[b]	30–70[b]
Steel	50	30
Rhenium	50	45
Lead	35	20 (liquid Pb)[a]
Glass	1	—
Brick	1	1

[a] 500°C is above the melting point of aluminium and lead, so the thermal conductivity values quoted refer to these metals in their liquid states.
[b] The thermal conductivity of graphite depends on the direction of measurement in relation to the sample, so a range of values of k is given.

We shall need to use the relationship

$$\frac{dQ}{dt} = kA\frac{(\theta_1 - \theta_2)}{l}$$

We must express all the known values in SI units:

Thermal conductivity, $k = 100$ Wm^{-1} K^{-1}

Cross-sectional area, $A = \pi r^2$, where $r = 2.5$ mm or 2.5×10^{-3} m

(radius is half the diameter)

$$= \pi \times 6.25 \times 10^{-6}$$

$$= 19.6 \times 10^{-6} \text{ m}^2$$

Temperature difference, $\theta_1 - \theta_2 = 2000 - 600$

$$= 1400 \text{ K}$$

Length of cylinder, $l = 30$ mm

$$= 30 \times 10^{-3} \text{ m}$$

So,

$$\frac{dQ}{dt} = kA\frac{(\theta_1 - \theta_2)}{l}$$

$$= \frac{100 \times 19.6 \times 10^{-6} \times 1400}{30 \times 10^{-3}}$$

$$= 91 \text{ W (corrected to two significant figures)}$$

Therefore, no more than about 90 W (i.e. 90 J s^{-1}) of energy will be conducted along the molybdenum rod.

Discussion. In Chapter 12, Section 12.4.1.3, we describe the design of a rotating-anode X-ray tube and refer to the component called the **anode stem**. The dimensions and material chosen for the metal cylinder in the preceding worked example closely match those of a typical X-ray tube anode stem, and the problem demonstrates how effectively a narrow anode stem protects the copper rotor to which it is attached, by limiting the conduction of heat from the white-hot anode disc. The 90 J of energy flowing through the stem each second represents roughly the same energy flow as is produced by a 100-W electric light bulb, hardly a major threat to the working of the X-ray tube! Note, however, that energy is also transferred to the rotor assembly by heat radiation.

2.4.2   *Convection*

In liquids and gases some conduction takes place but energy flow is mainly by convection. This is the movement of energy by circulation of the heated liquid or gas.

As the internal energy in the heated region of the fluid increases, circulation currents transport the heated material away and its energy is eventually spread throughout the entire volume of fluid. Meanwhile, the circulation currents replace the heated material which has been dispersed with cooler fluid (see Fig. 2.4). Energy transfer by convection is sometimes used as part of a heating system (e.g. a domestic central-heating system), but it can also be used as the basis of a cooling system (e.g. an air-conditioning system) when the circulating fluid is known as a **coolant**.

2.4.2.1   Characteristics of the convection medium

Whether for heating or cooling, to provide efficient energy transfer the circulating fluid should have a high specific heat capacity (enabling it to carry energy efficiently) and be of low viscosity (enabling it to flow easily). Water satisfies both these requirements and is often used as the fluid medium in both heating

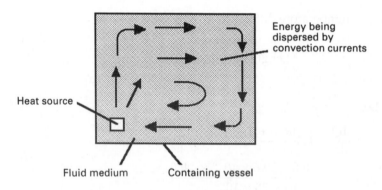

Fig. 2.4   Dispersion of energy by convection in a fluid.

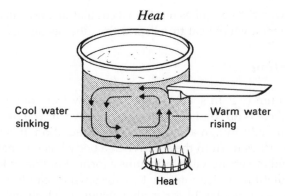

Fig. 2.5   Natural convection currents in a heated liquid.

and cooling systems. For some applications, water cannot be used, e.g. when temperatures above its boiling point are encountered or when its presence may pose electrical or corrosion problems. In these cases, an alternative medium such as a mineral oil may be employed. X-ray tubes and the high-voltage transformers used in radiography employ oil as a coolant (see Sections 10.7.5 and 12.7.3).

The circulation currents necessary for convection may occur naturally, or may be produced artificially.

2.4.2.2   Natural circulation

When a liquid (or gas) is heated, it becomes less dense (lighter) and rises to be replaced by cooler liquid (or gas). This is the reason why natural convection currents are set up. Figure 2.4 illustrates this process. Such convection currents are used in X-ray tubes to help disperse the heat produced when the tube is operating and we will be discussing this aspect of X-ray tube design in Chapter 12.

2.4.2.3   Artificial (forced) circulation

Circulation currents which occur naturally (Fig. 2.5) are not always sufficiently vigorous to provide a rapid energy transfer. In these circumstances convection may be improved by the introduction of a *pumping* system which forcibly circulates the fluid medium.

Heat exchangers
Pumped circulation systems often include a device known as a heat exchanger. Here, energy is efficiently transferred to or from the fluid before it is recirculated back around the system. Domestic central-heating systems, which distribute heat around the home, incorporate a heat exchanger to transfer energy from the water in the hot-water storage tank to that which circulates through the central-heating pipes and radiators. In radiography, X-ray film processors employ a heat exchanger in a forced circulation system which forms part of the developer temperature-control mechanism (Ball & Price, 1995). Additionally, some

high-powered X-ray tubes use forced circulation and a heat exchanger to accelerate the removal of heat from inside the tube casing (see Section 12.8.1).

2.4.3 Radiation

In a vacuum (e.g. in space) energy can flow from one place to another, even
though there is no solid, liquid or gas in between. The process by which energy
is transmitted through a vacuum is called radiation. It is the method by which
energy reaches us from the sun. When a body has internal energy, i.e. when its
atoms and molecules vibrate, it emits a form of radiation known as **electromagnetic radiation** or electromagnetic waves which can transport energy across a
vacuum (see Chapter 14 for further details of electromagnetic radiation). All
bodies possessing internal energy emit an *invisible* form of electromagnetic radiation known as **infrared**. If they are hot enough (e.g. red hot or white hot), they
also emit the *visible* form of electromagnetic radiation known as **light**. Only at
absolute zero (0 K), when it possesses no internal energy at all, would a body
cease emitting infrared radiation.

A body may be *absorbing* energy from an external source at the same time
as it is radiating energy. In such a situation, if the body gains more energy
than it releases, its temperature will rise. If it releases more than it absorbs,
its temperature will fall. If the energy absorbed *balances* the energy released,
thermal equilibrium is established and the temperature of the body will remain
constant. We have assumed here that latent heats of fusion or vaporisation are
not involved; i.e. the body does not melt, boil, condense or freeze (see Section
2.3.1). The rate at which a body radiates its thermal energy depends on its surface
colour and texture, its temperature and its area of surface.

2.4.3.1 Effect of surface colour and texture

A black and matt surface will radiate and absorb energy efficiently, while a white
and glossy surface will not. Years ago, X-ray tubes were encased in metal hous-
ings which had a black, dull finish so that the internal energy could be radiated
away more quickly. Modern tubes overcome the problem of heat dissipation
without resorting to this method.

It is possible to visualise a perfectly black object which is able to absorb 100%
of the radiation to which it is exposed and which also acts as a perfect emitter
of radiation. A body which possesses these characteristics is known as a **black-
body emitter**, or just a *black body*. While it is not possible to manufacture a
perfect black body, some components approach this ideal quite closely and are
very good emitters and absorbers of thermal radiation.

2.4.3.2 Temperature dependence

For a black-body emitter, the rate of emission of energy by radiation is *directly
proportional* to the fourth power of its temperature (T):

$$\frac{dQ}{dt} \propto T^4$$

2.4.3.3 Area dependence

For two black-body emitters of different sizes, but at the same temperature, the rate of emission of energy by radiation is *directly proportional* to the areas (A) of their emitting surfaces:

$$\frac{\mathrm{d}Q}{\mathrm{d}t} \propto A$$

A component whose purpose is to maximise the emission of thermal radiation should therefore

- Have a dull, blackened surface
- Operate at the highest possible temperature (Doubling the temperature, say, from 500 to 1000 K, increases the emission of energy by a factor of 2^4, i.e. 16 times.)
- Have the largest possible surface area (Doubling the surface area doubles the emission of energy.)

The anode disc of a rotating-anode X-ray tube is designed with these considerations in mind (see the worked example in the next section, and also Chapter 12).

2.4.3.4 Stefan's law

The relationships given in Sections 2.4.3.2 and 2.4.3.3 can be combined:

$$\frac{\mathrm{d}Q}{\mathrm{d}t} \propto AT^4$$

This can be written as an equation by introducing a *constant of proportionality*, in this case σ, the Greek letter sigma:

$$\frac{\mathrm{d}Q}{\mathrm{d}t} \propto \sigma AT^4$$

The relationship is known as **Stefan's law** and the constant σ is known as the **Stefan–Boltzmann constant**. Its value in SI units is 5.670×10^{-8} W m^{-2} K^{-4}.

Worked example
The anode disc of an X-ray tube has a diameter of 15 cm and runs at an operating temperature of 2000 K. Assuming that the anode disc approximates to a black-body emitter, estimate the rate at which it radiates thermal energy from its main emitting surfaces (i.e. ignore the emissions from its rim). Stefan's constant is 5.670×10^{-8} W m^{-2} K^{-4}.

We are probably justified in ignoring emissions from the rim of the disc because the surface area of the rim is very small compared with the combined area of the front and back surfaces of the disc.

From the diameter of the disc we can calculate its surface area:

$$\text{Area } (A) \text{ of } \textit{one} \text{ face of the disc} = \pi r^2 \text{ (where } r = 7.5 \text{ cm} = 0.075 \text{ m)}$$
$$= 0.018 \text{ m}^2$$
$$\text{Area of } \textit{both} \text{ faces} = 2 \times 0.018$$
$$= 0.036 \text{ m}^2$$

Using Stefan's law:

$$\frac{dQ}{dt} = \sigma AT^4$$
$$= 5.67 \times 10^{-8} \times 0.036 \times 2000^4$$
$$= 32\,700 \text{ W}$$
$$= 33 \text{ kW (corrected to two significant figures)}$$

Therefore at a temperature of 2000 K, a 'black-body' anode disc would be dissipating its energy in the form of radiation at roughly 33 000 J of energy per second! Compare this with the paltry 90 J of energy per second that we estimated was being *conducted* down its anode stem (Section 2.4.1.1). Assuming the figures we have used are typical, our calculations show that *less than 1%* of the energy transfer from the anode disc is by heat conduction and more than 99% by thermal radiation.

Warning

In this chapter, we have worked through a number of simple calculations. We hope these examples will have demonstrated how a knowledge of the science of heat is relevant to our understanding of the rationale behind different aspects of imaging equipment design. Our calculations involve a number of assumptions which were made primarily to reduce the complexity of the arithmetic; consequently, the results are at best only rough approximations to the truth. Nevertheless, the general conclusions we have drawn from our results, e.g. in relation to X-ray tube design, are valid.

In later chapters, we shall further consider how the various methods by which heat transfers energy from place to place are used to minimise problems of overheating in X-ray equipment. In the next chapter, however, we begin our study of the properties of electrical charges.

Chapter 3
Electricity

In this chapter we discuss some of the basic properties of electric charges. This will enable us to describe the structure of atoms in the next chapter with greater understanding and prepare us for later chapters.

3.1 Frictional electricity

Most radiographers will at one time or another have experienced the effects of so-called **static** electricity generated by friction of one material on another. A common example occurs during the removal of items of clothing such as a sweater particularly if it contains man-made fibres. Pulling off the sweater may be associated with crackling noises and tingling sensations, which may be quite unpleasant. Changing pillow cases is another example where such **frictional electricity** may be produced. Even walking around on certain types of floor coverings may cause an accumulation of electric charge on one's body, which could later discharge in a disturbing way. Such occurrences are common in the dry atmosphere of hospitals.

Although discharges of static electricity do not present a serious health hazard, they can have significant effects on some of the materials and equipment found in an imaging department. For example:

- Electrical discharge onto a photosensitive material such as an X-ray film produces image artefacts known as **static marks**, which are at best annoying and at worst may mean a radiograph has to be repeated, thereby increasing the radiation dose to the patient. Automated X-ray film handling and processing equipment sometimes gives rise to these effects, as well as manual handling of film in the darkroom (Ball & Price, 1995).
- Electronic components such as the **integrated circuits** and **field-effect transistors** used in computers and computerised imaging equipments are sensitive to static and may be irreparably damaged if subjected to this type of electrical discharge. Special precautions must be taken when handling these components.

- Television monitor and visual display unit **display screens** often acquire static electrical charges which tend to attract tiny dust particles from the air. The same process also occurs with domestic TVs and PCs in our own homes. Over a period of time, the accumulated dust may begin to interfere with our viewing of the image. Frequent cleaning of the display screens is therefore advisable, but *only* with suitable cleaning materials and *only* when the mains electrical supply is switched off!

From the above examples, it is clear that static or frictional electricity has a number of practical consequences in diagnostic imaging. For this reason, and as a first introduction to the broader concepts of electricity, we shall now consider frictional electricity in more detail.

3.1.1   *Generating frictional electricity*

To investigate the effects of static we need a rather more reliable method of generating frictional electricity. Some materials will allow electric charges to flow easily through them and are known as electrical conductors, e.g. metals such as iron, aluminium and copper. Other materials do not permit electric charges to flow through them. They are called electrical insulators, e.g. rubber, polythene, nylon and glass. Generally, the effects of frictional electricity are associated with insulators rather than conductors of electricity. Combing one's hair with a nylon comb will invariably enable the comb to attract small pieces of paper. Even better, if we rub a polythene rod with a nylon headscarf, the rod becomes capable of attracting small pieces of paper. In other words, the rubbing action has produced some change in the rod, giving it its property of attraction. We explain this by saying that the rod has become *charged* with electricity and it is the electric charge which is causing the attraction. It is also found that the nylon headscarf acquires the ability to attract things: the nylon, too, has become charged with electricity.

3.2   Types of electric charges

Experiments confirm that there are two kinds of electric charges. They are called **positive** (the type on the polythene rod) and **negative** (the type on the nylon). In its normal state, all matter contains lots of electric charges, but for every positive charge there is a corresponding negative charge and their effects balance exactly. Since there is no majority of either positive or negative charge, we say that the matter is **neutral**.

When some materials are rubbed together, the friction generated may cause some charges (particularly negative charges) to be transferred from one material to the other. In the case of the polythene rod and the nylon headscarf, negative charges are transferred from the rod to the headscarf. The state of neutrality is then disturbed, and the rod will have a majority of positive charges, while the nylon will possess a majority of negative charges (Fig. 3.1). It is usually the negative charge which is transferred because it is less firmly fixed than the positive charge.

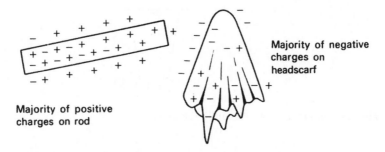

Majority of negative charges on headscarf

Majority of positive charges on rod

Fig. 3.1 Charged polythene rod and nylon headscarf.

3.3 Electric force

We have explained that electrically charged objects are able to attract small pieces of paper. This implies that forces must be involved, forces which are not evident when the objects are in a neutral state. Experiments can be carried out to investigate the properties of these electric forces. Because the forces are very weak, only light objects will be affected enough for the forces to be demonstrated adequately unless an extremely sensitive detector is available.

Consider, therefore, two small balls made of crumpled aluminium foil (the 'silver paper' found wrapped around blocks of chocolate is ideal), each about 1 cm in diameter, suspended on fine thread (e.g. nylon fishing line).

3.3.1 *Effect of type of charge*

If both balls are given a positive charge by touching them with a charged polythene rod, a force of *repulsion* will be seen to exist between them, pushing the balls apart. Charging both balls with a negative charge produces the same effect (Fig. 3.2). In other words, two bodies carrying the *same* type of electric charge will repel each other; i.e. 'like charges repel'.

However, if one ball is given a positive charge and the other a negative charge, a force of *attraction* will be demonstrated, pulling the balls together (Fig. 3.3). Thus two bodies carrying different types of electric charges will attract each other; i.e. 'unlike charges attract'.

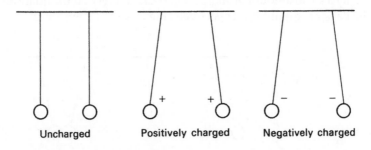

| Uncharged | Positively charged | Negatively charged |

Fig. 3.2 Repulsion between like charges.

Fig. 3.3   Attraction between unlike charges.

3.3.2   *Effect of separation*

If we separate the points of attachment of the supporting threads so that the balls are placed further apart, the electric forces will weaken and the deflection of the balls will reduce.

Bringing the balls closer together causes the forces to increase and the balls may even stick together for a time (Fig. 3.4).

From this we deduce that the magnitudes of the forces of attraction and repulsion are related to the *separation distance* between the charged objects. In fact, it has been found that the force (F) between two charges is inversely proportional to the square of the distance (d) between them; i.e.

$$F \propto \frac{1}{d^2}$$

This is an example of the relationship known as the inverse square law, which we shall discuss again in Section 8.3 and Chapter 14. Hence, if we double the separation, the force would be four (2^2) times weaker. If we treble the separation, the force would be nine (3^2) times weaker, and so on.

As we have already explained, electric forces are generally very weak, but they may become strong enough to be significant when the separation distances are very small.

3.3.3   *Effect of quantity of charge*

We can also influence the strength of the electric forces between charged objects by varying the *quantity* of charge involved. If aluminium-foil balls are given a large quantity of charge, they will attract or repel each other more strongly than if only a small amount of charge had been involved. If the quantities of charge on the balls are q_1 and q_2, respectively, the force (F) between them is proportional

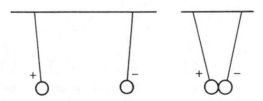

Fig. 3.4   The effect of distance on electric force.

to the product of the charges,

$$F \propto q_1 q_2$$

If we double *one* of the charges, the force is doubled; if we double *both* of the charges, the force increases by a factor of four (2×2).

The SI unit of electric charge is a derived unit known as the **coulomb** (C). Reference to Table 1.1 in Section 1.2.3 shows that one of the seven SI base units is an electrical unit called the **ampere** (A). The ampere, which we discuss further in Chapter 7, is a measure of **electric current**, which is the *rate of flow* of electric charge. Charge and current are therefore closely related:

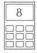

Current = rate of flow of charge (sometimes written in the form dq/dt)

= quantity of charge passing a given point in one unit of time

i.e.

$$\text{Current} = \frac{\text{charge}}{\text{time}}$$

which can be rearranged as:

Charge = current × time

The SI unit of charge is then seen to be the **ampere second** (A s), to which the coulomb is equivalent:

1 coulomb = 1 ampere second

Notice that the radiographic exposure factor known as **mA s** or **milliampere second** is actually a unit of electric charge. In fact,

$$1 \text{ mA s} = 10^{-3} \text{ C (i.e. } 1 \text{ mA s} = 1 \text{ mC)}$$

3.3.4   *Effect of the intervening medium*

The relationships discussed in Sections 3.3.2 and 3.3.3 can be combined into a single relationship, known as **Coulomb's law**:

$$F \propto \frac{q_1 q_2}{d^2}$$

or

$$F = k\frac{q_1 q_2}{d^2}$$

where k is a constant of proportionality.

When the force is measured between two charges in a vacuum or in air, the value of k is found to be 8.99×10^9 N m^2 C^{-2} (newton metre squared per square coulomb). However, when the force is measured between two charges in *other* media (oil, water, glass, etc.), k takes on different values, which are characteristic of the medium concerned. Our experiment with aluminium-foil balls (Section 3.3) was carried out in air. If it were practical to replace the air with some other medium, we would find that the magnitude of the electrical forces is different. In other words, the electric force between two charges depends not only on the magnitude of the charges and the distance separating them, but also on the *nature of the intervening medium.*

3.3.4.1   Consequences of the value of *k*

The very high value of *k* tells us that very strong electric forces operate even between small charges when the distances between them are small. These are the sorts of conditions which exist inside atoms and *between* the atoms in solids. For example, a hydrogen atom consists of two charged particles (see Section 4.3). One particle (the proton) is positively charged and the other (the electron) is negatively charged. They are about 5×10^{-11} m apart and the magnitude of the charge they each carry is 1.6×10^{-19} C. Using:

$$F = k \frac{q_1 q_2}{d^2}$$

the value of F, the force of attraction between the particles, works out at about 8×10^{-8} N. Bearing in mind the incredibly small mass of these particles, this is a very large force, producing tremendous accelerations, of the order of 10^{22} (ten thousand billion billion) times greater than g, the acceleration due to Earth's gravity! Try using the relationship $F = ma$ (Section 1.3.2) to confirm this for yourself: assume the mass of the particle (an electron) is about 9×10^{-31} kg (see Section 4.3).

Permittivity
For reasons which are partly historical, it is more usual to express the constant of proportionality *k* in terms of a different constant known as **permittivity**, represented by the symbol ε (the Greek letter epsilon), where

$$k = \frac{1}{4\pi\varepsilon}$$

The equation for the force between charges then becomes:

$$F = \frac{q_1 q_2}{4\pi\varepsilon d^2}$$

For forces acting in a vacuum, the value of ε is known as the **permittivity of free space**, represented by the symbol ε_0. Its numerical value is 8.85×10^{-12} $C^2 \, N^{-1} \, m^{-2}$. We shall see in Section 6.3.2 that this SI unit is equivalent to the **farad per metre** ($F \, m^{-1}$). Other media have different values of permittivity, but this property is often expressed in *relative* terms, by comparing the **absolute permittivity** of a medium with that of free space. The **relative permittivity** (ε_r) of the medium is then defined as:

$$\varepsilon_r = \frac{\varepsilon}{\varepsilon_0}$$

Relative permittivity has no units because it is a simple ratio of two quantities (ε and ε_0) having the same units. Table 3.1 shows values of absolute permittivity and relative permittivity for a range of different media. From the table it is clear that the permittivity of air is almost identical to that of a vacuum. Note also that the electric force between charges is reduced from its value in a vacuum (or in

Table 3.1   Approximate values of relative permittivity and absolute permittivity for a range of media

Medium	Relative permittivity (ε_r)	Absolute permittivity (ε) (F m^{-1})
Vacuum	1	8.85×10^{-12}
Air	1.00059	8.85×10^{-12}
Oil	2.2	20×10^{-12}
Benzene	2.3	20.4×10^{-12}
Glass		
(minimum value)	5	44×10^{-12}
(maximum value)	7	62×10^{-12}
Mica	6.0	53×10^{-12}
Water	80	710×10^{-12}

air) by a factor equal to the relative permittivity of the medium concerned; e.g. the electric force in oil is roughly half that in a vacuum (or in air).

3.4   Electric fields

To help us to explain the behaviour of electric charges we employ the concept of an electric 'force field' surrounding electric charges. We can define an electric field as being an area or region in which an electric charge experiences an electric force.

3.4.1   *Lines of force*

To indicate the direction of the electric force, we use the idea of a *line of force*. This is defined as the path a positive electric charge would follow if it were free to move. Figure 3.5 illustrates the lines of force around a fixed positive electric charge. They point *away* from the fixed charge because a free positive charge would be *repelled* in these directions. The lines of electric force around a fixed negative charge would point *towards* the charge because a free positive charge would be *attracted* towards it.

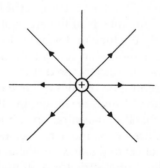

Fig. 3.5   Lines of force around a positive charge.

3.4.2   *Electric field strength*

In Section 1.3.2.2 we introduced the concept of a **force field**, and we defined gravitational field strength at a point as the magnitude of gravitational force acting on a unit mass placed at that point; i.e. gravitational field strength was the gravitational force *per unit mass*. In SI units it was expressed in newtons per kilogram ($N\,kg^{-1}$).

In a similar way, we can apply the general concept of field strength to *electric* fields and define **electric field strength** at a point as the magnitude of electric force acting on a unit of positive electric charge or, more correctly, the electric force *per unit positive charge*.

We must specify the *type* of charge (i.e. whether positive or negative) because it is this which determines whether the force acting is one of attraction or of repulsion. In the case of gravity there is no corresponding complication because gravitational forces are always attractive. If electric field strength is represented by E, then

$$E = \frac{F}{q}$$

where F is the force acting on a charge q. In SI units, electric field strength is therefore expressed in newtons per coulomb ($N\,C^{-1}$), although as we shall see in Section 5.2.7, this unit is equivalent to the volt per metre ($V\,m^{-1}$). We can now estimate the electric field strength experienced by an electron in a hydrogen atom. In Section 3.3.4.1 we established that a force of about 8×10^{-8} N acts on the electron. We also quoted the charge carried by an electron as 1.6×10^{-19} C. The electric field strength (E) is therefore given by

$$E = \frac{F}{q}$$
$$= \frac{8 \times 10^{-8}}{1.6 \times 10^{-19}}$$
$$= 5 \times 10^{11} \, N\,C^{-1}$$

Hence, the electric field strength experienced by a hydrogen electron is about 5×10^{11} N C^{-1}. There are also strong electric fields operating inside an X-ray tube, as we shall see in Chapter 12. The electric field strength between the anode and cathode of an X-ray tube is of the order of 10^7 N C^{-1}, powerful enough to accelerate electrons in the tube to the fantastic speeds, sometimes approaching half the speed of light, needed to generate X-rays.

We can also indicate the electric field strength by the concentration of lines of force. If a high concentration of lines of force exists, the electric field is strong. If a low concentration of lines is shown, the field is weak. Referring again to Fig. 3.5, we can see that the concentration of lines of force is greatest close to the fixed charge and reduces as we move further away. This confirms what we have already seen of the effect of distance on the magnitude of electric forces. Thus, the pattern of the lines of electric force around a charge maps out the electric field.

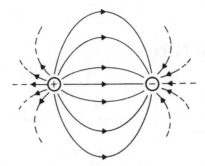

Fig. 3.6   Electric field between two unlike charges.

3.4.3   *Examples of electric field patterns*

The electric field produced by more than one charge is rather more complicated, but it is still defined in the same way, by deducing what a free positive charge would do if placed in the electric field. An example is given in Fig. 3.6. This shows that a free positive charge would always be drawn towards the negative charge: it is guided there by the electric field. If a free negative charge were put in the field, it would similarly be guided, but to the positive charge. This use of an electric field to guide or focus charges is used in the X-ray tube and will be discussed in Chapter 12.

Chapter 4
Atomic Structure

Later in this book, in Chapters 17 and 18, we shall examine what happens when a beam of X-rays is directed at matter, particularly living tissue. To explain the processes which take place we need to have a basic knowledge of the way in which matter is constructed. This knowledge will also help us to understand how electricity flows through matter, how X-rays are produced in the X-ray tube and how gamma rays are produced by radioactive materials.

4.1 Elements and compounds

All matter is made up of chemical substances of two basic kinds:

Elements. These are chemicals that cannot be broken down into simpler chemical forms. Examples include hydrogen, carbon, oxygen and nitrogen.

Compounds. These are the result of two or more elements linking together chemically; e.g. water is a compound of the elements hydrogen and oxygen; the anaesthetic gas nitrous oxide is a compound of the elements nitrogen and oxygen.

We may also find matter composed of a *mixture* of elements or compounds; e.g. air is a mixture of the elements nitrogen and oxygen, which are not chemically linked together.

4.2 Atoms and molecules

4.2.1 Atoms

From what we have learnt so far it follows that an element is the simplest form in which matter exists. If we have a sample of an element, e.g. a strip of lead, and cut it into two, the resulting pieces will still be made of lead, the same element. If we go on doing this repeatedly so that our samples get smaller and smaller, we will eventually reach the stage where it would be impossible to cut the samples into smaller pieces. We would have reached the smallest particle of the element which can exist and still retain all the properties of the element. This particle is known as an **atom**. The original strip of lead which we used as an example is made up of millions upon millions of atoms. In fact, *all* matter is composed of atoms.

An atom is defined as the smallest part of an element which retains the chemical properties of the element. Atoms are incredibly small – about one ten-millionth of a millimetre across (10^{-10} m).

4.2.2 Molecules

If we cut up a sample of a *compound* rather than an element, we will eventually reach a stage where to cut any further would separate the compound into the individual elements of which it is made.

A **molecule** is defined as the smallest part of a compound which retains the chemical properties of the compound. A molecule comprises a number of atoms linked together; e.g. a molecule of water is formed when two hydrogen (H) atoms and one oxygen (O) atom combine together (H_2O). This is a very simple molecule, but some molecules such as the proteins found in living organisms are highly complex and may contain many thousands of atoms. It is also possible for atoms of the *same* element to combine together to form a molecule of an element; e.g. nitrogen (N) gas normally exists in the form of molecules, each consisting of two nitrogen atoms combined together (N_2).

To understand the behaviour of matter we need to examine the way in which atoms themselves are made.

4.3 The structure of the atom

Early in the twentieth century, a Danish scientist, Niels Bohr, developed a concept or *model* to explain how an atom is constructed. We shall use the Bohr model as the basis of our explanation. Bohr thought of the atom as being essentially electrical in nature. He visualised an atom consisting of minute particles – the so-called fundamental or **elementary particles** – held together by electric forces.

At the centre of an atom is the **nucleus**, about one ten-thousandth of the diameter of the atom. Circulating around the nucleus at varying distances, like planets around the sun, are even smaller particles, the **electrons**. The nucleus carries a positive electric charge and the electrons possess a negative electric charge. The

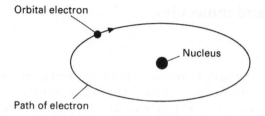

Fig. 4.1   An atom of hydrogen.

electric force of attraction between the nucleus and the electrons prevents the smaller particles from escaping. The approximately circular paths taken by the electrons around the nucleus are called orbits or shells, representing 'layers' at different distances from the nucleus. The element whose atoms have the simplest structure is hydrogen. As Fig. 4.1 illustrates, a hydrogen atom comprises a central nucleus with a single electron circulating around it. It was this arrangement on which we based our calculations in Sections 3.3.4.1 and 3.4.2. The atoms of all the other elements have *more than one* electron circulating around the nucleus. For example, an atom of the element carbon has *six* electrons circulating around its nucleus, at various distances from it. Figure 4.2 shows this arrangement, but we must remember that an atom is a three-dimensional structure, which we have tried to represent in two dimensions in this diagram.

In general, the nucleus is not a single particle, but consists of two types of particle packed together, and they are:

Protons which each carry a *positive* charge equal and opposite to the charge on an electron ($= 1.6 \times 10^{-19}$ C).
Neutrons which are *neutral*, having no net electric charge.

If positive protons are packed together, the electric forces between them will be very strong and will tend to cause the protons to fly apart. ('Like charges repel'.) The number of neutrons present seems to be crucial in overcoming this tendency, but what *kind* of binding forces do the neutrons provide? One possible attraction force is gravity; however, it has been found that although the distances between nuclear particles are very small, their masses are insufficient for gravitational attraction to play a significant role in holding the nucleus together. In fact, a new kind of force has had to be conceived to explain why, despite the presence of powerful electrical forces of repulsion, nuclei are able to remain intact. The force is known as the **strong nuclear force** and it provides a powerful attraction between *all* the particles inside the nucleus. For some atoms, the strong nuclear forces provide permanent nuclear stability, but in other cases stability is not achieved or is of short duration only (see also Section 4.3.3 and Chapter 20). Figure 4.3 shows how we might picture the arrangement of protons and neutrons in a typical nucleus.

To summarise, the Bohr model visualises three types of particles in atoms: *protons* and *neutrons* (collectively known as **nucleons**) in the nucleus, and *electrons* in orbit around the nucleus. Protons, neutrons and electrons are the **fundamental** (or **elemental**) **particles** in the Bohr model of the atom.

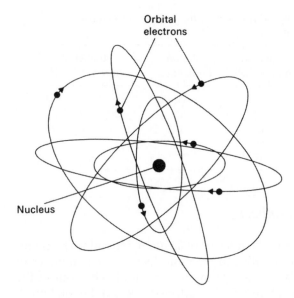

Orbital electrons

Nucleus

Fig. 4.2 An atom of carbon.

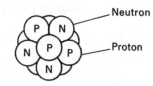

Neutron

Proton

Fig. 4.3 The nucleus of an atom.

Most of the mass of an atom is concentrated in its nucleus. Protons and neutrons have about the same mass, whereas an electron is nearly 2000 times lighter (proton mass $= 1.66 \times 10^{-27}$ kg; electron mass $= 9.11 \times 10^{-31}$ kg).

As we said in Section 3.2, matter is generally electrically neutral. This is because its atoms are neutral, having equal numbers of positive protons and negative electrons.

4.3.1 Proton number (atomic number)

The chemical behaviour of atoms is determined by the number and arrangement of orbital electrons around the nucleus. This, in turn, depends on the number of protons in the nucleus (which is *equal* to the number of electrons). We call the number of protons the **proton number** (Z), formerly known as **atomic number**. So the chemical behaviour of an atom is determined by its proton number. Each element has a different proton number and therefore each element also has a different group of chemical properties. For example, for the following elements:

Hydrogen, $Z = 1$
Helium, $Z = 2$
Carbon, $Z = 6$
Oxygen, $Z = 8$
Lead, $Z = 82$

A complete sequence of elements is known, having proton numbers ranging from 1 to well over 100. However, the elements with proton numbers above 92 do not occur naturally but have to be manufactured artificially; e.g. plutonium ($Z = 94$) is produced in a nuclear reactor.

Table 4.1   Chemical symbols and nuclear configurations of the most common form of five elements

Element	Chemical symbol	Nucleon number (A)	Proton number (Z)	Number of neutrons ($A - Z$)
Hydrogen	H	1	1	0
Helium	He	4	2	2
Carbon	C	12	6	6
Oxygen	O	16	8	8
Lead	Pb	207	82	125

4.3.2   Nucleon number (mass number)

Although the number of *protons* in the nucleus of an atom determines its chemical properties, the number of neutrons in an atom does not. The number of neutrons can vary without in any way altering the chemical behaviour of the atom. However, the *mass* of the atom *would* be affected. We call the total number of nucleons in the nucleus (i.e. the number of protons plus the number of neutrons) the **nucleon number** (A), formerly the **mass number** of the atom. Table 4.1 lists some examples of different elements together with their nucleon numbers.

4.3.3   Isotopes

Although, by definition, all atoms of a single element have the same proton number, they do not necessarily all have the same nucleon number; e.g. some atoms of hydrogen have a nucleon number of two instead of one. (These atoms of hydrogen are heavier than the usual kind because they contain a neutron in the nucleus and are called 'heavy hydrogen' or **deuterium**. However, they combine with other chemicals in exactly the same way as 'normal' hydrogen.) Atoms such as these, having the same proton numbers but different nucleon numbers are called **isotopes** of an element.

There is a useful 'shorthand' notation for writing down the numbers of particles in the nucleus of an atom, using the chemical symbol and two prefixes; e.g. $^1_1$H represents normal hydrogen and $^2_1$H heavy hydrogen. The upper prefix indicates the nucleon number, while the lower prefix shows the proton number. The letter is the chemical symbol for the element. Other examples are $^4_2$He, $^{16}_8$O, $^{12}_6$C and $^{207}_{82}$Pb. Specific arrangements of the nucleons in a nucleus are called **nuclides**.

Sometimes the electric forces of repulsion inside a nucleus are not completely overcome by the strong nuclear force. Sooner or later such nuclides break up, ejecting particles and/or radiation energy as they do so. We call this process of nuclear disintegration **radioactivity** and the unstable nuclides are known as **radionuclides**. We shall be studying radioactivity in more detail in Chapter 20.

4.3.4   *Electron shells*

So far, we have been concentrating on the features of the *nucleus* of an atom but, as we have said, it is the number and arrangement of electrons orbiting around the nucleus which determine how an atom will form links with other atoms.

Electrons move in shells around the nucleus, at particular distances from it. The different shells represent different energy states or levels of potential energy, just as different heights above the ground represent different levels of gravitational potential energy. The further above the ground we go, the greater is the potential energy we are storing. In a similar way, the further an electron shell is from the nucleus, the greater is the potential energy of the electrons in that shell. However, in an atom, only certain specified energy levels, known as **orbitals**, are allowed; electrons cannot exist between these levels. The situation is similar to that of cars in a multi-storey car park; cars cannot be parked between floors, and electrons cannot be 'parked' between shells.

The electron shells are identified by letters: the K shell is the level closest to the nucleus, the next farthest is the L shell and then M, N, and so on. Again, as in a car park, each shell has a limited capacity for electrons and the inner shells are always occupied first. For example:

(a) The K shell can accept up to two electrons.
(b) The L shell can accept up to eight electrons.
(c) The M shell can accept up to eighteen electrons, etc.

Note, however, that the *outermost* shell of an atom cannot accept more than eight electrons. Table 4.2 shows how the electrons are arranged in the first 12 elements in the list of elements.

Table 4.2   Electron arrangement of atoms

Element	Proton number	Number of electrons in shell		
		K	L	M
Hydrogen	1	1		
Helium	2	2		
Lithium	3	2	1	
Beryllium	4	2	2	
Boron	5	2	3	
Carbon	6	2	4	
Nitrogen	7	2	5	
Oxygen	8	2	6	
Fluorine	9	2	7	
Neon	10	2	8	
Sodium	11	2	8	1
Magnesium	12	2	8	2

4.3.5   *Electron energy states*

We commented near the beginning of Section 4.3.4 that each electron shell represents a different electron energy level or energy state. In many respects, viewing the electron configuration of atoms (and molecules) from an *energy-state* perspective is more fruitful than picturing the physical location of electrons orbiting at different distances from the atomic nucleus. For example, the conduction of electricity through metals (see Section 6.1.1.3), the behaviour of semiconductors (Section 6.1.1.2) and the processes of luminescence (Section 15.3.2) can be explained by reference to the energy states of electrons. For this reason, we will now develop further our understanding of this concept.

4.3.5.1   Pauli exclusion principle

It has been found that no two electrons in an atom can occupy exactly the same energy state at the same time: each electron must occupy a different energy state. The principle underlying this statement, known as the **Pauli exclusion principle**, is fundamental to our understanding of the electron configuration of atoms and therefore the chemical behaviour of the different elements (Hey & Walters, 2003). One consequence of the exclusion principle is that each electron shell (K, L, M, etc.) must represent a cluster of *slightly different* energy states rather than a single energy state: for example, the K shell embraces two different electron energy states, the L shell eight states, the M shell eighteen states, and so on.

4.3.5.2   Quantum numbers

The possible energy states of electrons in an atom are specified by four discrete values called **quantum numbers**, each of which defines a different aspect of an electron's condition. The four quantum numbers are known as follows:

- The **principal quantum number** (n) defines the main energy state, or *shell*, of an orbiting electron. For the K shell, $n = 1$; for the L shell, $n = 2$; for the M shell, $n = 3$, etc.
- The **azimuthal quantum number** (l) describes the *angular momentum* of the orbiting electron. The azimuthal quantum number can have the values 0, 1, 2, 3, ..., up to a maximum value of $n- 1$. Thus for the M shell ($n = 3$), l can have only three possible values: 0, 1 or 2.
- The **magnetic quantum number** (m) describes the *spatial orientation* of the plane of the orbiting electron; m can have whole-number values, ranging from $-l$ through zero to $+l$. Thus for the M shell, when $l = 0$, m is 0; when $l = 1$, m can be -1, 0 or $+1$; and when $l = 2$, m can be -2, -1, 0, $+1$ or $+2$, giving a total of *nine* possible energy states.
- The **spin quantum number** (m_s) describes the *direction of spin* of the electron.

Electrons behave like tiny magnets, and we explain their magnetism by imagining that they are rotating like a spinning top. (A rotating electric charge produces a magnetic field.) Whether electrons are *actually* spinning is quite another matter, which is beyond the scope of this book, but the concept is

Table 4.3 The 18 possible electron energy states in the M shell of an atom

Quantum number[a]		
Azimuthal (*l*)	Magnetic (*m*)	Spin (*m*$_s$)
0	0	$+\frac{1}{2}$
0	0	$-\frac{1}{2}$
1	−1	$+\frac{1}{2}$
1	−1	$-\frac{1}{2}$
1	0	$+\frac{1}{2}$
1	0	$-\frac{1}{2}$
1	+1	$+\frac{1}{2}$
1	+1	$-\frac{1}{2}$
2	−2	$+\frac{1}{2}$
2	−2	$-\frac{1}{2}$
2	−1	$+\frac{1}{2}$
2	−1	$-\frac{1}{2}$
2	0	$+\frac{1}{2}$
2	0	$-\frac{1}{2}$
2	+1	$+\frac{1}{2}$
2	+1	$-\frac{1}{2}$
2	+2	$+\frac{1}{2}$
2	+2	$-\frac{1}{2}$

[a] Principal quantum number, $n = 3$.

nevertheless a useful one (see also Section 23.1). The spin of an electron can be in one of two directions, known as **spin up** and **spin down**, and m_s can have only two values: $+\frac{1}{2}$ or $-\frac{1}{2}$. For the M shell, each of the nine states referred to above can have one or other of these two spin states, giving 18 different electron energy states altogether, which confirms the statement made in Section 4.3.4 that the M shell can accept up to 18 electrons.

Table 4.3 summarises the 18 different combinations of values of *l*, *m* and m_s for the M shell. It is possible to establish the maximum number of electrons permitted in *any* electron shell of an atom by carefully examining how many different combinations of values exist for quantum numbers *l*, *m* and m_s.

Note that the maximum electron capacity of the *n*th shell can also be determined from the following formula:

Electron capacity $= 2n^2$

e.g. for the M shell, where $n = 3$,

$$2n^2 = 2 \times 3^2$$
$$= 18$$

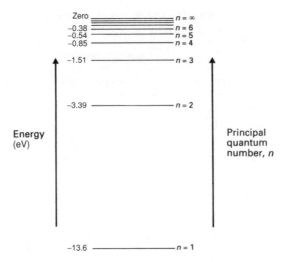

Energy
(eV)

Principal
quantum
number, n

Fig. 4.4   Electron energy levels in a hydrogen atom.

But note that this formula tells us nothing about the *detailed* energy states of electrons in that particular shell. Let us see how we can illustrate the energy levels in an atom in diagrammatic form.

4.3.5.3   Energy-level diagrams

We usually represent the energy levels in an atom as a series of horizontal lines forming what is known as an **energy-level diagram** (Fig. 4.4). Each line represents a different energy level characterised by its principal quantum number (n) shown at the right-hand end of the line. The lowest level has $n = 1$, the next $n = 2$, etc. The energy of the level where $n = \infty$ (∞ means infinity) is zero. This is the *baseline* or reference level from which the other energy levels are measured. If an electron is raised to this level, it becomes free of the atom. The *actual* values of energy are shown at the left-hand end of each horizontal line. Two further conventions are adopted:

- Electron energy levels are expressed not in SI units (joules), but in **electronvolts** (eV), where $1\,\text{eV} = 1.6 \times 10^{-19}$ J. Electronvolts are particularly appropriate and convenient units when dealing with particle energies. The derivation of the electronvolt is discussed in Section 5.3.
- Electron energy levels have *negative* values. Electron energy levels are levels of **potential energy** and as we found in Section 1.3.4.1, potential energy is a *relative* quantity which is always quoted by reference to a baseline level. In the present case, the electron energy levels are *below* the chosen baseline value of zero and are therefore negative.

Figure 4.4 is the energy-level diagram for the hydrogen atom. As we discovered earlier (Fig. 4.1), hydrogen has only one electron, normally occupying the lowest energy level, which we referred to as the K shell whose principal quantum number, *n*, is 1. When an atom of hydrogen is in this condition, it is said to be in its **ground state**.

4.3.5.4   Excitation

If an atom in its ground state absorbs energy (e.g. by colliding with another particle or by absorbing electromagnetic radiation), one of its electrons may be shifted into one of the higher energy levels. (We can think of this as being moved to an orbit further from the nucleus.) The atom, which is then, unstable is said to be in an **excited state**. However, soon afterwards, the electron 'falls' back to its former energy level and the atom returns to its ground state, at the same time releasing in the form of electromagnetic radiation the energy that was originally absorbed. Atoms do not remain in their excited states for long (often for less than 1 μs), but because the process is a random one, we cannot predict the precise moment when any individual atom will revert to its ground state.

4.3.5.5   Ionisation

If an atom absorbs sufficient energy, an electron may be raised to the level where $n = \infty$ and will be completely freed from the atom. An atom which has lost an electron is said to be **ionised** and Fig. 4.4 tells us that the minimum energy needed to ionise a hydrogen atom in its ground state is 13.6 eV. Forms of electromagnetic radiation, such as X-rays and gamma rays, which are capable of ionising atoms are known as **ionising radiations**.

4.3.5.6   Ionisation energies

The *minimum* energy needed to ionise an atom which is in its ground state (i.e. to remove its most loosely bound electron) is called the **first** (or **principal**) **ionisation energy** of the atom. Thus the first ionisation energy of hydrogen is 13.6 eV. The minimum energy to remove the *next* most loosely bound electron is the **second ionisation energy**, and so on. Because hydrogen has only one electron, it has no ionisation energies higher than the first. The first ionisation energy of an atom is often simply known as its ionisation energy; i.e. if no qualifying adjective (first, second, etc.) is present, we can safely assume that reference is being made to the first ionisation energy.

4.3.5.7   Excitation energies

Similarly, the energy required to *excite* an atom from its ground state is called the **excitation energy** of the atom. To excite the atom by raising its most loosely bound electron to the next available energy level is called the **first excitation energy** of the atom. To raise it one level further is the **second excitation energy** of the atom, and so on. Referring back to Fig. 4.4 we can see that the first excitation energy of hydrogen is 10.2 eV (i.e. 13.6 – 3.39), while its second excitation energy is 12.1 eV (i.e. 13.6 – 1.51).

4.3.6   *The characteristic nature of electron energy levels*

We have been using a hydrogen atom to illustrate the features of electron energy-level diagrams. We chose hydrogen because it is the simplest example available. All atoms of hydrogen have exactly the same set of permitted energy levels. In fact, all the atoms of *any* given element have exactly the same set of energy levels (e.g. each atom of lead has the same set of energy levels as every other atom of lead, each atom of carbon has the same set of energy levels as every other atom of carbon, and so on). However, no two *different* elements have the same set of energy levels; each element has its own unique characteristic set. Each set of energy levels therefore acts as a sort of fingerprint, different for each different element, thus announcing the identity of the element concerned. So, for example, the set of energy levels for lead atoms is different from that for carbon atoms, and different again from that for hydrogen, or indeed from those for the atoms of any of the other elements. Moreover, the sets of **ionisation energies** (Section 4.3.5.6) and **excitation energies** (Section 4.3.5.7) are also uniquely characteristic of the individual elements.

4.4   The chemical behaviour of atoms

The chemical properties of the different elements are determined by the configuration of the *outermost* electron shells of their atoms. When atoms link together to form molecules, it is their *outer* electron shells which interact with each other, while the shells deeper in the atoms, nearer to their nuclei, remain undisturbed. The outermost shell of an atom is known as its **valence shell**, and the electrons found there are known as **valence electrons**. Referring back to Table 4.2 we can see, for example, that the valence shell for elements 1 and 2 (hydrogen and helium) is the K shell; for elements 3–10 (lithium to neon) it is the L shell; for elements 11 and 12 (sodium and magnesium) it is the M shell; and so on.

The lowest energy state for an atom (and therefore its most stable state) is achieved when its valence shell contains either two electrons (if it is the K shell) or eight electrons (for the L shell and beyond). Of the examples listed in Table 4.2, only helium and neon satisfy this condition. Helium has *two* electrons in its K shell (its valence shell), and neon has *eight* electrons in its L shell (its valence shell). The elements helium and neon are therefore chemically very stable, and it is exceedingly difficult to get them to react with other elements. The elements argon, krypton, xenon and radon also have eight electrons in their valence shells, and therefore exhibit the same inherent chemical stability. These six most stable elements, all gaseous at normal temperatures, are known as the **inert** or **noble gases**.

4.4.1   *Periodic table*

Elements whose atoms have similar electron configurations in their valence shells can be expected to have similar chemical properties. The inert gases are an example of this phenomenon. If we work systematically through a list of the elements, arranged in order of proton number, we will find that similar valence-shell configurations keep reappearing as each new valence shell is reached. Thus similar (but not identical) sets of chemical properties are found periodically as we work our way down the list of elements. For example, the elements fluorine, chlorine, bromine and iodine have a valence shell containing *seven* electrons. They all share similar chemical properties and are collectively known as the **halogen elements** or the **halogens**.

It is possible to set out all the elements in a **periodic table**, grouping together the elements with similar chemical characteristics. Knowing in which group an element is situated enables us to predict with some confidence what chemical behaviour it is likely to exhibit.

4.4.2   Chemical bonding

Atoms whose valence shells do not normally match the inert configuration described in Section 4.4 may achieve a lower energy state by combining with other atoms. For example, an atom of fluorine needs just one more electron in its valence shell to enable it to achieve greater stability. If it could combine with another atom (such as lithium) which would like to relinquish an electron, the result would be a molecule (of lithium fluoride) in which each participating atom has been able to achieve a lower energy state than it had before. Indeed, both the elements fluorine and lithium are highly reactive chemicals, but the compound lithium fluoride is quite stable.

There are two ways in which atoms can bond together to form compounds, ionically and covalently.

4.4.2.1   Ionic bonding

In ionic bonding, an electron is donated by one atom to another as a means of achieving a lower energy state. In doing so, the atom which donates an electron loses its electrical neutrality and becomes a *positively* charged **ion**. The atom which gains an electron also loses its electrical neutrality and becomes a *negatively* charged ion. The two ions are then held together by the electric force of attraction between their opposite electric charges. The atoms of metallic elements are able to donate electrons easily, and therefore readily form **ionic bonds**. For example, the metallic element *silver* (Ag) forms an ionic bond with the halogen element *bromine* (Br) to form the compound **silver bromide** (AgBr), which is of great importance in the manufacture of photographic and X-ray film. A molecule of silver bromide comprises a positive silver ion (Ag^+) linked to a negative bromine ion (Br^-).

4.4.2.2   Covalent bonding

In covalent bonding, atoms *share* electrons rather than permanently donating them. Consider, for example, the elements carbon and oxygen. An atom of carbon has *four* electrons in its valence shell; it needs another four to achieve a more stable state. An atom of oxygen has *six* electrons in its valence shell; it needs another two to achieve stability. As Fig. 4.5 shows, if a carbon atom links with

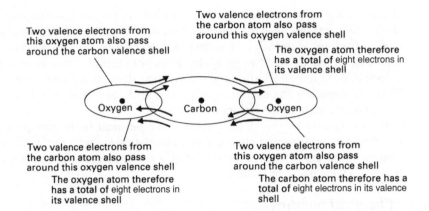

Two valence electrons from
this oxygen atom also pass
around the carbon valence shell

Two valence electrons from
the carbon atom also pass
around this oxygen valence shell

The oxygen atom therefore
has a total of eight electrons in
its valence shell

Two valence electrons from
the carbon atom also pass
around this oxygen valence shell
The oxygen atom therefore
has a total of eight electrons in
its valence shell

Two valence electrons from
this oxygen atom also pass
around the carbon valence shell
The carbon atom therefore has a
total of eight electrons in its valence
shell

Fig. 4.5 Covalent bonding between a carbon atom and two oxygen atoms to form a molecule of carbon dioxide. By sharing electrons, all three atoms achieve a stable valence-shell configuration. Note that for greater clarity, only the valence shells of the atoms are shown.

two oxygen atoms and the three atoms share some of their valence electrons, each atom can achieve a state in which eight electrons are present in its valence shell. The result is a molecule of the stable compound **carbon dioxide** (CO_2). In covalent bonding, it is the interlinking of valence shells, rather than electric attraction, which holds the atoms together. Each shared pair of electrons forms one covalent bond, so in CO_2 the carbon atom has four bonds, two with each oxygen atom. This arrangement may be symbolically expressed as O=C=O, in which each single line ($-$) linking the chemical symbols represents a *single* covalent bond and a double line ($=$) represents a *double* bond. This method of representation is more informative than using traditional chemical formulae (e.g. CO_2) because it tells us something about the spatial relationships between the atoms in a molecule, albeit in two dimensions only (see Table 4.4).

4.4.3   Polar and non-polar molecules

Both the positive and negative electrical charges in a single isolated atom are centred on the nucleus. Positive charge is centred on the nucleus because the protons which carry the positive charge are found in the nucleus. Negative charge is centred on the nucleus because the paths of the electrons, which carry the negative charge, are centred on the nucleus. In other words, viewed from outside the atom, both the positive and negative charges appear to be centred on the nucleus; i.e. *the centres of positive and negative charge coincide.* This is described as a **non-polar** distribution of charge.

When an atom forms covalent bonds with other atoms, the centres of positive and negative charge in the molecule may not coincide. This is because the positive charges are in a number of different locations (the individual nuclei of the atoms), and the negative charge distribution is complicated by the sharing of electrons that occurs; electrons may spend more of their time near one of the atoms than the other. The result is that the molecule may exhibit *polar* properties, with its positive charge centred in one position within the molecule, while its

Table 4.4   Covalent bonding: some examples of symbolic representations of the structure of covalent molecules together with the traditional chemical formulae

Molecule	Chemical formula	Symbolic representation
Hydrogen	H_2	H—H
Chlorine	Cl_2	Cl—Cl
Sulphur	S_2	S=S
Carbon dioxide	CO_2	O=C=O
Methane	CH_4	H—C—H with H above and H below
Butane	C_4H_{10}	H—C—C—C—C—H with H above and below each C

negative charge is centred in another position (Fig. 4.6). The molecule acts as a tiny electrical **dipole**, with its positive charge at one end and its negative charge at the other. Such **polar molecules** are influenced by the presence of external electric fields; for example, they may try to rotate to align themselves with the direction of the electric field. This property may lead to phenomena such as **piezoelectricity**, which has applications in diagnostic ultrasound imaging (see Section 22.3). Not all covalent molecules are polar; e.g. a hydrogen molecule (H—H) is non-polar because it is symmetrical.

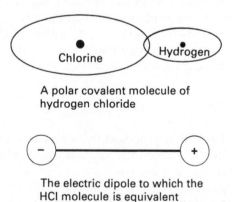

A polar covalent molecule of
hydrogen chloride

The electric dipole to which the
HCl molecule is equivalent

Fig. 4.6   The polar covalent molecule hydrogen chloride. The shared valence electrons spend more of their time around the chlorine atom than they do around the hydrogen atom. The effect is to place the centre of negative charge at the chlorine end of the molecule and the centre of positive charge at the hydrogen end. The molecule behaves like an electric dipole. Note that only the valence shells of the atoms are shown in the diagram.

4.5   Post-Bohr ideas on the structure of the atom

As we explained in Section 4.3, the description of atomic structure in this chapter is based largely on the model conceived by Niels Bohr in 1913. The Bohr model provides a useful starting point when studying atomic structure, and many of the properties of atoms can be explained by reference to this model. Over the past 90 years, however, experiments have brought to light observational evidence which has required the original Bohr model to be refined and modified, often in quite fundamental ways. While it is beyond the scope of this book to explore these post-Bohr developments in any detail, we can justify a brief look at some of them. For a readable account of modern ideas on atomic structure, we refer the student to sources such as Hey and Walters (2003) and Hawking and Mlodinow (2005).

4.5.1   *Elementary particles*

The Bohr model required the existence of just three elementary particles: the *proton*, the *electron* and the *neutron* (Section 4.3). This model, in which the whole of the universe and everything in it is made from just three different kinds of particles, is a persuasively simple concept. Not surprisingly perhaps, reality is far more complex: several *hundred* elementary particles are now known experimentally (Close, 1992). The proton and neutron are no longer truly fundamental particles, because they themselves are made up of even smaller particles known as **quarks** (usually pronounced to rhyme with 'bark'). Furthermore, there are at least six different types of quarks (known by physicists as *up-, down-, strange-, charmed-, bottom-* and *top-quarks*), and each type of quark can have three characteristics (known as *red, green* or *blue*). A proton contains two up-quarks and one down-quark, while a neutron has two down-quarks and one up-quark. Clearly, the particle physicists who dreamt up such labels have more fertile imaginations and a more bizarre sense of humour than those who, a century ago, named the alpha and beta particles described in Chapter 20! Other elementary particles and groups of particles include photons (see Section 14.5.2), bosons, baryons, leptons, mesons, gluons, muons and neutrinos (Section 20.2.3.2).

4.5.2   *Antiparticles*

In the 1930s, Paul Dirac proposed that every elementary particle has a corresponding **antiparticle**. Soon afterwards, scientists discovered the antiparticle of the electron (known as a **positron**) which carries a *positive* charge rather than a negative charge (see Sections 17.2.4 and 20.2.3.1). Other antiparticles have since been found, and it is now known that the Dirac prediction is valid for *all* elementary particles, although in some cases (such as the photon) a particle may be its own antiparticle. Physicists generally place a bar '⁻' above the symbol for a particle to indicate its antiparticle; e.g. $\bar{e}$ represents an antielectron or positron. The existence of antiparticles raises the possibility of antiatoms and antimolecules forming **antimatter**.

Taking this concept even further, one can imagine, with the science fiction writers, whole planets to be made of antimatter, perhaps inhabited by antimatter intelligent life-forms, even entire universes made of antimatter. However, a major problem arises when antimatter undergoes a close encounter with 'normal' matter: they annihilate each other in a burst of energy! Fictional 'antimatter drives' employ this principle to provide an energy source with which to power the starships that *'boldly go where no one has gone before'*. These ideas may seem very far removed from our everyday experience, but it is worth remembering that antiparticles are a *normal* by-product of some radioactive decay processes (Section 20.2.2) and may also arise when high-energy X- or gamma radiation interacts with matter (Section 17.2.4). The matter–antimatter annihilations accompanying such events are disappointingly unspectacular and usually go completely unnoticed.

4.5.3   *Electron clouds and the uncertainty principle*

The Bohr model pictures electrons moving around the nucleus of an atom like the planets of the solar system moving around the sun. However, it has been known for over 70 years that it is not possible to define precisely both the position and the motion of an electron in an atom at the same instant of time. This fundamental constraint on our knowledge of the position and motion of a particle was discovered by Werner Heisenberg and is known as the **Heisenberg uncertainty principle**. The uncertainty remains, no matter how accurate our measurement techniques. Consequently, we no longer picture electrons in well-defined orbits but rather in nebulous clouds around the nucleus. The position of an electron is now defined in terms of the *probability* of finding it at some distance from the nucleus (see Fig. 4.7). This **probability-cloud** view of the atom has superseded the original solar-system model (Arnold, 1994).

4.5.4   *Matter waves*

Traditionally, a clear distinction has been made between particles and waves. They seem quite different concepts with different properties. For example, particles possess mass, inertia and momentum, while waves display reflection, refraction, interference and diffraction. However, since early last century, scientists (notably Albert Einstein and Max Planck) found that light, which had previously been described as a wave phenomenon, exhibited some properties that were better explained if light was thought of as a stream of particles. We now call these particles **photons**, and we explore the **dual nature of light** (and other electromagnetic radiations) in Chapter 14.

If a wave phenomenon such as light can behave like particles of matter, is the reverse also true? Can matter behave like waves? Does matter have a dual nature, too? In 1924, the scientist Louis de Broglie (pronounced 'de Broy') stunned the scientific establishment by suggesting exactly that. He proposed that particles of matter such as electrons, and indeed *all* matter, should display some wave-like behaviour. It has since been shown that the de Broglie hypothesis was correct, and that matter *does* have wave properties; e.g. a beam of electrons suffers

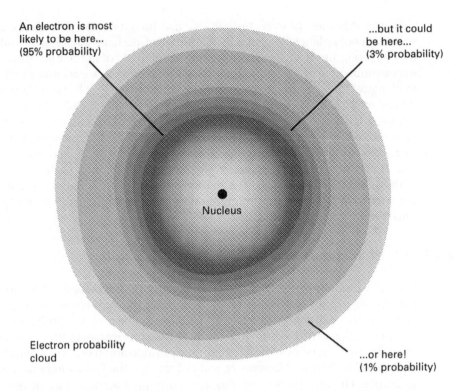

An electron is most
likely to be here...
(95% probability)

...but it could
be here...
(3% probability)

Nucleus

Electron probability
cloud

...or here!
(1% probability)

Fig. 4.7   The electron probability cloud around a hydrogen nucleus. The varying density of the cloud represents the way in which the probability of finding an electron changes at different locations in the atom. The most likely location (95% probability) corresponds with the position of the K shell, but the electron may be elsewhere!

diffraction, a characteristic of waves (Arnold, 1994). These **matter waves** are sometimes known as **de Broglie waves** in his honour.

It may seem paradoxical that we have to attribute particle properties to a phenomenon such as radiation, previously considered to be a wave, and to attribute wave properties to a phenomenon such as matter, previously thought of as a collection of particles. We must remember, however, that these are merely different *conceptual models* or *tools* which help us to explain and predict the behaviour of radiation and matter. Rather than pondering over an apparent paradox, it is perhaps more helpful to think of the two models as *complementary* rather than contradictory. The important point is to know which model is the more appropriate one in any given situation or problem (see also Section 14.2).

We have now completed, at least for the present, our discussion of the structure of matter. We shall be returning to this topic in Chapter 20 when we explore radioactivity, but our task in the next few chapters is to develop further our understanding of electricity.

Chapter 5

Electric Charge and Potential

5.1   Electric charges

As we saw in Chapter 4, the protons and electrons in an atom carry minute electric charges: electrons negative and protons positive. When we speak of a body being charged with electricity we mean it has a surplus or deficiency of electrons so that its atomic charges no longer balance. A surplus of electrons would produce a net negative charge and a deficiency of electrons would give a net positive charge.

A possible (and logical) way of measuring electric charges would be to specify the *number* of electrons in surplus or deficit, i.e. to specify charge in terms of electronic charge units. For many practical purposes this would be rather inconvenient because the electron charge is so very small. It would be rather like measuring the distance from London to Paris in inches (about 14 million), rather than in miles (about 220). We therefore require a larger unit in which to measure quantities of electric charge. The SI unit of electric charge is called the **coulomb** (C), which we introduced in Section 3.3.3.

5.1.1   Unit of charge

The coulomb (C) is the ampere second. It is defined as the quantity of charge which passes a given section of a conductor in 1 s when a current of 1 A is flowing through the conductor. The charge on one electron is 1.60×10^{-19} C, so 1 C of charge is equivalent to the charge on about 6×10^{18} electrons. Even this amount of charge is not large in practical terms; e.g. 4 C of charge passes through a one-bar electric fire *every second*.

5.1.2   Properties of electric charge

In Chapter 3, we saw that:

- Like charges repel each other and unlike charges attract.
- The force between two charges is inversely proportional to the square of the distance between them.
- The force between two charges is directly proportional to the product of the magnitudes of the charges.

We also noted that charges can flow easily through electrical conductors, but cannot flow through electrical insulators. We can therefore deduce that:

- Charges (e.g. electrons) applied to a *conductor* will spread over its surface. They will not move inside the conductor because of the mutual repulsion between them. Each charge moves as far away as possible from its neighbours (see Fig. 5.1).
- Charges deposited on the surface of an *insulator* remain where they are placed because they cannot move through an insulator.

The charge on a pointed conductor tends to concentrate around the point, generating a stronger electric field around a curved or pointed surface (Fig. 5.2). The field may become strong enough to ionise the air surrounding the point if electrons from the atoms of air are repelled away and electrons from the charged conductor replace them. In such a case, the electric charge on the conductor will gradually leak away and we say an electric discharge is occurring. Sometimes the discharge may be rapid and violent, causing a spark or an **arc** to be produced. If the conductor is smooth and rounded rather than having sharp points or edges, discharge is less likely to occur. High-voltage electrical components may have to be manufactured with smooth contours in order to reduce the risk of electrical breakdown due to arcing. This is one of the considerations in the design of the X-ray tubes and high-voltage transformers used in radiography.

The powerful electric field which surrounds a pointed conductor does not always create problems. In some cases it can have useful applications. For example,

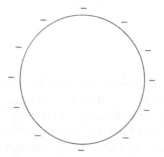

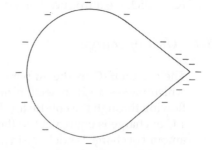

Fig. 5.1   Charge on the outside of a conductor.   Fig. 5.2   Charge concentrated on a *pointed* surface.

the pointed tip of a lightning conductor ionises the air around it and enables the electric charge being generated by storm clouds to drain away harmlessly. Without the lightning conductor, the charge might build up and eventually discharge violently as a lightning strike.

5.2   Electrical potential and potential difference

When a charge is moved from one point to another in an electric field, a net change of potential energy may be involved and work may have to be done to overcome the electric forces experienced by the charge (see Fig. 5.3). To help explain why work may have to be done to move the electric charge, we assign a property known as **electrical potential** (often just called **potential**) to the two points in the electrical field. If the potential energy of a charge changes when it moves from one point to the other and work has to be done to achieve the move, the two points are said to be at *different* electrical potentials. However, if a charge experiences *no* net change in potential energy when it moves from one point to the other and no work has to be done, the two points are said to be at the *same* electrical potential.

Note that electrical potential is a property *of the electric field only*, whereas the potential energy of a charge depends on both the electric field *and* the size of the charge.

Definition. The electrical potential at a point in an electric field is numerically equal to the work done in moving a unit positive charge from infinity to the point. (The term *infinity* here just means a point far enough away to be removed from all electrical influences.)

Definition. The potential difference between two points in an electric field is numerically equal to the work done in moving a unit positive charge from one point to the other.

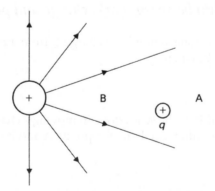

Fig. 5.3   A small positive charge *q* in an electric field. To move the charge from A to B requires work to be done against the electric field. The potential energy of the charge would therefore increase as it moves from A to B. The points A and B are said to be at different potentials. The potential difference between them is the work done in moving a unit charge from A to B.

5.2.1   *Earth potential*

From the first definition, it follows that the potential at a point at infinity is zero. Because the concept of a point at infinity is rather difficult to realise in practice, for most purposes the potential of the earth is assigned zero potential. The earth is chosen because its potential is known to be constant, and of course the earth is always near at hand. This **ground** or **earth potential** becomes the baseline to which the potentials of other points may be referred.

5.2.2   *Positive and negative work*

The work done in moving a charge can be positive or negative because the electric force on a charge can be one of attraction or repulsion.

- If the work done is positive, energy must be *given to* the charge for it to move; i.e. the charge is being moved *against* the force produced by the electric field. As a result of the move, the potential energy of the charge increases.
- If the work done is negative, energy is *released* as the charge moves; i.e. the charge is accelerating or 'falling' under the influence of the electric field. Its potential energy is decreasing and being converted, for example, into kinetic energy.

5.2.3   *Potential difference*

Although we can specify the *absolute* potential at a point in an electric field (by referring it to earth potential or to the potential at infinity), we are more often concerned only with the *difference* in potential (or potential difference, **PD**) between two points in an electric field. We argued along similar lines in our discussion of potential energy in Section 1.3.4.1, where differences in potential energy were our main consideration.

5.2.4   *Relationship between work, charge and potential*

If W is the work done in moving a charge Q from infinity to a point, the potential at the point is V, where:

$$V = \frac{W}{Q}$$

Furthermore, if W is the work done in moving a charge Q from point A to point B, the potential difference between points A and B is V, where:

$$V = \frac{W}{Q}$$

5.2.5   *Unit of potential*

In SI units, work is measured in joules (J) and charge is measured in coulombs (C), so the SI unit of electrical potential (and potential difference) is the joule per coulomb ($J\,C^{-1}$), which is known as the **volt** (V).

Definition. A potential difference of 1 V exists between two points if 1 J of work is done in moving 1 C of charge from one point to the other.

Because the unit of potential difference is the volt, potential difference is commonly known as **voltage**.

Let us now apply our knowledge to a simple problem.

Worked example

As will be described in Chapter 12, when we make an X-ray exposure, electrons in an X-ray tube are accelerated across the vacuum between a negatively charged cathode and a positively charged anode. Assuming that the potential difference between the cathode and the anode is 50 kV, estimate the work done by the electric field as it accelerates *one* electron from cathode to anode. (The charge on an electron is 1.6×10^{-19} C.)

We shall apply the relationship between work (W), charge (Q) and potential difference (V):

$$V = \frac{W}{Q}$$

In this problem, we know the values of Q (=1.6×10^{-19}C) and V(=5×10^4 V), but we need to calculate W. Rearranging the expression gives:

$$W = VQ$$
$$= 5 \times 10^4 \times 1.6 \times 10^{-19}$$
$$= 80 \times 10^{-15}$$
$$= 8 \times 10^{-14} \text{ J}$$

The electric field therefore does 8×10^{-14} J of work on each electron as it accelerates them from cathode to anode, so each electron acquires about 8×10^{-14} J of energy by the time it reaches the anode. While this may not sound a great deal of energy, during a typical X-ray exposure (e.g. of a hand), between 10^{16} and 10^{17} electrons may cross the X-ray tube! The total energy (E) carried by these electrons is then as much as:

$$E = 10^{17} \times 8 \times 10^{-14}$$
$$= 8000 \text{ J (i.e. 8 kJ)}$$

which is a *much* more significant amount of energy!

5.2.6 *Potential gradients*

Let us consider further the conditions described in our worked example. We noted that a potential difference of 50 kV existed between the cathode and the anode, setting up a strong electric field in the space between them. Figure 5.4 illustrates that the cathode and anode are positioned about 1 cm apart. Across this gap, the electrical potential gradually changes from its value at the cathode to its value at the anode, a total change of 50 kV in 1 cm. If the electric field was uniform, we could infer that the electrical potential changes at a constant rate of 50 kilovolts per centimetre (50 kV cm^{-1}), 5 kilovolts per millimetre (5 kV mm^{-1})

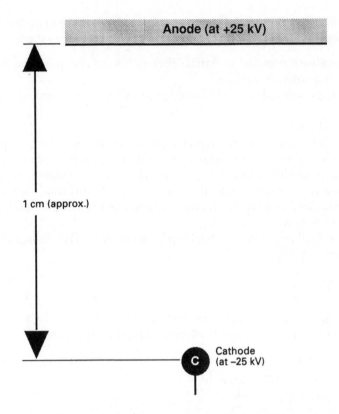

Fig. 5.4   The arrangement of the cathode and anode in an X-ray tube when a potential difference of 50 kV is applied. Electrons leaving the cathode are accelerated towards the anode by an electric field in the space between the two electrodes. In this gap, the potential changes gradually, but non-uniformly, from −25 kV at the cathode to +25 kV at the anode, a total change of 50 kV.

or 500 000 volts per metre (V m^{-1}). This quantity is known as the **potential gradient**. It represents the *rate* at which potential changes with distance, and it is an important factor in determining both the direction and the rate of flow of electric charge. In many respects, the concept of potential gradient parallels that of *temperature gradient*, which determines the direction and rate of energy flow through a thermal conductor (Section 2.4.1).

5.2.7   *Electric field strength*

In Section 3.4.2, we specified the strength of an electric field by quoting the force acting on unit charge, expressed in newtons per coulomb (N C^{-1}). We have now established an alternative method: we can quote the potential gradient. In SI units, we would express electric field strength in **volts per metre** (V m^{-1}). Thus, the newton per coulomb is the same as the volt per metre; i.e.

$$1 \, N \, C^{-1} = 1 \, V \, m^{-1}$$

5.2.8 *Equipotential lines*

In Section 3.4.2, we explained how lines of electric force can be used to map out the pattern of an electric field, and we used Figs 3.5 and 3.6 to illustrate the

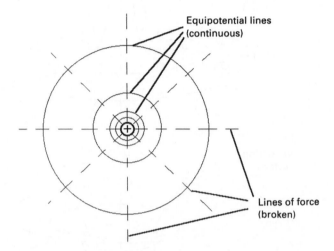

Fig. 5.5 The electric field around a single isolated positive electric charge. Here, the field is mapped by equipotential lines as well as lines of force. Note that the spacing of the equipotential lines decreases with increasing distance from the central charge. This reflects the reduction in potential gradient, which characterises the progressively weakening electric field.

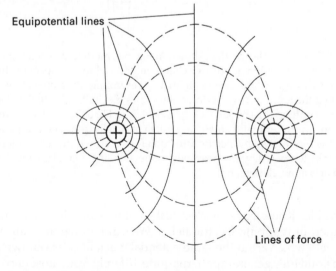

Fig. 5.6 The electric field between two unlike charges. The pattern of the electric field is shown both by lines of force (as in Fig. 3.6) and by equipotential lines. The potential rises from a negative value around the negative charge (right) to a positive value around the positive charge (left). Note that equipotential lines intersect lines of force at right angles.

(a)

Wandering positive
charge

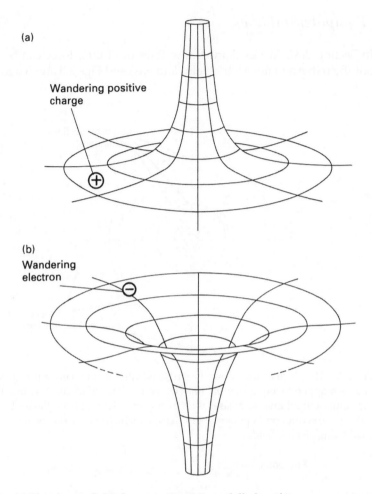

(b)
Wandering
electron

Fig. 5.7 (a) The electric field shown in Fig. 5.5, modelled as if it were a geographical landform. A wandering positive charge might find the prospect of climbing the peak (i.e. moving *against* the electric field) a rather intimidating one. However, having reached the top, the descent down the slopes (i.e. 'falling' *with* the electric field) would be exhilarating! (b) The same electric field as in Fig 5.7(a), but seen from the point of view of a wandering *negative* charge such as an electron. The charge would be drawn into the central well by electric attraction forces. Any initial excitement the electron feels might be tempered by the possibility of never being able to escape. This type of electric field acts as an electron trap.

principle. Knowledge of electrical potential provides us with an alternative method of mapping electric fields. We can join together all points in an electric field which are at the same potential. Such lines are known as **equipotential lines**, and they generate patterns quite different from those encountered in Chapter 3. Figures 5.5 and 5.6 show how the electric fields previously illustrated by lines of force in Figs 3.5 and 3.6 can be represented by patterns of equipotential lines. It is helpful to think of equipotential lines as similar to the *contour* lines used by geographers when mapping landforms. Contour lines join together all points at the same *height*, while equipotential lines join together all points at the same *electric potential*. As with contour lines, if equipotential lines are placed close together, we know that a steep potential gradient exists. One can even visualise what kind of three-dimensional landform a particular electric field pattern might mimic. For example, to a wandering positive charge, the electric field in Fig. 5.5 would seem to represent a high mountain peak. The charge would need to acquire a large input of energy to conquer the peak (Fig. 5.7a). To a wandering *negative* charge, the same electric field would represent a deep hollow like a black hole (Fig. 5.7b), into which it might fall and remain trapped! Figure 5.8a shows the electric field between the cathode and the anode of an X-ray tube. Try to visualise what kind of terrain this would represent to an electron and thereby predict how the electron might behave (see Fig. 5.8b).

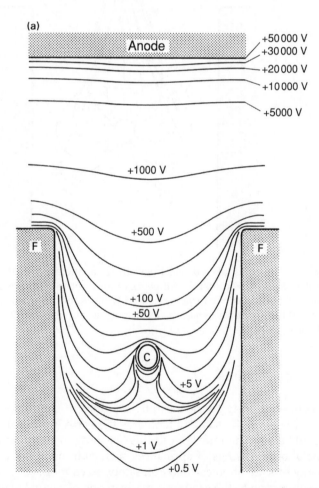

Fig. 5.8   (a) The electric field between the cathode (C) and the anode of an X-ray tube. The field is illustrated using equipotential lines and shows the effect of the focusing hood (F) in which the electron-emitting cathode filament is seated. The figures indicate the potential (relative to cathode potential) assigned to different equipotential lines. Notice that the potential gradient is greatest in the region adjacent to the anode surface.

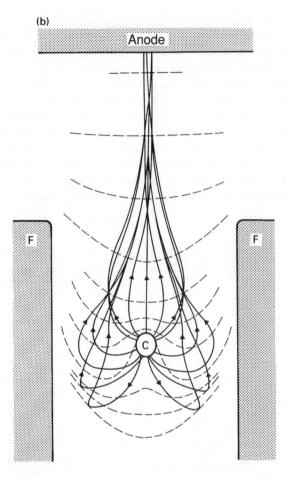

Fig. 5.8 (b) The paths taken by electrons as they accelerate from the cathode (C) to the anode of an X-ray tube under the influence of the electric field shown more fully in part (a). The field created by the focusing hood (F) guides the electrons onto a small area of the target of the anode known as the focal spot (see also Section 12.3.1.3). (Data adapted from Thorpe, 1949.)

5.2.9 Earth connections

If we connect a body to the earth by an efficient conductor of electricity, the body will take on the same potential as the earth (i.e. zero). This will make it electrically safe to handle. We call this 'earthing' or 'grounding' a component. The metal outer casings of appliances such as irons, vacuum cleaners, fridges and X-ray sets are often earthed as a safety precaution.

The connection to the ground is made in one of several ways:

(1) **Special earthing plates**. These are metal conducting plates buried beneath the earth, having a large area of contact with moist soil. The electrical symbol for an earth connection is derived from this idea (Fig. 5.9).

Fig. 5.9   Electrical symbol for an earth connection.

(2)   **Connections to water pipes**. The mains cold-water supply is usually provided through metal piping, which enters a building from below ground. This can be used as an efficient earth connection.

What happens if an appliance is not earthed?

- If it is working normally, nothing happens.
- *But*, if a fault occurs, and a live (electrified) component comes into contact with the metal casing, the casing becomes 'live'; i.e. its potential will not be zero. If we touch the casing, *we* become its earth connection and electrons flow through *us*, giving us an electric shock, which may be mild or severe according to the rate of flow of electrons.
- *However*, if the appliance had been properly earthed, the electrons would have run down to earth via the earth connection rather than through us because the human body is not a very efficient conductor of electricity. The usual result, in practice, is that a fuse blows, switching off the supply and making the appliance safe.

5.3   The electronvolt

If we were to rearrange the definition of the volt, we could arrive at a new definition of the unit of energy (the joule). For example, we could say that 1 J of work is done if a charge of 1 C is moved through a potential difference of 1 V. This is not an accepted definition, because it defines the joule in terms of units which are derived from the joule. In other words, we are using the joule to define the joule. However, it is a useful idea, which is worth developing further.

Suppose that instead of moving 1 C of charge, we move an electron charge (i.e. we move an electron) through a potential difference of 1 V. Clearly, the energy involved would be less than a joule because the charge on the electron is so much smaller than 1 C. The quantity of energy thus defined is called an electronvolt (eV). It is a very small unit of energy:

$$1\,eV = 1.602 \times 10^{-19} J$$

Definition. An electronvolt is the work done in moving an electron through a potential difference of 1 V.

For example, if an electron 'falls' (is accelerated) through a potential difference of 1000 V, it gains 1000 eV of kinetic energy, or 1 kiloelectronvolt (keV). A larger unit is the megaelectronvolt (MeV), where:

$$1\,MeV = 1\,million\,eV$$

Using the electronvolt as the unit of energy greatly simplifies many calculations. For example, we can immediately see that the electrons accelerated across the X-ray tube in the worked example of Section 5.2.5 each gain 50 keV of energy (because they have moved through a potential difference of 50 kV). Thus, the electronvolt is a very useful unit when working with vacuum tubes in which electrons are accelerated and is generally used to describe the energy of the radiation produced in such devices.

Chapter 6

Conduction and Storage of Electric Charges

In this chapter we shall extend our knowledge of the electrical properties of materials and examine some methods of using these materials to store electric charges.

6.1 Electrical conductors and insulators

In Section 3.1 we defined electrical conductors as materials through which electric charges move easily. Electrical insulators were said to be materials through which electric charges are not able to move.

Why do materials have these properties? To explain this demands that we explore further the electrical nature of matter that we studied in Chapter 4. In particular, we need to understand how the close spacing of individual atoms, especially in metals, creates conditions in which electrons can move freely through the material. Our explanation is based on the presence of **energy bands**, rather than discrete energy levels, for the electrons around atoms.

6.1.1 Band theory of conduction

We saw in Section 4.3.5.3 that the electrons in an atom can exist only in certain specified energy states, and we showed how these energy states could be represented on energy-level diagrams. In Fig. 4.4 we illustrated the permitted electron energy levels for a hydrogen atom. The energy states shown were those in a single *isolated* atom. However, when two atoms are in close proximity (e.g. when they form a covalent bond), their permitted energy levels become modified because their electrons are now influenced by the electric fields of *both* atoms. In fact, each previously single energy level splits into *two*, with the outermost energy levels being split more than the inner ones (Fig. 6.1).

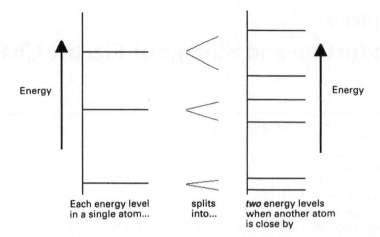

Fig. 6.1   The left-hand energy-level diagram shows the discrete electron energy states in a single isolated atom. The close presence of another atom modifies these levels by splitting them into pairs as shown in the right-hand diagram.

If *large numbers* of atoms are closely spaced, each single electron energy level splits not into two, but into many different energy levels, producing what is termed an *energy band* (Fig. 6.2). Within each band, the individual energy levels are so close together that a continuous range of energy states is available to electrons in that band. As before, the outer energy levels are affected more than the inner levels. The energy bands are separated from each other by regions

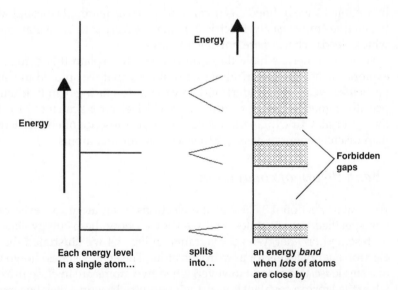

Fig. 6.2   When many atoms are close by, as in a solid material, discrete energy levels are replaced by broad energy bands, which are illustrated in the energy band diagram on the right. Note the forbidden gaps which separate the energy bands.

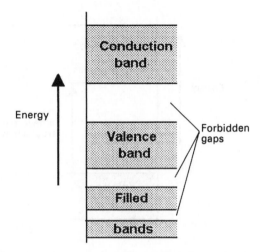

Fig. 6.3   An energy band diagram showing the different categories of energy band found in a solid.

known as **forbidden gaps**, in which there are *no* permitted electron energy states. There are *three* categories of energy bands, shown in Fig. 6.3 and described below:

- **Valence band.** This is the highest energy band whose electrons are still tied to a particular atom. It corresponds to the valence shell of a single isolated atom.
- **Filled bands.** These are energy bands *below* the valence band. They possess a full complement of electrons. Because the filled bands do not contribute to electrical conduction, we normally omit them from energy band diagrams.
- **Conduction band.** This represents an energy band *above* the valence band. Electrons in the conduction band are often called **free electrons** because they are no longer tied to a particular atom and can move freely within the material. Electrons in the conduction band are therefore available as charge carriers, enabling an electric current to flow if a potential gradient is present.

The conduction properties of different materials largely depend on the existence and the size of the forbidden gap between the valence and conduction bands. Materials can therefore be divided into three groups called **insulators**, **semiconductors** and **conductors**, according to whether the forbidden gap is large, small, or absent.

6.1.1.1   Electrical insulators

In insulators, such as oil, glass, rubber, plastic and ceramic materials, the forbidden gap between the valence and conduction band is *large* (of the order of 5 eV, but varying for different materials; Fig. 6.4). In normal circumstances it is rare for a valence electron in an insulator to receive enough energy to enable it to climb into the conduction band. The conduction band of an insulator is therefore

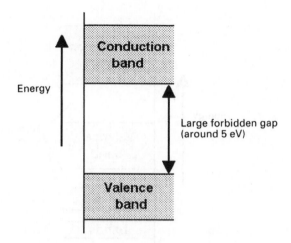

Fig. 6.4 An energy band diagram of an electrical insulator. The large energy gap prevents electrons entering the conduction band and flow of current through the material cannot take place.

practically empty; there are very few free electrons, and an electric current will not flow. At high temperatures however, or in very strong electric fields, significant numbers of electrons may gain sufficient energy to enter the conduction band and the insulating properties of the material then begin to break down. Thus, as well as temperature and type of material, the point at which a particular insulator breaks down depends on the *potential difference* applied and on the *thickness of insulator* because these are the factors which determine the potential gradient and therefore the electric field strength (Sections 5.2.6 and 5.2.7). This is why the **high-tension cables** attached to an X-ray tube employ a thick layer of insulation.

6.1.1.2 Semiconductors

In a *pure* semiconducting material such as silicon, the forbidden gap is *small* (of the order of 1 eV, but varying for different materials; Fig. 6.5). At very low temperatures, approaching 0 K, no electrons gain enough energy to enable them to cross the forbidden gap, the conduction band remains empty and there are no free electrons. Under these conditions, therefore, a semiconductor behaves like an insulator and does not conduct electric current. At room temperature, however, there is sufficient internal (thermal) energy in the material for some of the valence electrons to gain the 1 eV or so needed to cross the forbidden gap into the conduction band, and the material begins to conduct, albeit in a limited way. If the temperature is raised further, the number of free electrons increases and the conduction properties improve. When electrons are promoted from valence band to conduction band, they leave behind vacancies known as **holes**. Under some conditions, holes rather than electrons act as the charge-carrying agents for electric current flow (see Section 13.1). The limited amount of conduction which occurs in a *pure* semiconductor is known as **intrinsic conduction**.

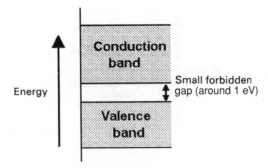

Fig. 6.5 An energy band diagram of a pure semiconductor. At room temperature, background thermal energy is sufficient to promote a number of electrons across the forbidden gap and into the conduction band, allowing a small current to flow in the presence of a potential gradient across the material.

Doping

It is possible, during the manufacture of a semiconductor, to modify its conduction properties by incorporating a minute quantity of a carefully chosen 'impurity' or **doping agent** whose effect is to create additional energy levels in the forbidden gap. In the type of doped semiconductor known as an **n-type**, these extra energy levels act as 'steps' which enable many more electrons to climb from the valence band to the conduction band, thereby enhancing the ability of the semiconductor to conduct electricity. In a **p-type** semiconductor, the extra energy levels enable *holes* to become mobile, which also enhances the conducting properties of the material. Conduction which occurs in a *doped* semiconductor (whether n-type or p-type) is called **extrinsic conduction**. Even in extrinsic semiconductors, electric current flow is still constrained by the limited availability of free charge carriers. The composition, properties and applications of n-type and p-type semiconductors are discussed further in Chapter 13.

6.1.1.3 Conductors

In conducting materials such as metals, there is *no* forbidden gap between the valence band and the conduction band. In fact, the two bands *overlap*, enabling electrons to move easily between valence and conduction bands (Fig. 6.6). The conduction band therefore has an almost unlimited supply of electrons and the flow of electric current is no longer constrained by a shortage of free electrons. However, as we shall see in the next chapter, *other* constraints may be present which limit current flow in a conductor.

The direction of movement of a free electron in a conducting material is entirely random. Just as many electrons move to the left as to the right; just as many move upwards as downwards and so on. This is illustrated in Fig. 6.7. If, however, an electrical potential difference is applied across the conductor, all the electrons will tend to drift in the same direction – from the low potential to the high potential. Thus electric charge is flowing through the conductor and we say an electric current is flowing (Fig. 6.8). Although all metals are good electrical conductors, silver, copper and aluminium are particularly efficient.

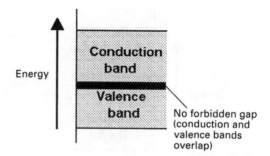

Fig. 6.6   An energy band diagram of a good electrical conductor. There is no forbidden gap because the valence and conduction bands overlap. Electrons move freely into the conduction band, providing an ample supply of free electrons, which gives the material its excellent conducting properties.

6.2   Storing electric charge

Now that we have an idea of the nature of conducting and insulating materials we can examine methods of using them to store electric charges. When, in Section 3.1.1, we separated electric charges by rubbing a polythene rod with a nylon headscarf, the charges were stored on the polythene and nylon until we were ready to use them. We might imagine that if we had a very large rod and a big scarf, we could store a lot more charge. In this case we would be storing the charge on insulating materials. We could also store charge on a conductor, such as a metal sphere, by transferring charge onto it from the polythene rod, as long as the conductor was insulated from the ground so that the charges could not flow away to earth (Fig. 6.9).

    If we use this method to transfer charge onto a conductor, the process of transfer becomes progressively more difficult because of the repulsion forces caused by the charges we have already deposited there. Because more and more work has to be done to transfer each charge, we know that the electrical potential of the conductor must be rising. Eventually, the potential of the conductor becomes *equal* to the potential on the polythene rod. Once this point is reached, no more charge can flow onto the conductor because there is no longer a

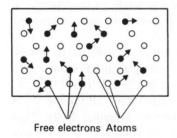

Free electrons Atoms

Fig. 6.7   Random movement of free electrons in a conductor.

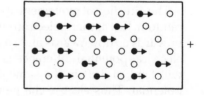

Fig. 6.8   Free electrons in a conductor drifting towards a positive potential.

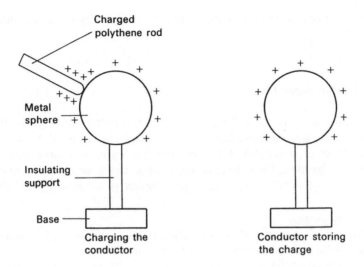

Fig. 6.9   Storing charge on a conductor.

potential gradient to drive it. The only way to store more charge would be to raise the potential of the rod in some way, e.g. by rubbing it more vigorously with the nylon. However, if the conducting sphere was bigger, we could store more charge on it, without having to increase the rod potential. This is because on a large conductor, the charge already deposited can move further away from the point where new charge is being added and the repulsion effect is then weaker.

A useful analogy to consider is the storage of oxygen gas in the familiar black-and-white steel pressure cylinders, which you will have seen in hospitals. Oxygen can be forced into the cylinder under pressure until the pressure of the gas inside the cylinder is equal to the pressure being applied to introduce the gas. The only way to store more oxygen is either to increase the pressure being applied or to use a bigger cylinder. It is sometimes quite helpful to visualise potential as a kind of electrical *pressure*.

6.2.1   *Capacitance*

We can compare the electrical storage capacities of different conductors by applying the same potential to each and seeing how much charge each conductor accepts at that potential. The quantity of charge which can be stored on a conductor *per unit potential* is called the **capacitance** of the conductor.

Thus if Q is the amount of charge a conductor is able to store at a potential V, its capacitance C is given by:

$$C = \frac{Q}{V}$$

Capacitance also represents the amount of charge that can be transferred either onto or off a conductor per unit *change* in its potential, so if V is the change in the potential of a conductor resulting from the addition (or removal) of an amount of charge Q, its capacitance (C) is given by the same relationship:

$$C = \frac{Q}{V}$$

6.2.1.1 Unit of capacitance

Because the SI units of charge and potential are the coulomb and the volt, respectively, the unit of capacitance is the *coulomb per volt* ($C\ V^{-1}$), which is known as the **farad** (F). Unfortunately, the farad is an extremely large unit, and in practice we are far more likely to encounter capacitance measured in **microfarads** (μF), where $1\ \mu F = 10^{-6}$ F, or even in **picofarads** (pF), where $1\ pF = 10^{-12}$ F.

Worked example
The capacitance of a 30-cm-diameter metal sphere is 15 pF. What potential must be applied to enable it to store 1 C of charge?
  We are told that $C = 15$ pF and $Q = 1$ C. Rearranging the relationship:

$$C = \frac{Q}{V}$$

gives

$$V = \frac{Q}{C}$$

Knowing the values of charge (Q) and capacitance (C), we can find the value of potential (V), but first we must convert capacitance from picofarads to farads:

$$C = 15\ pF = 15 \times 10^{-12}\ F$$

Then

$$V = \frac{Q}{C}$$
$$= \frac{1}{15 \times 10^{-12}}$$
$$= 6.7 \times 10^{10}\ V \quad \text{(corrected to two significant figures)}$$

This may seem a rather surprising result. To persuade a 30-cm-diameter metal sphere to store just 1 C of charge would require a potential of nearly *70 billion* volts! In other words, we would need to do *70 billion* joules of work to deposit 1 coulomb of charge on the sphere. Furthermore, we know from Section 5.1.1 that 1 C is hardly a great amount of charge in everyday terms. Clearly, using a metal sphere is *not* a very effective way of storing electric charge!

N.B. We hope you were not confused by the use of the letter C as an algebraic symbol representing the capacitance of the conductor and the use of the same letter as an abbreviation for the coulomb, the SI unit of charge. Throughout this book, we have adopted the common practice of using italic script for algebraic quantities in an attempt to minimise such confusion.

6.3 Capacitors

We have described the storage of charge on a spherical conductor, but *all* conductors, no matter what their size, shape and design, possess some capacitance. In many cases capacitance is an *incidental*, and sometimes, undesirable consequence of the design of a component. For some purposes, however, a device is designed for the sole purpose of storing electric charge. Such a device is known as a **capacitor**.

6.3.1 *Mode of operation of capacitors*

Capacitors essentially consist of two conductors (electrodes) separated by an insulator. One type, known as a **parallel-plate capacitor**, has a thin layer of insulation (known as a **dielectric**) sandwiched between two flat metallic electrodes or **plates**. As Fig. 6.10 shows, one plate is charged positively and the other negatively. The presence of the positively charged right-hand plate makes it very much easier to transfer negative charges onto the left-hand plate. This is because the *repulsion* effect of charges already on the left-hand plate is weakened (but not completely neutralised) by *attraction* from the opposite (positive) charges on the right-hand plate. For every negative charge (free electron) deposited on the left-hand plate, a negative charge departs from the right-hand plate, leaving it positively charged (Fig. 6.11). The closer together the two plates are placed, the more effective the second plate becomes at easing the charging process.

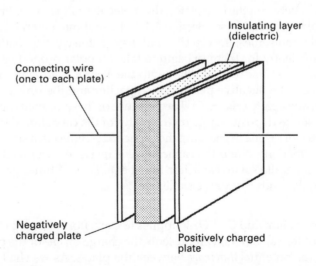

Fig. 6.10   A parallel-plate capacitor shown with its left-hand plate charged negatively and its right-hand plate charged positively. The plates are shown separated from the dielectric material for clarity, although in an actual capacitor the plates would be touching the dielectric.

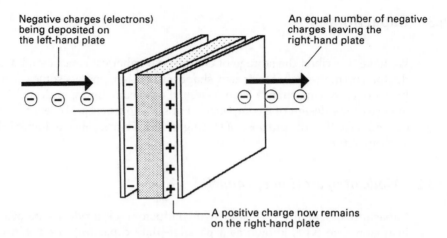

Negative charges (electrons)
being deposited on
the left-hand plate

An equal number of negative
charges leaving the
right-hand plate

A positive charge now remains
on the right-hand plate

Fig. 6.11   A parallel-plate capacitor shown during the process of charging. As negative charges are deposited on the left-hand plate, an equal number of negative charges are drained from the right-hand plate, leaving it positively charged. The presence of the positive charges makes it easier for the left-hand plate to acquire its negative charge and therefore increases the capacitance of the device.

6.3.1.1   Functions of the insulating layer

- *To prevent the two plates from touching each other.* If they touched, charge would flow between them, neutralising and thereby losing all the stored charge.
- *To increase the capacitance of the capacitor.* Under the influence of the electric field between the two plates, the molecules of the insulating material display **polar** properties (see Section 4.4.3). Even if the material is formed from *non-polar* molecules, the electric field distorts the electron paths in the molecules sufficiently for them to begin to take on polar properties.. The result is that the molecular dipoles align with the electric field, with their positive poles facing the negative plate of the capacitor and their negative poles facing its positive plate (Fig. 6.12). The presence of these aligned dipoles makes it even easier to deposit charge on the plates of the capacitor. Furthermore, because the work done in charging the capacitor is reduced, a smaller rise in potential is experienced and the capacitance is increased. In practice, the capacitance of a parallel-plate capacitor may be *millions* of times greater than that of a single conductor of the same size.

The relationship $C = Q/V$ applies to capacitors as well as to a single conductor, but for capacitors, Q represents the charge on *one* of the plates and V represents the potential *difference* between the plates. As we shall see in the worked examples which follow, for some purposes the relationship is rearranged and written in the form

$$Q = CV$$

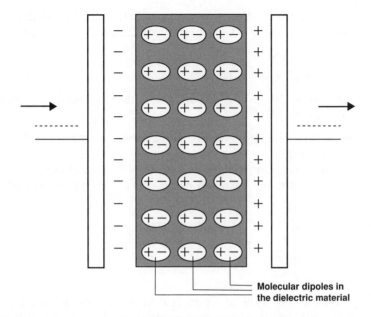

Molecular dipoles in the dielectric material

Fig. 6.12   The action of the insulating dielectric material in a parallel-plate capacitor. The electric field between the two plates has a polarising effect on the dielectric, creating alignment of its molecular dipoles. The positive charges on the left-hand edge of the dielectric layer make it easier for negative charges to be deposited on the left-hand plate. A similar effect occurs on the right-hand side of the capacitor. This results in a substantial increase in the capacitance of the device. Of course, in practice, there would be many millions of polarised molecules present in the dielectric material.

Worked examples

(1)   A capacitor with a capacitance of 1 pF is charged to a potential difference of 100 V. How much charge will be stored at this potential?

   Before simply inserting the values of capacitance (*C*) and potential (*V*) into $Q = CV$, we must pause and recall that *Q*, *C* and *V* should be in SI units, i.e. coulombs, farads and volts, respectively, so we must first convert 1 pF into farads:

$$1\,pF = 10^{-12}F$$

then

$$Q = CV$$
$$= 10^{-12} \times 100$$
$$= 10^{-10}C$$

Answer: The capacitor will store 10^{-10} C of charge at 100 V.

(2)   A capacitor is charged to a potential difference of 250 V and has a capacitance of 0.5 μF. How much charge should be added to raise the potential difference to 300 V?

We require this time to produce a change of 50 V in the potential difference. So we use $Q = CV$ and put $V = 50$ and $C = 0.5 \times 10^{-6}$ F. Then

$$Q = 0.5 \times 10^{-6} \times 50$$
$$= 25 \times 10^{-6} C \ (25 \ \mu C)$$

Answer: A charge of 25 μC must be added to raise the potential difference
from 250 to 300 V.

(3)   What potential difference would be needed to make a 1-μF capacitor store
1 C of charge?
This time we are told the values of $C (=10^{-6}$ F) and $Q (=1$ C). We therefore
need to rearrange the relationship $Q = CV$ to enable us to calculate V.

$$V = \frac{Q}{C}$$
$$= \frac{1}{10^{-6}}$$
$$= 10^6 \ V$$

Answer: One million volts (10^6 volts) would be needed to make a
1-microfarad capacitor store 1 coulomb of charge! Clearly, no ordinary capacitor would survive that sort of treatment, but this example is useful in
showing that only comparatively small quantities of electric charge can, in
practice, be stored in capacitors.

6.3.2   *Factors affecting capacitance*

Various design features of capacitors can be used to improve their storage
capacity:

(1)   If the conducting plates are made larger in area, the capacitance will be
increased.
(2)   If the distance separating the conducting plates is decreased, the capacitance will be increased.
(3)   If a better dielectric material is used between the plates, the capacitance
will be increased. A capacitor could be used with nothing (i.e. a vacuum)
between its plates. Inserting a dielectric material between the plates would
increase its capacitance by a factor equal to the **relative permittivity** (ε_r) of
the material used (see also Section 3.3.4.1). In other words,

$$\varepsilon_r = \frac{C}{C_0}$$

where C is the capacitance when the *dielectric material* is between the plates
and C_0 is the capacitance when there is a *vacuum* between the plates. For
example, the relative permittivity of waxed paper is approximately 4. Thus
if the vacuum between the plates of a capacitor is replaced by waxed paper,
its capacitance will be increased by about four times.
We saw in Table 3.1 that the relative permittivity of air is almost identical
to that of a vacuum, so a capacitor which has air between its plates has the

Table 6.1   Approximate values of relative permittivity (dielectric constant) for typical dielectric materials.

Dielectric	Relative permittivity (ε_r)[a]
Vacuum	1 (exactly)
Air	1.0
Teflon	2.1
Polythene	2.3
Waxed paper	3.2–4.7
Polyvinyl chloride (PVC)	2.8–3.2
Neoprene	5.7–6.5
Mica	7.0
Strontium titanate	200

[a] Because it is a simple ratio, relative permittivity has no units. Note that apart from the value for a vacuum, values of relative permittivity of dielectric materials are not constant, but vary according to the precise conditions (e.g. temperature, frequency, etc.) under which they are used.

same capacitance as it would if it had a vacuum between its plates. Table 6.1 shows the values of relative permittivity for some of the dielectric materials used in capacitors. Note that the relative permittivity of a dielectric material is sometimes known as its **dielectric constant**.

For the parallel-plate type of capacitor we can say *exactly* how these design features influence capacitance:

(1)   Capacitance (C) is directly proportional to plate area (A):

$$C \propto A$$

(2)   Capacitance is inversely proportional to plate separation (d):

$$C \propto \frac{1}{d}$$

(3)   Capacitance is directly proportional to relative permittivity (ε_r):

$$C \propto \varepsilon_r$$

Combining these three factors gives:

$$C \propto \varepsilon_r \frac{A}{d}$$

This is a *proportional* relationship. In fact, the constant of proportionality is ε_0, the permittivity of free space, and the relationship becomes:

$$C = \varepsilon_0 \varepsilon_r \frac{A}{d}$$

Note that the rearrangement of this equation provides us with an alternative SI unit for absolute permittivity, because:

$$\varepsilon_0 = \frac{Cd}{\varepsilon_r A}$$

where *C* is in farads, *d* is in metres, *A* is in square metres and ε_r has no units because it is a simple ratio. The units of ε_0 are therefore farad metres per square metre (F m m^{-2}), which simplifies to **farads per metre** (F m^{-1}). Thus, the C^2 N^{-1} m^{-2}, which is the SI unit of absolute permittivity previously described in Section 3.3.4.1, is equivalent to the farad per metre (F m^{-1}).

6.3.3   *Types of capacitors*

Frequently, capacitance is increased by having more than one pair of conducting plates. A whole series of plates may be used, effectively increasing the total plate area. Such devices are called multi-leaf capacitors and their capacitance is proportional to the number of plates employed.

If a thin metal foil is used to form the conduction layers and thin, wax-impregnated paper to form the dielectric, the whole 'sandwich' may be rolled up into a 'Swiss roll' arrangement. In this way a large plate area can be combined with a small plate separation and made into a tiny electrical component which has a reasonably large capacitance.

To produce very large values of capacitance, a device called an electrolytic capacitor may be used. Although it may have a large capacitance, e.g. 1000 µF, it can easily be damaged if it is wrongly connected in an electrical circuit.

Capacitors are one of the components found on printed circuit boards (see Fig. 6.13) and in integrated circuits:

- **Printed circuit boards** (PCBs) provide physical support for, and electri-cal connection between, electronic components, using conductive pathways etched from copper sheets laminated onto a non-conductive substrate.

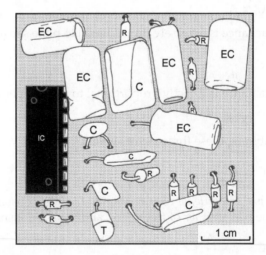

Fig. 6.13   A selection of miniaturised electronic components mounted on a printed circuit board. The components include the following: capacitors (C), electrolytic capacitors (EC), resistors (R), an integrated circuit (IC) and a transistor (T). The size of the components can be judged by reference to the 1-cm scale in the bottom right corner of the diagram.

- **Integrated circuits** (ICs or "chips") are miniaturised electronic circuits consisting mainly of semiconductor devices (Chapter 13), deposited in the surface of a substrate of thin semiconducting material. A single integrated circuit may contain more than a million electronic components, including capacitors.

6.3.4 *Charging and discharging capacitors*

When a capacitor is being charged, we find that the charge builds up rapidly at first, but after a while slows down, until eventually no more charge is being added. This is due to the changing potential of the capacitor. As we saw earlier in this chapter in our analogy with the oxygen cylinder, we can continue to 'charge' the cylinder only as long as the pressure we are applying to put the oxygen in is greater than the pressure inside the cylinder. As the pressure inside builds up, we find it more and more difficult to force in any more oxygen. Similarly, the process of *discharging* a capacitor (releasing its stored charge), though rapid initially, becomes progressively slower as the potential difference across the plates of the capacitor falls.

The precise behaviour of charging or discharging capacitors depends greatly on the electrical circuit to which they are connected. For this reason, we shall delay any further discussion of these processes until the end of Chapter 7, in which we describe the essential features of electrical circuits.

Chapter 7
Current Electricity

7.1   Electric current

In Section 6.1 we referred to the *movement* of electric charge as **electric current**.

If we make one end of a conductor positive and the other end negative, electrons move towards the positive end. It is this flow of electrons which constitutes the electric current.

The action of making one end of a conductor positive and the other negative is known as 'applying a potential difference'.

7.1.1   Direction of current flow

We have established that electrons (electric current) flow from negative to positive, but when electric current was first observed, physicists did not know about electrons, so they guessed (wrongly) that current flowed from positive to negative. Since this convention was used as the basis for some of the laws of physics, we must differentiate between the two types of current, so we call flow from negative to positive **electron current** and flow from positive to negative **conventional current** (Fig. 7.1). In the rest of this book the word **current** should be taken to mean *electron current*, unless stated otherwise. In Section 3.3.3, we derived the relationship

$$\text{Current} = \frac{\text{charge}}{\text{time}}$$

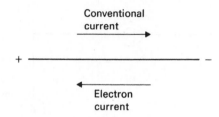

Fig. 7.1   Conventional current flow and electron flow.

7.1.2   *Unit of current*

The SI unit of current is the **ampere**, often abbreviated to 'amp', or just 'A'. An 'amp', therefore, represents a certain amount of charge, or number of electrons, flowing per unit time. If we express charge in terms of the number of electrons, the figures involved would be very large, so we instead use the *coulomb*. (1 coulomb represents the charge on 6×10^{18} electrons; see Section 5.1.1.)

We sometimes need to talk about currents smaller than 1 amp, so the term 'milliamp' (mA) is used, where:

$$1 \text{ milliamp} = 10^{-3} \text{ amp}$$

or

$$1000 \text{ mA} = 1 \text{ amp}$$

A device used to measure the flow of current is called an ammeter (or milliammeter).

The amount of electric charge which flows through an X-ray tube during an exposure is obtained from the product of tube current expressed in milliamps (mA) and exposure time expressed in seconds (s). A typical chest radiograph may require an exposure of 5 mA s, which represents 5×10^{-3} C of charge.

7.2   Circuit symbols

When we draw electrical circuits (circuit diagrams) we use a selection of symbols, each of which represents a component, as shown in Fig. 7.2. For a current to flow it is always necessary to have a *complete* circuit, i.e. a continuous path for the electrons to flow along. Thus the lamp in the diagram will light up only when the switch in the circuit is closed. A battery is used in the circuit as a source of potential difference, to drive the current around the circuit.

7.3   Potential difference

This can be thought of as the difference in *electrical pressure* between any two points in the circuit. The relationship between potential, charge and work done was discussed in detail in Section 5.2.

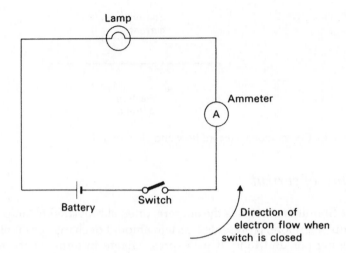

Fig. 7.2   Simple electrical circuit.

7.4   Resistance

Resistance, as the word suggests, is the 'opposition' experienced by an electric current. For example, if you imagine walking down a wide corridor, there would be very little 'opposition' to your progress. Now imagine trying to walk down a crowded narrow corridor. This would be much harder; i.e. the narrow corridor would offer a higher resistance.

As this analogy suggests, energy is lost or used up in overcoming a resistance (electrical or otherwise). Resistance (R) is defined as the ratio of the potential difference (V) applied across a conductor to the current (I) flowing through it:

$$R = \frac{V}{I}$$

The circuit symbol for resistance is ⊑⊒ (The symbol may include the letter R or have a numerical value alongside.) The factors affecting resistance will be discussed in Section 7.4.4.

7.4.1   *What causes electrical resistance?*

We mentioned above that resistance is the 'opposition to the flow of current'. What produces this opposition?

If we imagine looking closely at a piece of wire, we would see all the atoms vibrating and free electrons moving around at random. When we apply a potential difference across the wire, the free electrons tend to move towards the positive end, but on the way they collide with some of the vibrating atoms; this effect is **resistance**.

7.4.2 *Ohm's law*

The German physicist Georg Simon Ohm investigated the relationship between the current flowing through a metallic conductor and the potential difference applied across it. His findings are summarised in **Ohm's law**, which can be applied to many electrical circuits and is best demonstrated by an experiment (Fig. 7.3). (Because charge is not lost anywhere in the circuit, the current leaving the battery must be the same as the current returning to it. Therefore the ammeter can be placed anywhere between the battery and the resistance.)

In this experiment, as with most, we will assume that the wires joining the components together have *no* resistance. (This is of course not strictly true, as all conductors have some resistance.) By altering the values of voltage supplied by the battery the following values of current were obtained:

V	1.0	2.0	3.0	4.0	5.0	6.0	(volts)
I	1.1	2.2	3.3	4.4	5.5	6.6	(amps)

When these values are plotted in the form of a graph we get a straight line (Fig. 7.4). Note that in practice, experimental errors would result in the plotted points deviating slightly from the straight line.

From similar results Ohm concluded that I was proportional to V and Ohm's law is derived from this conclusion. (**Note.** Ohm's law applies only to metallic conductors, sometimes referred to as **ohmic conductors**. **Non-ohmic conductors**, such as crystals and gases, may result in a curve rather than a straight-line graph.) Examples of non-ohmic conductors found in X-ray equipment include the X-ray tube itself and light-emitting diodes.

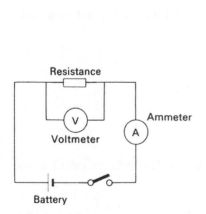

Fig. 7.3 Ohm's law circuit.

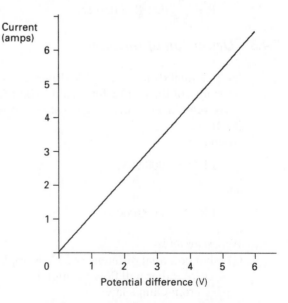

Fig. 7.4 Results of Ohm's law experiment displayed as a graph of current against voltage.

7.4.2.1   Definition of Ohm's law

Ohm's law states that the current flowing through a conductor is directly proportional to the potential difference between its ends, so long as all physical conditions (e.g. temperature) remain constant; i.e.

$$I \propto V$$

Therefore

$$V = I \times \text{constant}$$

This constant is known as *resistance* (R); i.e.

$$V = I \times R$$

and

$$R = \frac{V}{I}$$

The SI unit of resistance is the **ohm** (Ω). Thus if V is in volts and I is in amps, then R is in ohms. Looking back at the Ohm's law experiment, we can check whether this relationship is confirmed. If we take the readings at 1.0, 3.0 and 5.0 volts, we obtain from $R = V/I$:

$$R = \frac{1}{1.1} \text{ (i.e. } R = 0.91 \; \Omega)$$

$$R = \frac{3}{3.3} \text{ (i.e. } R = 0.91 \; \Omega)$$

and

$$R = \frac{5}{5.5} \text{ (i.e. } R = 0.91 \; \Omega)$$

7.4.3   *Definition of the ohm*

If a potential difference of 1 V drives a current of 1 A through a conductor, the resistance of the conductor is said to be 1 Ω.

We often need much larger values, so we use **kilohms** (kΩ) and **megohms** (MΩ),
where:

$$1 \, \text{k}\Omega = 1000 \; \Omega$$

and

$$1 \, \text{M}\Omega = 1\,000\,000 \; \Omega$$

Worked examples
(1)   If a potential difference of 6 V is applied to a 3-kΩ resistance, calculate the current that will flow through it.
        From Ohm's law:

$$I = \frac{V}{R}$$

Therefore

$$I = \frac{6}{3000}$$

$$= \frac{1}{500} \, \text{A}$$

$$= 2 \, \text{mA}$$

(2) If a current of 4 A flows through a resistance of 60 Ω, calculate the potential difference across it.
From Ohm's law:

$$V = IR$$

Therefore

$$V = 4 \times 60$$

$$= 240 \, \text{V}$$

7.4.4 Factors affecting resistance

These can be discussed by comparing electric current flow with the flow of water through a pipe, as shown in the following examples.

7.4.4.1 Length (*l*)

A long pipe will obstruct the flow of water more than a short one. This is analogous to a long conductor, which has a greater resistance than a short one; i.e.

$$R \propto l$$

7.4.4.2 Cross-sectional area (*A*)

A narrow pipe will obstruct the flow of water more than a wide one. This is analogous to a thin conductor, which has a greater resistance than a thick one; i.e.

$$R \propto \frac{1}{A}$$

Combining the above two relationships gives:

$$R \propto \frac{1}{A}$$

or

$$R = \frac{\rho l}{A}$$

where ρ is a constant. We call the constant ρ **resistivity**. It is a measure of the opposition a particular substance exhibits to the passage of electric current. The resistivity of different materials is defined under standard conditions of length and cross-sectional area. It is defined as the resistance in ohms, measured between opposite faces of a cube with a side length of 1 m. For example, the resistivity of copper is 1.55×10^{-8} Ωm at 0°C, for silver $\rho = 1.47 \times 10^{-8}$ Ωm and for gold $\rho = 2.05 \times 10^{-8}$ Ωm. Thus, pieces of wire with the same length and cross-sectional area, if made of different materials, will have different values of resistance.

7.4.4.3 Temperature

At a higher temperature the atoms in a conductor vibrate more actively; thus, it is more likely that the flowing electrons will collide with the vibrating atoms; i.e. the resistance is *increased*. For this reason it is usual to quote resistance values at a standard temperature (in practice, 20°C).

Consider this analogy. Imagine you are in a room half full of people and you are trying to walk from one side to another. If the people are moving slowly, your path to the other side would be fairly easy and this is comparable with low resistance. If, however, all the people were rushing around very actively (with lots of energy), it would be quite hard to reach the other side and this is comparable with high resistance.

It is worth noting here that increasing the temperature of insulators and semi-conductors *reduces* their resistance. This is because at higher temperatures more electrons will be raised into the conduction band, improving their ability to conduct electric current (see Sections 6.1.1.1 and 6.1.1.2).

Temperature coefficient of resistance
The effect of temperature on the resistance of a conductor can be expressed in terms of a temperature coefficient. The **temperature coefficient of resistance** (α) is defined as the fractional change in resistivity per unit change in temperature. If the resistance (R_0) of a conductor at a standard temperature (e.g. 20°C) is known, its resistance (R) at a different temperature can be estimated from the formula:

$$R = R_0(1 + \alpha t)$$

where t is the difference between the required temperature and the standard temperature.

Worked example
The resistance of the tungsten filament of a 60-W mains electric light bulb is 300 Ω at 20°C. Calculate its resistance at its operating temperature of 1500°C. Assume that the temperature coefficient of resistance of tungsten is 5.8×10^{-3} K^{-1}.

In the formula, $R_0 = 300$ Ω, $\alpha = 5.8 \times 10^{-3}$ K^{-1} ($=5.8 \times 10^{-3}$°C^{-1}) and $t = 1500 - 20 = 1480$°C. Therefore using $R = R_0 (1 + \alpha t)$:

$$R = 300(1 + 5.8 \times 10^{-3} \times 1480)$$
$$= 300(1 + 8.6)$$
$$R \approx 2900 \text{ } \Omega$$

The resistance of the filament is increased by a factor of nearly ten times. Note, however, that we have used this merely as an illustration of how temperature affects the resistance of a component. Strictly, the formula $R = R_0 (1 + \alpha t)$ is not appropriate for large temperature changes such as this.

7.4.4.4 Summary

The factors affecting the resistance of a conductor can be remembered by the mnemonic MALT (**m**aterial, **a**rea of cross section, **l**ength and **t**emperature).

7.4.5 *Superconductivity*

It is worth mentioning briefly a property known as **superconductivity**, which is possessed by some materials. At very low temperatures these **superconductors** exhibit *zero* electrical resistance, permitting an electric current flow to be maintained without the need for a potential difference. Metal alloys such as niobium–titanium, which become superconducting below 10 K (−263°C), are used in some magnetic resonance imaging (MRI) equipment (see Section 23.2.1). Cooling is achieved by immersion in liquid helium (temperature 4.2 K).

Some recently discovered ceramic metal-oxide compounds become superconductors at relatively high temperatures, e.g. yttrium–barium copper oxide (at 93 K) and thallium–calcium–bismuth copper oxide (at 125 K). This enables them to be cooled by liquid nitrogen (temperature 77 K), which is a cheaper and more effective coolant than liquid helium.

7.5 Combinations of resistances

Resistors in electrical circuits may be combined *either*

- **in series** – where they are connected end to end so that the current flows through each resistor in turn, *or*
- **in parallel** – where the potential difference across each resistor is the same, but the current divides so that only a proportion of the current passes through each individual resistor.

7.5.1 *Resistors in series*

Let us look first at a circuit with three resistors in *series* (Fig. 7.5). We have already said that resistance is the 'opposition to the flow of current'. It follows,

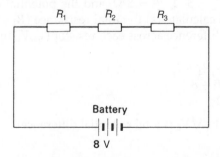

Fig. 7.5 Resistors in series. (R_1, R_2 and R_3 are three resistors in series.)

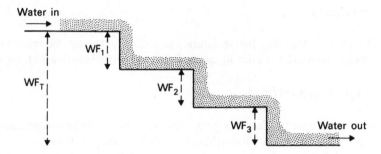

Fig. 7.6   Waterfall analogy of resistances in series.

then, that if we put three resistors in series, the *total* value of these resistors can be calculated by *adding* their individual values. This is a very important idea and we will illustrate it with a numerical example in a moment.

It is first worth considering the potential at various points in this circuit. Because the current in the circuit is the same in all places, it follows that the current through each of the resistors is the same. From Ohm's law, it is therefore possible to calculate the total potential difference or voltage drop across each resistor, namely:

$$V_1 = IR_1$$
$$V_2 = IR_2$$
$$V_3 = IR_3$$

with the total potential difference $V_T = IR_T$. To help understand what is happening, let us imagine a waterfall (Fig. 7.6).

The amount of water flowing in at the top is the same as the amount of water flowing out at the bottom ('current'). The total height difference is WF_T, which is in turn made up of WF_1, WF_2 and WF_3. In this analogy we are comparing a drop in height with a drop in electrical potential.

The total effective resistance (R_T) of three resistors (of values R_1, R_2 and R_3) connected in series is found from the equation:

$$R_T = R_1 + R_2 + R_3$$

Worked example
If $R_1 = 3\ \Omega$, $R_2 = 5\ \Omega$, $R_3 = 8\ \Omega$, and the potential difference supplied by the battery is 8 V, calculate (a) the total resistance (R_T), (b) the current (I), and (c) the potential difference across each resistor (V_1, V_2 and V_3).

(a) $R_T = R_1 + R_2 + R_3$
$R_T = 3 + 5 + 8$
$R_T = 16\ \Omega$

(b) $I = \frac{V_T}{R_T}$ (where V_T is total potential difference)

$I = \frac{8}{16}$

$I = \frac{1}{2}$ amp

(c) $V_1 = I R_1$
$V_1 = \frac{1}{2} \times 3$
$V_1 = 1\frac{1}{2}$ V
$V_2 = I R_2$
$V_2 = \frac{1}{2} \times 5$
$V_2 = 2\frac{1}{2} V$
$V_3 = I R_3$
$V_3 = \frac{1}{2} \times 8$
$V_3 = 4$ V

If we add the individual potential differences, we would expect to get the total potential difference across all three resistors (i.e. the PD supplied by the battery); i.e. $1\frac{1}{2} + 2\frac{1}{2} + 4 = 8$ V.

7.5.2   *Resistors in parallel* (Fig. 7.7)

As with the previous circuit, the current leaving the battery is the same as that returning to it, but in this case the current divides, some current passing through each resistor.

Because the potential difference across all the resistors is the same, the current divides up in a manner *inversely proportional* to their values. Common sense suggests that this will be the case because, given the choice of three routes, the majority of the current chooses the path of least resistance.

The total value of three resistors connected in parallel can be found from the equation:

$$\frac{1}{R_T} = \frac{1}{R_1} + \frac{1}{R_2} + \frac{1}{R_3}$$

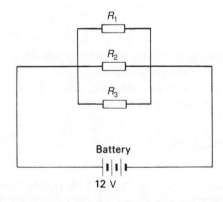

Fig. 7.7   Resistors in parallel. (R_1, R_2 and R_3 are three resistors in parallel.)

Worked example

Let us now calculate the total resistance of the three resistors shown in Fig. 7.7. If $R_1 = 2\,\Omega$, $R_2 = 3\,\Omega$, and $R_3 = 4\,\Omega$,

$$\frac{1}{R} = \frac{1}{R_1} + \frac{1}{R_2} + \frac{1}{R_3}$$

$$\frac{1}{R} = \frac{1}{2} + \frac{1}{3} + \frac{1}{4}$$

$$\frac{1}{R} = \frac{6 + 4 + 3}{12}$$

$$\frac{1}{R} = \frac{13}{12}$$

$$R = \frac{12}{13} = 0.92\,\text{V}$$

Therefore the current in the circuit will be

$$I = \frac{V}{R}$$

$$I = \frac{12}{12/13}$$

$$I = 13\,\text{amps}$$

We can check our calculation by working out the current through each of the individual resistors:

$$I_1 = \frac{V}{R_1} \quad I = \frac{12}{2} \quad I = 6\,\text{amps}$$

$$I_2 = \frac{V}{R_2} \quad I = \frac{12}{3} \quad I = 4\,\text{amps}$$

$$I_3 = \frac{V}{R_3} \quad I = \frac{12}{4} \quad I = 3\,\text{amps}$$

By adding these currents together, we get $6 + 4 + 3 = 13$ amps, which equals the current we calculated using the total resistance value (see above).

7.5.2.1   Summary

(1)   The current approaching resistors in parallel divides in inverse proportion to the value of the resistances.

(2)   The total resistance of resistors connected in parallel is always less than the value of any individual resistor.

7.6   Variable resistors

A **variable resistor** is a component whose resistance value can be altered, either manually or mechanically. One such device, sometimes known as a **rheostat**, is used to provide a continuously variable control of electrical current.

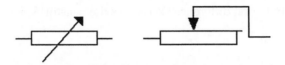

Fig. 7.8 Two alternative circuit symbols representing a variable resistor.

Because for a given potential difference, current (I) is inversely proportional to resistance (R) :

$$I \propto \frac{1}{R}$$

increasing the resistance of the variable resistor will reduce the current flowing in the circuit. Figure 7.8 shows two alternative circuit symbols representing a variable resistor.

7.6.1 *The potential divider*

Two resistors connected in series may be used to provide a given proportion of the total applied potential difference. This arrangement is known as a **potential divider**. Figure 7.9a shows a potential divider with two resistors (R_1 and R_2) connected in series, with a potential difference (V_0) applied across them. The current (I) flowing through the resistors is given by:

$$I = \frac{V_0}{R_1 + R_2}$$

The potential difference across each individual resistor can be found from

$$V = IR$$

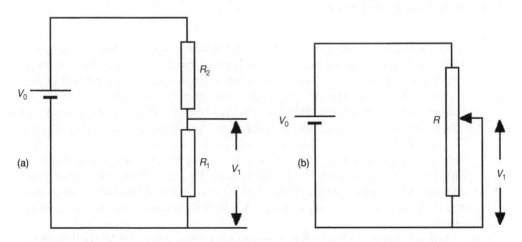

Fig. 7.9 (a) A potential divider using two fixed resistors R_1 and R_2, and (b) a potential divider using a variable resistor R.

e.g. the potential difference (V_1) across the resistor R_1 is

$$V_1 = IR_1$$

If a *variable* resistor is used, as in Fig. 7.9b, the circuit provides a voltage (V_1) which can be varied from zero up to a maximum equal to the applied potential difference (V_0).

7.7   Kirchhoff's laws

The equations we have considered in this chapter can be used to calculate the total value of resistors combined in various ways. From such considerations, Gustav Kirchhoff developed two laws which enable the current in any part of a circuit to be calculated.

Law 1 states that at a junction of two or more conductors, the total current flowing towards the junction is equal to the total current flowing away from it.

This helps us to understand parallel resistor arrangements and it is logical that, because charge cannot build up anywhere in a circuit, the current leaving the negative terminal of the battery will be the same as the current returning to the positive terminal.

Law 2 states that in a complete circuit the sum of the products of current and resistance in each part of the circuit is equal to the total available electromotive force (emf).

This applies to series resistor combinations, where the total applied potential difference divides across each individual resistor in proportion to the product of the current and resistance.

7.8   Internal resistance

If we measure the voltage of a battery when it is not connected in a complete circuit, and then again when it is supplying current, we find in the latter case that there is a drop in voltage. This is because all sources of electrical energy possess **internal resistance**. Why is this voltage drop noticeable only when the battery is in a *complete* circuit? This is because there will be a voltage drop only when *current is flowing* (through the internal resistance). This voltage drop is proportional to the current flowing and is therefore greater and more noticeable with larger currents. For example, if you try to start a car when the headlights are on, you will notice the lights dim. This is because the starter motor draws a very large current (about 200 A) and this will produce a large voltage drop across the battery (about 2 V), which produces the dimming of the lights.

An experiment to show internal resistance is shown in Fig. 7.10. (In this circuit, we have represented the internal resistance by an imaginary resistor in between the plates of the battery.)

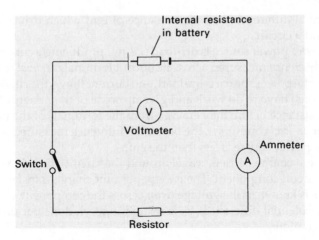

Fig. 7.10 Experiment to illustrate the internal resistance of a battery.

The readings taken were:

(a) Voltage – open circuit (switch off): 6 V
(b) Voltage – complete circuit (switch on): $5\frac{1}{2}$ V
(c) Current – 5 A

From Ohm's law:

$$R = \frac{V}{I}$$

so

$$R_{int} = \frac{V_{drop}}{I}$$

$$R_{int} = \frac{1/2}{5}$$

$$R_{int} = 0.1\ \Omega$$

The internal resistance of the battery is found to be 0.1 Ω.

The magnitude of internal resistance varies considerably between different sources of electrical energy, depending on their size and construction. For example, small chemical batteries generally have a higher internal resistance than larger ones. The *type* of battery also influences internal resistance (e.g. lead–acid, mercury, nickel–cadmium, dry or wet cell, etc.).

7.9 Electromotive force

The **electromotive force** generated by a source of electrical power is the energy per unit charge which is transferred by the source to the charge carriers. Electromotive force, often referred to as '**emf**', is measured in the same units as potential difference. It is the presence of emf which drives an electric current around a circuit.

When a power source is **off-load** (i.e. not producing a current flow), the potential difference measured across its output terminals is *equal* to the emf. However, when the power source is **on-load**, and current flows, the charge carriers (usually electrons) have to do work and give up some of their energy to overcome internal resistance before they emerge from the terminals of the power source. Thus under *on-load* conditions, the potential difference measured across the terminals of the power source is *less* than the emf.

As the charge carriers travel around the circuit, they do work in negotiating each circuit component. The energy per unit charge transferred at each of these stages is known as the **voltage drop** across the component. As we saw in Section 5.2.4, potential difference (V) is related to work done per unit charge (W/Q) by the equation:

$$V = \frac{W}{Q}$$

and because work done means energy transferred

$$V = \frac{E}{Q}$$

It is helpful to visualise the charge-carrying electrons in a circuit 'falling' down the potential gradient created between the terminals of the battery or other power source, like the water down the waterfalls in our analogy illustrated in Fig. 7.6.

Note that the emf generated by each single cell in a battery depends on its chemical constituents rather than on the size of the cell. For example, both a small (MN 2400 size) alkaline dry cell and a large (MN 1300 size) alkaline dry cell produce an emf of 1.5 V.

7.10   Electrical energy and power

7.10.1   *Electrical energy*

We know that energy is the ability to do work, but how can we calculate how much work *electricity* can do?

Reference to the previous section, and to Section 5.2, reminds us that the potential difference (V) between two points is the work done (or energy transferred) per unit charge in moving charge from one point to the other; i.e.

$$V = \frac{E}{Q}$$

from which:

$$E = VQ$$

where E is the energy released when a charge (Q) is moved through a potential difference (V). This relationship therefore enables us to calculate the energy released by the movement of electric charge.

For example, if 5 mC of charge is moved through a potential difference of 50 kV, the energy released is given by:

$$E = 50 \times 10^3 \times 5 \times 10^{-3}$$
$$= 250 \text{ J}$$

(This is roughly the energy released when making a chest X-ray exposure of 5 mA s at 50 kV.) The equation $E = VQ$ can be expressed in a different form, because we know from Section 3.3.3 that charge (Q) represents the product of current (I) and time (t); i.e.

$$Q = It$$

Therefore, $E = VQ$ can also be written in the form:

$$E = VIt$$

Worked example
An electric torch is operated for 60 s. If the torch is powered by a 3-V battery and passes a current of 100 mA, calculate the energy consumed.
Using $E = VIt$:

$$E = 3 \times 100 \times 10^{-3} \times 60$$
$$= 18 \text{ J}$$

Slightly less than 20 J of electrical energy is converted (into light and heat) during the time the torch is switched on.

7.10.2 Electrical power

Power is defined as the rate of doing work, or the rate of conversion of energy (Section 1.3.5). In other words:

$$P = \frac{E}{t}$$

However, in electrical terms we have seen that $E = VIt$. Therefore, electrical power (P) is given by:

$$P = \frac{VIt}{t}$$
$$= VI$$

i.e. electrical power is the product of potential difference (V) and current (I).If V is in volts and I in amperes, then power will be expressed in watts, but note that when large amounts of power are being considered, it is usual to express power in kilowatts (1 kW = 1000 W) or megawatts (1 MW = 1 000 000 W).

Worked examples
(1) Calculate the power ('wattage') of the torch bulb referred to in the previous worked example. The potential difference was 3 V and the current flow was

100 mA therefore,

$$P = VI$$
$$= 3 \times 100 \times 10^{-3}$$
$$= 0.3 \text{ W}$$

The torch bulb operates at a power of 0.3 W.

(2)   Calculate the power involved when an X-ray exposure of 50 kV and 5 mA s is made. Assume that the exposure time involved is 20 ms.

In this case we can employ the relationship:

$$P = \frac{VIt}{t}$$

Because $V = 50 \times 10^3$ V, $It = 5 \times 10^{-3}$ A s and $t = 20 \times 10^{-3}$ s,

$$P = \frac{50 \times 10^3 \times 5 \times 10^{-3}}{20 \times 10^{-3}}$$
$$= 12.5 \times 10^3 \text{ W}$$
$$= 12.5 \text{ kW}$$

Hence during the X-ray exposure, energy is being converted (mostly into heat) at the rate of 12.5 kW.

Summary
(1) Power = the 'rate of doing work' (watts or joules per second).
(2) Energy = 'work done' (joules or watt seconds).
(3) Power = current × voltage.
(4) Energy = power × time.

Worked example
A hair drier has a resistance of 115 Ω and is operated at a potential difference of 230 V. Calculate (a) the current flowing through it, (b) the charge flowing through it in 20 s, (c) the power consumption, and (d) the energy it consumes in 2 min.

(a) From Ohm's law:
$$I = \frac{V}{R}$$
$$= \frac{230}{115}$$
$$= 2 \text{ A}$$

(b) Charge = current × time

$$Q = 2 \times 20$$
$$= 40 \text{ C}$$

(c) Power = current × voltage

$$P = 2 \times 230$$
$$= 460 \text{ W}$$

(d) Energy = power × time

$$E = 460 \times 2 \times 60 \text{ (time in seconds)}$$
$$= 55\,200 \text{ J}$$

7.10.3 *Heating effect of an electric current*

When a current passes through a conductor energy is converted. This energy appears as *heat* (and sometimes light). The amount of energy can be found by using the equation $E = VIt$. By using Ohm's law we can modify this equation. Since

$$V = IR$$

then

$$E = IR \times It$$

or

$$E = I^2 Rt$$

This equation is important because it shows us that the heat generated is proportional to the square of the current; i.e. $H \propto I^2$. In other words, if the current flowing through a component is doubled, there will be four times as much heat produced.

We can use these equations to calculate how much energy an X-ray tube consumes during an exposure. Let us take a typical radiographic exposure, e.g. 100 kV, 50 mA s.

$$\text{Energy} = VQ$$
$$= 100\,000 \times \frac{50}{1000}$$
$$= 5000 \text{ J}$$

Because 99% of the energy consumed in an X-ray tube appears as heat, it is not surprising that the X-ray tube becomes very hot in use!

A very useful application of the heating effect of an electric current is found in a **fuse**. This is a piece of wire whose melting point is accurately known. If a fuse is incorporated into a circuit, and the current in that circuit reaches a dangerous level, the fuse will melt, thus breaking the circuit and preventing the risk of fire or damage to other components in the circuit.

7.11   A further look at capacitance

In Chapter 6 we described electrical storage devices known as capacitors. Having investigated some of the ways in which components may be connected together to form an electrical circuit, we can now explore further the behaviour of capacitors. In particular, we shall study the processes of *charging* and *discharging* capacitors.

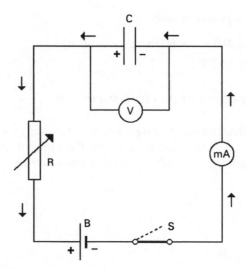

Fig. 7.11   The circuit used to investigate the process of charging a capacitor. The switch (S) is shown in the closed position. The short arrows indicate the flow of electrons around the circuit as the capacitor (C) is charged. The other components in the circuit are battery (B), variable resistor (R), voltmeter (V) and milliammeter (mA) (see text for operational details).

7.11.1   Charging capacitors

Figure 7.11 shows a simple circuit, which we could use to investigate the process of charging a capacitor. A number of different circuit components are included:

- a **capacitor** (C) – the subject of the study (Note that the circuit symbol for a capacitor is a stylised representation of a parallel-plate capacitor.)
- a **battery** (B) – which provides an emf to drive the circuit
- an **ON/OFF switch** (S) – with which we can open and close the circuit
- a **variable resistor** (R) – which enables us to control the current flowing in the circuit
- a **milliammeter** – with which we can monitor the current flowing around the circuit
- a **voltmeter** – which enables us to monitor the potential difference across the capacitor

N.B. To carry out this experiment in the laboratory requires the right equipment and proper preparation and planning. In particular, the circuit components must be carefully chosen to produce a very slow capacitor charging rate: otherwise, the whole charging process will be over in a fraction of a second, rendering the analysis impossible.

7.11.1.1 Initial conditions

Initially, there is no charge stored on the capacitor and the switch is open. The zero reading on the voltmeter shows that the potential difference (V) across the capacitor is zero. This confirms that the capacitor is empty of electric charge (Q), because from the relationship $Q = CV$, if V is zero then Q must be zero. The zero reading on the milliammeter assures us that no current is flowing around the circuit.

7.11.1.2 Charging process

(1) As soon as the switch is closed, the milliammeter detects a current flow (I) in the circuit. The direction of current flow tells us that negative charges are flowing *onto* the right-hand plate of the capacitor, while negative charges are *leaving* its left-hand plate. The left-hand plate is therefore becoming positively charged with respect to the right-hand plate.

(2) At the same time, the voltmeter reading (V) begins to rise. This tells us that the potential difference across the capacitor is rising, and because Q is directly proportional to V, the amount of charge on the capacitor is increasing. In other words, the capacitor is charging.

(3) As time passes, the reading on the milliammeter gradually falls towards zero. This tells us that the capacitor charging process is slowing down. At the same time, the rise in the voltmeter reading begins to slow down. This suggests that the potential difference across the capacitor is approaching some sort of limit.

(4) Eventually, the milliammeter reading settles on zero, indicating that the current in the circuit has stopped flowing. At the same time, the voltmeter reading reaches a final limiting value (V_F) and settles on this value, which we notice is equal to the emf generated by the battery.

The capacitor is now charged, but there are two important features of the capacitor charging process that need further consideration; these are the characteristic way in which

- the PD across the capacitor rises, and
- the current charging the capacitor falls.

7.11.1.3 Pattern of rise in potential difference

Remember that the potential difference across the capacitor started at zero and rose until it reached a final steady value equal to the emf produced by the battery. Why did it behave in this way? The potential difference (V) across the capacitor is merely a reflection of the amount of charge (Q) it contains:

$$V = \frac{Q}{C}$$

If we interpret the changes in potential difference as changes in stored charge, the pattern we observed indicates that:

(1)   Initially, there was no charge in the capacitor.
(2)   There was a *limit* to the amount of charge we could store in the capacitor. This follows from a point made during our discussion of capacitance in Sections 6.2 and 6.2.1: namely, the amount of charge that can be stored in a capacitor depends on the potential difference applied to it and on its capacitance. In our circuit, the potential difference we were able to apply to the capacitor was limited by the battery emf and this, in turn, limited the amount of charge we could store.

7.11.1.4   Pattern of fall in charging current

The current which charged the capacitor started at a high value, gradually decreased and eventually fell to zero. At the moment we switched on the circuit, there was *no* potential drop across the capacitor (the voltmeter reading was zero), so the whole of the potential difference (E) produced by the battery appeared across the resistor. The current flow at that instant was limited only by the value of resistance (R) in the circuit, i.e. by the setting we had chosen on the variable resistor. Ohm's law therefore enables us to determine the *initial* value of current (I_0), i.e. the current flowing at the instant we switched on:

$$I_0 = \frac{E}{R}$$

However, this value of current was not maintained. As the capacitor charged up, the potential difference across it increased and the difference between the battery potential and the capacitor potential fell. Thus, the potential gradient driving current into the capacitor eventually decreased to zero. Consequently, the charging current also decreased and eventually ceased to flow.

7.11.1.5   Effect of the resistor

We have deduced that the initial value of the charging current depends on the circuit resistance (R). For a given battery voltage, if we select a small value for R, a large initial charging current will flow and the capacitor will charge up rapidly. Conversely, if we select a large value for R, the initial charging current will be small and the capacitor will take longer to charge up. The variable resistor therefore provides a means of controlling the *rate* at which the capacitor charges.

7.11.2   *A quantitative approach to capacitor charging*

So far, we have employed a mainly qualitative approach to our analysis of the charging of capacitors. We must now quantify the process. A good starting point is to repeat the observations we have made, but this time record them for closer analysis. We therefore record the values of the circuit components (battery voltage, resistance and capacitance) and the readings (V and I) on the voltmeter and

Table 7.1 Voltmeter and milliammeter readings taken at 2-s intervals during the charging of a capacitor

Time (s)	Voltmeter reading (V)	Milliammeter reading (mA)
0	0.0	1.20
2	2.2	0.98
4	4.0	0.80
6	5.4	0.66
8	6.6	0.54
10	7.6	0.44
12	8.4	0.36
14	9.0	0.30
16	9.6	0.24
18	10.1	0.19
20	10.4	0.16
22	10.7	0.13
24	10.9	0.11
26	11.2	0.08
28	11.3	0.07
30	11.4	0.06

milliammeter. Because the meter readings were not constant, we record them at regular intervals of time, e.g. every 2 s. The meter readings are then tabulated and graphs plotted to show how the charging current and potential difference vary with time. Table 7.1 shows an example of the data that might be obtained, and Figs 7.12 and 7.13 show graphs drawn from the same data.

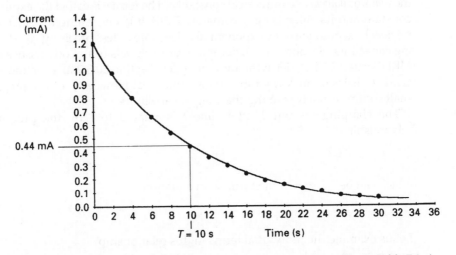

Fig. 7.12 A graph of charging current against time, drawn from data in Table 7.1. A curve has been drawn through the points plotted, showing the characteristic pattern of an exponential decay relationship. Note that after one time constant (in this case 10 s) the current has fallen to 0.44 mA, about 37% of its initial value (see Section 7.11.2.1).

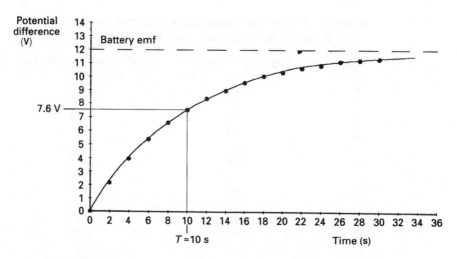

Fig. 7.13 A graph of capacitor potential against time, drawn from data in Table 7.1. The curve shows how the potential difference rises exponentially towards a limiting value equal to the applied emf (in this case 12 V). After one time constant (10 s), the potential difference has risen to 7.6 V, about 63% of its final value (see Section 7.11.2.1).

7.11.2.1   Exponential decay of current

Examination of Fig. 7.12 reveals the characteristic way in which the charging current decays during the charging process. Both theoretical analysis and experimental observations tell us that the decay of charging current with time always follows a precise mathematical **exponential relationship**. The relationship is described as *exponential* because the time variable (t) appears in the **exponent** (i.e. the *index* or *power*) of a numerical constant e. The term e is called the **exponential constant** and its value is approximately 2.718. It is interesting that many other physical phenomena obey exponential rules more or less precisely, e.g. discharging capacitors (Section 7.11.3), decaying radio signals from body tissues during MRI (Section 23.1.4), decaying radionuclides (Section 20.3.2.2), even the cooling characteristics of an X-ray tube and a cup of tea! However, for the present we shall confine ourselves to the charging of capacitors.

The charging current I after time t is related to t by the proportional relationship:

$$I \propto e^{-t/T}$$

which can be written in the form of an equation:

$$I = I_0 e^{-t/T}$$

Let us examine the individual terms in this relationship:

- The term I_0 is the initial value of charging current. As we saw in Section 7.11.1.4, the initial value of charging current $I_0 = E/R$.
- The term $-t/T$ is the exponent of e.

- The negative sign of the exponent indicates that the current decreases as time increases; i.e. it is *decaying*.
- The term T in the exponent is known as the **time constant** of the circuit.

Time constant
A time constant (T) is a fundamental characteristic of all exponential relationships that involve time as one of the variables. Because time constant always represents a quantity of time, its SI unit is the second. In electrical circuits the time constant tells us how rapidly the circuit responds to changing conditions. In the present context, the value of T indicates how quickly the capacitor charges. However, for reasons discussed in Worked Example 4 of Section 7.11.2.2, the time constant is *not* the total time taken for the capacitor to charge fully. T has a high value in circuits where the charging process takes place slowly and a low value in circuits where the charging process is rapid. We saw in Section 7.11.1.5 that the circuit resistance (R) influences charging rate. The capacitance (C) also has an effect because a large capacitor takes longer to charge than a small one. The time constant of a simple capacitor charging circuit depends only on the product of these two factors; i.e.

$$T = RC$$

7.11.2.2   Exponential rise in potential difference

Examination of Fig. 7.13 reveals the way in which the potential difference across the capacitor rises during the charging process. It is clear that the shape of this graph is similar, in some respects, to that for the decay of current, but the curve is inverted. This relationship can also be precisely defined by an exponential expression, but the expression is different from that in Section 7.11.2.1, reflecting the fact that potential difference *rises* with time.

The potential difference V after time t is related to t by the proportional relationship:

$$V \propto (1 - e^{-t/T})$$

and by the equation:

$$V = V_F(1 - e^{-t/T})$$

in which V_F represents the *final* value of the potential difference across the capacitor when the charging process is complete. As we saw in Section 7.11.1.3, V_F is equal to the applied potential difference; i.e. the emf (E) produced by the battery and $e^{-t/T}$ is the same exponential term that we discussed in relation to the decay of charging current (Section 7.11.2.1). The negative sign again tells us that the value of $e^{-t/T}$ decreases with time; it then follows that the value of $1 - e^{-t/T}$ and therefore the potential difference across the capacitor must be *increasing* with time, which is confirmation of the pattern of rising potential difference shown in Fig. 7.13.

Worked examples
Let us now see how these mathematical relationships can be applied to the numerical data we have recorded. The circuit components used to produce the data in Table 7.1 had the following values: capacitance $(C) = 1000$ µF $(=10^3$ microfarads $= 10^{-3}$ farads), resistance $(R) = 10\,000$ Ω $(=10^4$ ohms) and battery emf $(E) = 12$ V.

(1) Finding the time constant.
    We noted that the time constant (T) of the circuit is given by:

$$T = RC$$
$$= 10^4 \times 10^{-3}$$
$$= 10 \text{ s}$$

(2) Finding the initial charging current.
    We also noted that the initial current (I_0) was given by:

$$I_0 = \frac{E}{R}$$
$$= \frac{12}{10^4}$$
$$= 1.2 \times 10^{-3} A$$

(3) Finding the charging current after a given time.
    We can now use the relationship for the exponential decay of current to predict the value of charging current after any given time has elapsed. For example, what will be the value (I) of charging current after 20 s? We insert the values of I_0 and T into the equation.

$$I = I_0 e^{-t/T}$$
$$I = 1.2 \times 10^{-3} \times e^{-20/10}$$
$$= 1.2 \times 10^{-3} \times e^{-2}$$
$$= 1.2 \times 10^{-3} \times 0.135$$
$$= 0.162 \times 10^{-3} A$$
$$= 0.162 \text{ mA}$$

Reference to Table 7.1 shows that after 20 s, our milliammeter reading was 0.16 mA, which is in close agreement with the predicted value.

(4) Finding the total charging time.
    The same table shows that even after 30 s, when we took our final readings, the current had still not reached zero. We can use the exponential decay formula to try to predict how long it would have taken for the current to fall to zero (i.e. how long the capacitor would take to charge fully). In this case we need to rearrange the formula to enable us to find the value of t when I is zero.

$$t = T \log_e (I/I_0)$$
$$= 10 \log_e 0$$

Unfortunately, when we attempt to evaluate $\log_e 0$ with an electronic calculator an error message is displayed. This is because the value of $\log_e 0$ is *infinitely large*, indicating that we would have to wait an infinite length of time for the capacitor to charge fully! (It is a characteristic of all true time-based exponential phenomena that they take an infinite time to complete.) Although at first sight this may seem a great inconvenience, further calculations show that after a period equal to five time constants a capacitor will be more than 99% full of charge. We are probably justified in concluding that to wait any longer than this would serve no practical purpose. On reflection, therefore, perhaps during our experiment we should have continued taking milliammeter and voltmeter readings for a further 20 s (a total of 50 s, or five time constants) to enable us to claim that we had monitored over 99% of the charging process.

(5) Assessing the significance of the time constant.

We have seen that after a period of five time constants, a capacitor is over 99% charged, but by how much will it have charged after just *one* time constant? We can find this by working out the charging current when t is equal to the time constant; i.e. we make $t = T$. The exponent $-t/T$ then becomes $-T/T$, which has the value -1, so that

$$I = I_0 \, e^{-t/T}$$

becomes

$$I = I_0 \, e^{-1}$$
$$= I_0 \times 0.368$$

After a period equal to one time constant, the charging current has fallen to 0.368 (36.8%) of its initial value. In other words, it has fallen *by* 63.2% (100 − 36.8 = 63.2), so 63.2% of the charging process has already taken place.

We could have arrived at the same conclusion by considering the rise in potential difference instead of the fall in current. After one time constant, the potential difference across the capacitor would have *risen* to 63.2% of its final value. In fact, the time constant for *any* phenomenon which follows an exponential pattern can be shown to exhibit the same property: it represents the time taken for 63.2% of the change to have occurred.

7.11.3 *Discharging capacitors*

Having investigated the characteristic way in which a capacitor charging circuit behaves, we now move on to explore how capacitors can be **discharged**. The term *discharge* refers to the process by which the capacitor releases its stored charge. Capacitors can be discharged in a number of ways, e.g. by:

- **Leakage** across the dielectric. Any charged capacitor, if left long enough, will slowly lose its charge because the dielectric material between its plates is not a perfect insulator. A capacitor which discharges in this way is said to be *leaking*. The leakage rates of good-quality capacitors are very low if they

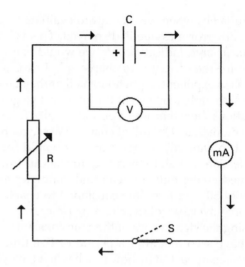

Fig. 7.14   A circuit used to investigate the process of discharging a capacitor. The switch (S) is shown in the closed position. The short arrows indicate the flow of electrons around the circuit as the capacitor (C) discharges. The other components in the circuit are variable resistor (R), voltmeter (V) and milliammeter (mA) (see text for operational details).

are used within their design limits (e.g. if they are not subjected to excessive potential differences).

- **Short circuit** across the terminals. If a conducting wire is connected, either deliberately or by accident, between the terminals of a capacitor, a *short circuit* occurs. Charge then rushes from the negative plate of the capacitor to its positive plate via the conductor and the stored charge is neutralised. The uncontrolled discharge current which occurs may be great enough to damage the conducting wire, the capacitor itself, or possibly both. A short circuit is therefore *not* a sensible way to discharge a capacitor.
- **Controlled discharge** through a resistor. This is the preferred method of discharging a capacitor, which we shall now investigate further.

Controlled discharge of capacitors
The circuit shown in Fig. 7.14 allows us to investigate the controlled discharge of a capacitor. The circuit is very similar to the one used for *charging* a capacitor, but a battery is no longer required and has been omitted. The circuit components include the following:

- A **capacitor** (C) – the subject of the study
- An **ON/OFF switch** (S) – to open and close the circuit
- A **variable resistor** (R) – to control the current flowing in the circuit
- A **milliammeter** – to monitor the current flowing around the circuit
- A **voltmeter** – to monitor the potential difference across the capacitor

7.11.3.1   Initial conditions

Initially, the switch (S) is open and no current is flowing, so the milliammeter reads zero. The capacitor has previously been charged and the voltmeter therefore reads the potential difference (V_0) across its terminals.

7.11.3.2   Discharging process

(1) As soon as the switch is closed, the milliammeter detects a current flow (I) in the circuit. The direction of current flow tells us that negative charges are leaving the negatively charged right-hand plate of the capacitor, while negative charges are arriving on the positively charged left-hand plate.

(2) At the same time, the voltmeter reading begins to fall from its initial value, reflecting the redistribution of charge in the capacitor.

(3) As time passes, the milliammeter reading gradually falls towards zero; the discharging process is slowing down. Meanwhile, the voltmeter reading also falls towards zero as the amount of charge stored in the capacitor drops.

(4) Eventually, both milliammeter and voltmeter readings settle on zero, indicating that the discharge process has ended.

The capacitor is now empty.

Figures 7.15 and 7.16 are graphical representations of the change of current and potential difference with time. Notice the similarities between this *discharge* process and the charging process discussed earlier. It is clear that we are again dealing with examples of **exponential decay**. As before, we will consider the

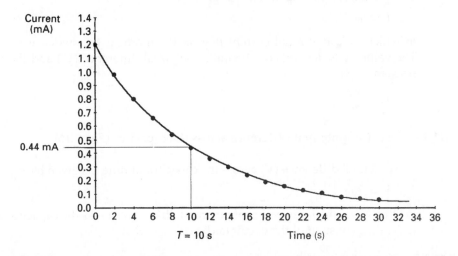

Fig. 7.15   A graph showing the exponential decay of current as a capacitor discharges through a resistor (Section 7.11.3.4). After one time constant (10 s), the current has fallen to 0.44 mA, about 37% of its initial value. The graph is identical to that shown for the charging capacitor in Fig. 7.12 because we have assumed the same values for potential difference (V), and for capacitance (C) and resistance (R), thereby defining the same time constant ($T = RC$).

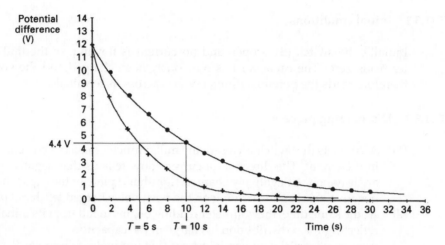

Fig. 7.16 A graph showing how the potential across a capacitor decays exponentially with time as the capacitor discharges through a resistor (Section 7.11.3.3). Two curves are shown, illustrating the two rates of discharge and two time constants (5 and 10 s), which are the result of two different values of circuit resistance. In both cases, after one time constant the potential difference has fallen to 4.4 V (about 37% of its initial value).

patterns of change in the current flow from the capacitor and the potential difference across it.

7.11.3.3   Decay of discharge current (Fig. 7.15)

The current (I) flowing at time t is given by:

$$I = I_0 e^{-t/T}$$

in which I_0 is the initial current flow at the moment the switch was closed. The value of I_0 depends on the initial potential difference (V_0) and the circuit resistance (R) :

$$I_0 = \frac{V_0}{R}$$

7.11.3.4   Decay of potential difference across the capacitor (Fig. 7.16)

The potential difference (V) across the capacitor at time t is given by:

$$V = V_0 e^{-t/T}$$

in which V_0 is the initial value of potential difference across the capacitor and T is the time constant of the circuit (as before, $T = RC$).

7.11.3.5   Effect of the resistor

The resistor controls the rate at which the capacitor discharges because it affects the value of the time constant and, as we have seen, it limits the initial flow of discharge current. A similar strategy can be used to control the *charging* rate of a capacitor. If R is extremely small, the discharge takes place very rapidly, which is what happens when a short circuit occurs. Figure 7.16 shows *two* rates of exponential voltage decay as a capacitor discharges, each one representing the effect of a different value of circuit resistance (R).

7.11.4　Similarities between charging and discharging

For both processes:

- The current flow follows a similar pattern of decay, described mathematically by the relationship $I = I_0 e^{-t/T}$.
- Time constant $T = RC$.

7.11.5　Differences between charging and discharging

- Potential difference *rises* when the capacitor charges:

    $V = V_F(1 - e^{-t/T})$

- Potential difference *falls* when the capacitor discharges:

    $V = V_0 e^{-t/T}$

- Charging a capacitor requires an *input* of energy. (*Work has to be done* to deposit charge on the capacitor.) A charged capacitor is therefore an energy store.
- Discharging *releases* energy from the capacitor. (A charged capacitor can *do work*.)

7.11.6　Combinations of capacitors in circuits

Just as with resistors, capacitors can be joined together in circuits.

When capacitors are joined together in series (Fig. 7.17), the following equation is used to calculate the total capacitance:

$$\frac{1}{C_T} = \frac{1}{C_1} + \frac{1}{C_2} + \frac{1}{C_3}$$

i.e. the total capacitance is less than that of any individual capacitor.

Figure 7.18 shows three capacitors connected in parallel. The total capacitance is found by the equation:

$$C_T = C_1 + C_2 + C_3$$

i.e. the total capacitance is the sum of the individual capacitors.

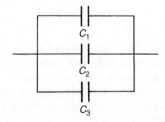

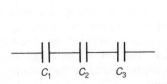

Fig. 7.17　Capacitors in series.

Fig. 7.18　Capacitors in parallel.

Note. Compare these formulae with those for resistance calculations in Sections 7.5.1 and 7.5.2.

7.11.7   *Applications of capacitors*

The circuits shown in Figs 7.11 and 7.14 were devised purely to demonstrate the charging and discharging characteristics of capacitors. They do not represent the practical uses of capacitors. However, certain aspects of the behaviour of capacitors may suggest possible applications in diagnostic imaging such as those outlined below.

7.11.7.1   Smoothing capacitors

Capacitors absorb, store and release electric charge rather in the manner that a spring absorbs, stores and releases energy. Springs are used in the suspension systems of motor cars, where they help to absorb the undulations in the road surface and provide us with a smoother ride. When a wheel drops into a pot-hole, the spring expands, releasing its stored energy and momentarily helps to support the frame of the car. This reduces any disturbance to the passengers. Conversely, when a wheel encounters a hump in the road, the suspension spring is compressed, preventing the frame of the car from rising. This again minimises the effect on the passenger.

Capacitors can have a similar *smoothing* effect in an electrical circuit. For example, unwanted variations in the potential difference of a *direct current* electrical supply to an appliance can be minimised by connecting a capacitor across the supply. If the supply voltage drops below its correct value, the capacitor makes up some of the deficit and the appliance is protected from the worst effects of the change in voltage (Fig. 7.19). Note, however, that a smoothing capacitor can

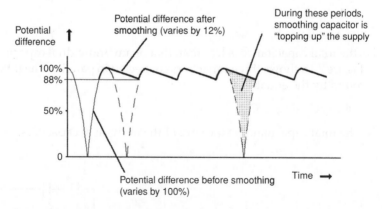

Fig. 7.19   The effect of a smoothing capacitor. In the example shown, the supplied potential difference varies between zero and a maximum (100%). The smoothing capacitor 'tops up' the supply, raising its minimum value from zero to (say) 88% of the maximum, thus providing a more constant potential difference, which varies only by 12% (i.e. it has a 12% ripple). A larger value of capacitance would produce an even more effective smoothing action and a reduced ripple factor.

compensate only for *momentary* variations in voltage. **Smoothing capacitors** are often used in modern X-ray units to provide a more constant high-voltage X-ray tube supply (see Section 13.2.2.1).

7.11.7.2   Capacitor timing

We have seen that the charging and discharging rates of capacitors can easily be controlled by selecting different values of circuit resistance (Sections 7.11.1.5 and 7.11.3.5). It is therefore a relatively simple matter to devise a circuit in which the potential difference across a charging capacitor rises to a given value in any predetermined time. In Fig. 7.13, for example, the potential difference across the capacitor reached 7.6 V after 10 s. When the voltmeter reading indicated 7.6 V, we would know that 10 s had elapsed. If we reduced the circuit resistance to half its former value, the time constant of the circuit would be halved and the potential difference would then reach 7.6 V in only 5 s. We can therefore employ the capacitor charging circuit as a basis for measuring time. Such an arrangement is known as a **time-base circuit** and it provides a very reliable and accurate method of timing certain events, even for times as short as thousandths of seconds (*millisecond* timing). The control of the duration of a radiographic exposure is sometimes based on the charging of such a **timing capacitor**.

Chapter 8
Magnetism and Electromagnetism

Laws of magnetic force
Force between magnetic poles
Magnetisation
Dia-, para- and ferromagnetism
Magnetic fields
Magnetic flux and flux density
Magnetic effect of electric current
Force on a current-carrying conductor
Moving-coil meter

8.1 Introduction

The effect known as magnetism was first observed more than 2000 years ago, but perhaps the most common example of a magnet is the magnetic compass which was invented by the Chinese in the eleventh-century AD as an aid to navigation. It was discovered that one end of the compass needle points towards the north pole of the earth and the other end towards the south pole. It was subsequently discovered that the magnetic effect appears to arise from two specific regions known as the **poles**, near the ends of the magnet. The north-seeking end of a magnet is called its **north pole** and the south-seeking end, its **south pole**.

8.2 Law of magnetic force

If two bar magnets are suspended so that they are free to rotate, we find that two south magnetic poles repel each other and two north magnetic poles repel each other, but a south pole attracts a north pole. These observations are summarised in the **law of magnetic force**, which states that *like poles repel and unlike poles attract*.

It is now known that *all* magnetism is the result of the movement of electric charge and we shall consider the links between electricity and magnetism later in this chapter. The effects of magnetism, however, were first described without this knowledge.

8.3 Force between magnetic poles

The force of attraction (or repulsion) between two magnetic poles depends on a number of factors: specifically, the *strength* of the individual magnetic poles, the *distance* separating them and the material or *medium* occupying the space between them.

We can estimate the magnetic force between two poles in a similar way to the method previously described to estimate the *electric* force between two charges (Section 3.3). Note, however, that whilst the concept of magnetic poles is in some ways very similar to that of electric charges, there is a fundamental difference between them: namely, that a single magnetic pole cannot exist in isolation (see Section 8.4.3.2).

The force (F) between two magnetic poles is given by the inverse square law relationship:

$$F \propto \frac{m_1 m_2}{d^2}$$

where m_1 and m_2 are the pole strengths and d is the distance between them.

From this proportional relationship, we can derive the equation:

$$F = \frac{m_1 m_2}{4\pi \mu d^2}$$

where $1/4\pi \mu$ is the constant of proportionality. The SI unit of pole strength is the **weber** (Wb). The quantity μ is known as **permeability**.

8.3.1 *Permeability*

The **absolute permeability** (μ) of a medium is a characteristic of the medium which is the magnetic equivalent of the electrical permittivity (ε) discussed in Section 3.3.4.1. For forces acting in a vacuum, the **permeability of free space** is represented by the symbol μ_0, where:

$$\mu_0 = 1.26 \times 10^{-6} \text{ weber per ampere metre (Wb A}^{-1} \text{ m}^{-1})$$

Note that the SI unit of permeability, the **weber per ampere metre**, is equivalent to the **henry per metre** (H m^{-1}). The value of μ_0 may therefore be quoted as 1.26×10^{-6} H m^{-1}. We shall encounter the SI unit known as the **henry** (H) in Chapter 9.

Reference if often made to the **relative permeability** of a medium (μ_r), which is the ratio of the absolute permeability of a medium to the permeability of free space,

$$\mu_r = \frac{\mu}{\mu_0}$$

Note that relative permeability has no units because it is a simple ratio of two similar quantities. Table 8.1 shows the values of relative permeability for a range of different media.

8.4 **Magnetisation**

The magnetisation of materials depends largely on the presence of **atomic dipoles**, which arise from the various orbital and spin magnetic moments of

Table 8.1 Values of relative permeability

Medium	Relative permeability (μ_r)
Water	0.99999
Vacuum (by definition)	1
Air	1.0000004
Platinum	1.0001
Iron	5500
Stalloy	5500
Mumetal	80 000

the atomic electrons. The dipoles in most materials are arranged randomly, resulting in no net magnetic effect.

8.4.1   Diamagnetism

Diamagnetic materials possess no inherent dipoles, but their electron orbits can be distorted by the application of an external magnetic field or magnetising force. Removal of the external field results in the loss of alignment and no residual magnetism remains. The relative permeability of diamagnetic materials (e.g. water) is always less than 1 because the induced magnetism *opposes* the external field (see Lenz's law, Section 9.3). Diamagnetic effects are always very weak.

8.4.2   Paramagnetism

Atoms in paramagnetic materials possess inherent magnetism, resulting from the spin and orbiting of electrons around the atomic nucleus. Each atom resembles a very small bar magnet. Application of an external magnetic field causes some alignment of these atomic 'bar magnets' and the sample becomes magnetised. The effect is relatively weak, and at normal temperatures the alignment is quickly destroyed by the background internal energy in the material. Thus the induced magnetism decays rapidly after removal of the external magnetic field.

8.4.3   Ferromagnetism

Ferromagnetic materials contain groups of aligned atomic dipoles known as **domains**. Each domain may be less than 1 mm^3 in size. In a non-magnetised sample, the domains are randomly orientated (Fig. 8.1) and there is no net magnetic effect.

Under the influence of an external magnetic field the domains become aligned, resulting in a considerable degree of magnetisation (Fig. 8.2). Examples of ferromagnetic materials include iron, nickel, stalloy and mumetal.

8.4.3.1   Magnetic saturation

Application of a strong magnetising force to a ferromagnetic material eventually results in the complete alignment of all the domains. Increasing the magnetising

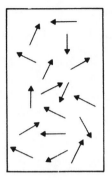

Fig. 8.1 Random arrangement of domains in a non-magnetised ferromagnetic material. ↑ indicates north pole.

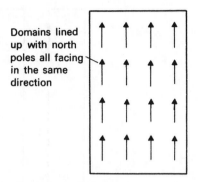

Domains lined up with north poles all facing in the same direction

Fig. 8.2 Arrangement of domains in a magnetised ferromagnetic material.

force beyond this point does not result in any further increase in magnetisation. **Magnetic saturation** has been achieved (Fig. 8.3). Removal of the magnetising force still leaves the material with some residual magnetism or **remanence**, because many of the domains remain aligned. A reversed magnetising force called **coercive force** must be applied to destroy the alignment and achieve complete demagnetisation. This magnetic inertia, or resistance to changes in magnetisation, exhibited to a greater or lesser degree by all ferromagnetic materials, is known as **hysteresis**.

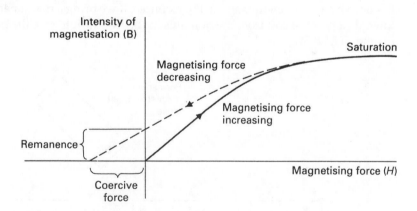

Fig. 8.3 Graphical representation of remanence and coercive force.

8.4.3.2 What happens if we try to isolate one magnetic pole?

If we cut a small piece off the end of a magnet to try to isolate the north pole, we find that there is always a south pole associated with it. Thus it is impossible for a magnetic pole to exist on its own (Fig. 8.4).

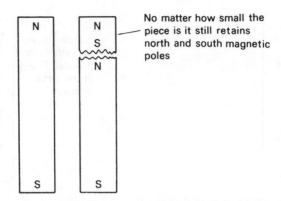

Fig. 8.4   An attempt to isolate the north pole of a magnet.

8.4.3.3   Permanent magnets

Compass needles and other devices manufactured to retain their magnetism for a very long time are known as permanent magnets. They are made of hard ferromagnetic iron and retain their magnetism because the domains find it difficult to turn, and once they are facing in one direction, they are reluctant to alter their arrangement.

8.4.3.4   Temporary magnets

In contrast, some ferromagnetic materials become *temporary magnets* when influenced by a permanent magnet. For example, if we bring a permanent magnet towards a piece of soft iron, the domains in the iron turn to face the permanent magnet (Fig. 8.5).

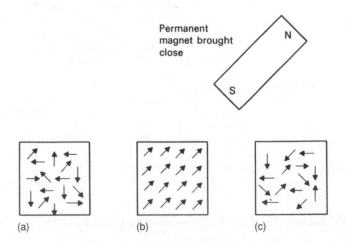

Fig. 8.5   (a) Non-magnetised piece of soft iron; (b) soft iron becomes temporary magnet under the influence of approaching permanent magnet; (c) soft iron returns to non-magnetised state, after permanent magnet is removed.

However, when the permanent magnet is taken away, the domains return to their random arrangement again. This is because the domains are free to rotate.

8.5 Magnetic fields

Just as electric charges are surrounded by an electric field (Section 3.4), so too are magnets surrounded by a magnetic field. A magnetic field is an area around a magnet in which a magnetic effect is noticed.

8.5.1 Lines of force

Magnetic fields are mapped out with **lines of force**. A line of force can be defined as the path taken by an independent north pole moving from the north pole of a magnet to the south. The total number of lines of force can be used to express pole strength and is known as **magnetic flux**.

Lines of force can be observed in two ways:

(1) A bar magnet is placed under a sheet of paper and lots of small particles of soft iron (iron filings) are sprinkled on top. When the paper is tapped, the iron filings line up in the paths of the lines of force (Fig. 8.6).
(2) The lines of force can be plotted, as in Fig. 8.6, but by using small compass needles. This method also illustrates their direction (Fig. 8.7).

8.5.1.1 Observations

(1) A line of force originates at the north pole and ends at the south pole.
(2) No two lines of force cross each other.
(3) The strength of a magnetic field is greatest near its poles. This is shown by the concentration of lines of force (flux density – see Section 8.5.2).

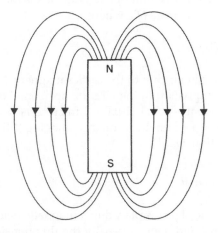

Fig. 8.6   Magnetic field around a bar magnet.

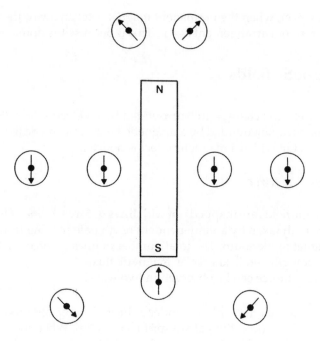

Fig. 8.7   Compass used to illustrate the direction of lines of force.

It is worth noting that magnetic fields are three dimensional; only two dimensions are illustrated for simplicity.

8.5.2   *Magnetic flux and flux density*

The term **magnetic flux** is often used to indicate the total number of lines of magnetic force, and the term **flux density** (B) is used to represent the magnetic flux per unit area. The SI unit of magnetic flux is the **weber** (Wb) and the SI unit of flux density is the **tesla** (T), where

$$1\,\text{T} = 1\,\text{Wb m}^{-2}$$

The flux density in air due to the *earth's* magnetic field has both a vertical and a horizontal component. In the UK, the horizontal component is 19 μT and the vertical component is 43 μT (1 μT = 1 microtesla = 10^{-6} T). By comparison, the magnetic field in a magnetic resonance imaging (MRI) unit may be 30 000 times this value (Section 23.2.1).

8.5.3   *Field distortion*

If a ferromagnetic object is placed in a magnetic field, the effect is to *concentrate* the lines of force and hence intensify the flux density within and immediately around the object (Fig. 8.8).

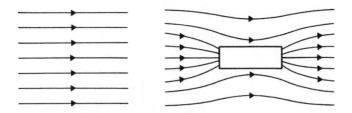

Fig. 8.8   Distortion of magnetic field using ferromagnetic material.

8.5.4   *The horseshoe-shaped magnet*

A horseshoe-shaped magnet is used in the construction of moving-coil milliammeters (Section 8.6.4.1).

This is really just a bar magnet that has been bent into a horseshoe shape (Fig. 8.9). It does however offer two important advantages over a conventional straight bar magnet:

(1)   The strength of the magnetic field is greater because the poles are closer together.
(2)   By adding specially shaped soft-iron pole pieces, we can produce a magnetic field in which most of the lines of force are parallel to each other.

This effect will be used later when we look at the construction of meters (Section 8.6.4.1).

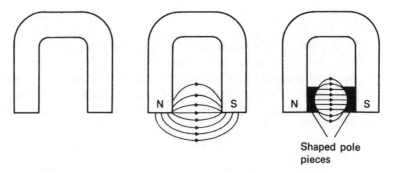

Fig. 8.9   Horseshoe-shaped magnet.

8.6   Magnetic effect of an electric current

In 1820, Oersted discovered that there was a magnetic effect associated with the passage of an electric current. (This is logical because magnetism in temporary and permanent magnets is the result of electron movement around atoms.) When a compass needle is placed near a current-carrying conductor, a deflection is noticed when the current is switched on.

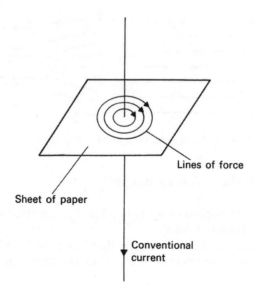

Fig. 8.10   Magnetic field around a current-carrying conductor.

8.6.1   *Observations*

(1)   The magnetic field is present only when the current is switched on.
(2)   The lines of force around the conductor are circular (Fig. 8.10).
(3)   Their direction (clockwise or anticlockwise) depends on the direction of the current.

The direction of the lines of force can be predicted by using Maxwell's corkscrew rule (which applies to conventional current). If the current is *in* to the paper, the magnetic field is *clockwise*, and if the current comes *out* of the paper, the magnetic field is *anticlockwise*. Compare this with screwing a corkscrew into a cork; when the corkscrew is going into the cork, the direction of rotation is clockwise (Fig. 8.11).

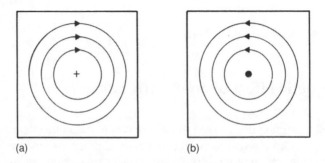

Fig. 8.11   Direction of lines of force around a straight current-carrying conductor: (a) current *in* to page (away from us); (b) current *out* of page (towards us).

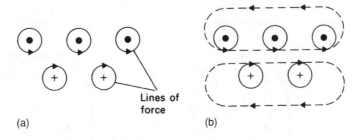

(a)   (b)

Fig. 8.12 Lines of force around the turns of a current-carrying coil: (a) cross section through coil; (b) the combined effect of the lines of force.

The dot (·) in the centre indicates that the current is coming out towards us, and the cross (+) indicates that the current is going away from us. The magnetic fields produced by this method are, however, too weak to be of any practical use.

8.6.2   *Coils and solenoids*

If the conductor is wound into the shape of a **coil** (**solenoid**), we find that the magnetic effect is much stronger. This is because each of the turns produces a magnetic field which reinforces the next (Figs. 8.12 and 8.13). (Note the similarity to the magnetic field produced by a bar magnet.)

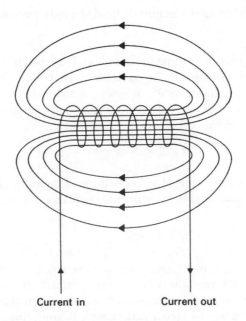

Current in   Current out

Fig. 8.13   The resultant magnetic field around the coil.

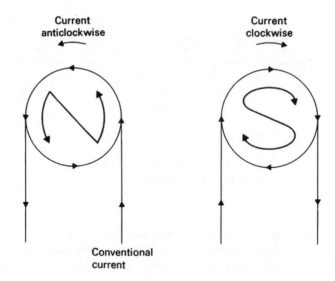

Fig. 8.14   Magnetic poles associated with the ends of the coil.

8.6.2.1   How do we know which end of the coil is a north pole?

A simple way is to look at the coil from the end; if a letter N can be drawn with its 'legs' representing the direction of current, it is a north pole. Conversely, S represents a south pole (Fig. 8.14).

8.6.2.2   Factors affecting the magnetic field strength produced by a coil

Presence of a core
Inserting a piece of ferromagnetic material (e.g. soft iron), known as a **core**, inside the coil greatly increases the strength of the field it generates because the core becomes magnetised. As the magnetic domains in the core become aligned, the resulting magnetisation of the core reinforces the magnetic field produced by current flow in the coil.

Current
For a coil with *no* core, the magnetic field strength (H) produced by a coil is directly proportional to the **current** (I) flowing through the coil:

$$H \propto I$$

In a coil with a ferromagnetic core, the vast majority of the field strength it creates arises from magnetisation of the core material itself. Increasing the current flowing through such a coil increases field strength significantly until *all* the domains in the core are aligned (**core saturation**). Beyond this stage, further increases in current result in much smaller increases in field strength (Fig. 8.15).

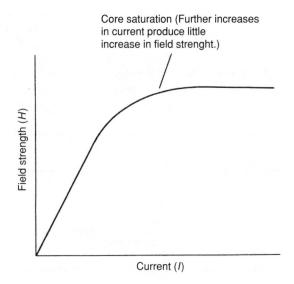

Fig. 8.15   Effect on field strength when the volume of current is increased.

Number of turns (n)
Increasing the **number of turns** of wire on the coil increases the field strength
(*H*) because for each extra turn of wire, additional lines of force are produced.
For a coil with no core,

$$H \propto n$$

A solenoid with a soft-iron core is known as an **electromagnet**. The soft-iron core acts as a temporary magnet and therefore does not retain much of its magnetism after the current has been switched off. Thus, we have a magnet which can be switched on and off as required.

8.6.2.3   Practical applications

(1)   Equipment for removing metallic foreign bodies from the eye
(2)   Brakes on X-ray equipment, e.g. to hold X-ray tubes in position
(3)   Remotely operated switches, known as relays, use electromagnets to open and close electrical contacts
(4)   Underpinning principle of MRI (see Chapter 23)

8.6.3   *Force on a current-carrying conductor in a magnetic field*

Because we know that there are always forces of attraction or repulsion between magnets (magnetic fields), it would be reasonable to assume that such a force would exist between a permanent magnet and a current-carrying conductor. This is known as the **motor effect** (see Fig. 8.16).

When a current flows through the conductor, it moves at right angles to the magnetic field; in this example it moves downwards. (There is *no* movement towards either of the poles.)

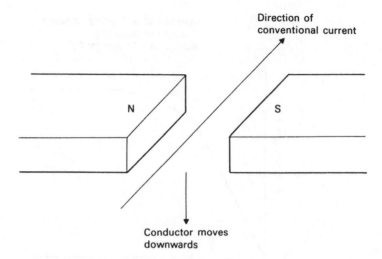

Fig. 8.16   Force on a current-carrying conductor in a magnetic field.

If the direction of current is reversed, we find that the movement of the conductor is reversed; i.e. it moves upwards. Similarly, if the direction of the magnetic field is reversed, the movement is again reversed. The reason for this movement is illustrated in Fig. 8.17.

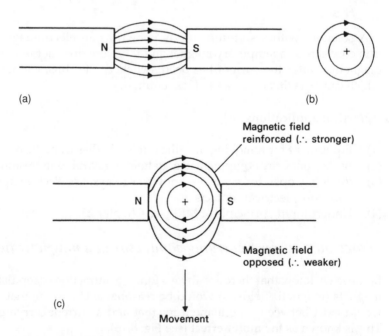

Fig. 8.17   Reason for the movement: (a) magnetic field produced by permanent magnets; (b) magnetic field produced by current-carrying conductor; (c) result of interaction of these two magnetic fields.

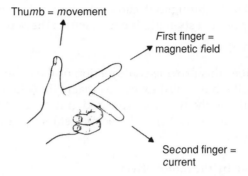

Thumb = *movement*

First finger = magnetic field

Second finger = current

Fig. 8.18   Fleming's left-hand rule.

The rule which determines the direction of motion of the conductor is **Fleming's left-hand rule** (Fig. 8.18). This states that 'if the first three fingers of the left hand are extended at right angles to each other, so that the first finger indicates the direction of the magnetic field and the second finger indicates the direction of the current, then the thumb will indicate the direction of movement of the conductor'. An easy way to remember this is:

> **First finger = Field**
> **Second = Current**
> **Thumb = Movement**

By applying this rule we can see why the direction of movement is reversed if either the field or the current is reversed. If both the field and the current are reversed, the direction of movement remains the same.

It should be realised that the interaction is between the field produced by the magnet and the field produced by the current. The conductor plays no part except as a carrier of the current.

8.6.3.1   Biot–Savart law

If the angle of the conductor to the external magnetic field is θ, then the force (F) on the conductor is given by:

$$F = BIl \sin \theta$$

where B is flux density, I is current and l is length of conductor.

This relationship is known as the **Biot–Savart law**. Note that if the conductor is *parallel* to the magnetic field, the angle θ is zero and the conductor will experience no force.

The link between the tesla and electrical units
Rearranging the above relationship gives:

$$B = \frac{F}{Il \sin \theta}$$

Inserting SI units throughout leads us to the conclusion that the tesla (the unit of flux density or field strength) is equivalent to the newton per ampere metre; i.e.

$$1\,T = 1\,NA^{-1}\,m^{-1}$$

Not only does this provide confirmation of the close link between magnetism and electricity, but it also expresses magnetic field strength in terms of *force*. This is similar to the way we expressed gravitational field strength as *force* per unit mass (Section 1.3.2.2) and electric field strength as *force* per unit charge (Section 3.4.2).

8.6.3.2   Work done by the motor effect

The work done by the current in moving the conductor may be calculated from the following relationship:

Work done = force × distance moved in the direction of the force (see Section 1.3.3)

8.6.3.3   The ampere

The next logical conclusion is that the magnetic fields arising from *two* current-carrying conductors will interact in a similar way. This application of the motor effect is used to define the ampere, the SI unit of electric current.

Definition
A current of 1 A flows in one infinitely long straight wire if an equal current in a similar wire placed 1 m away in a vacuum produces a mutual force of $2 \times 10^{-7}\,N\,m^{-1}$.

8.6.4   *Applications of the motor effect*

There are many applications of the motor effect in X-ray equipment. For example, it is used to deflect electron beams in television cameras and monitors, and also in electric motors. However, we shall illustrate an application of the motor effect by describing the sensitive current-measuring instrument known as a moving-coil milliammeter. At one time, this analogue instrument was a common sight on the control panels of X-ray units to monitor X-ray tube current, but it has largely been replaced by various forms of digital display.

8.6.4.1   Moving-coil meter

Components
(1)   A horseshoe-shaped magnet with curved pole pieces, with a cylindrical soft-iron core (Fig. 8.19)
(2)   An aluminium former (frame) with a coil of thin (insulated) wire wound on it (Fig. 8.20)
(3)   A spindle attached to the former and held in place with spiral springs and jewelled bearings
(4)   A pointer attached to the former and moving over a linear scale

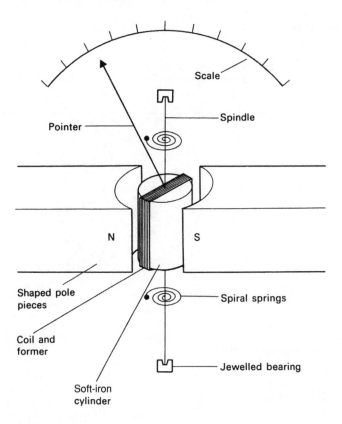

Fig. 8.19 Moving-coil meter.

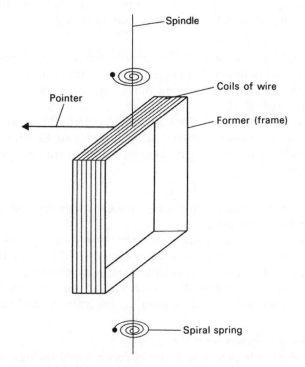

Fig. 8.20 Moving parts of a moving-coil meter.

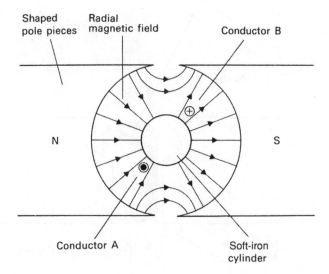

Fig. 8.21   Plan view of a moving-coil meter, showing lines of force between poles of a horseshoe-shaped magnet.

Principle of operation
The principle depends on the motor effect. (It is important to remember that if the conductor is parallel to the magnetic field, it will experience no force.)

Looking at Fig. 8.21, we can assume that the coil is made up of a single turn of wire. (In practice, this is not normally the case.)

(1)   **Looking at wire A.** This is carrying (conventional) current up, toward us, and the magnetic field is left to right. Applying Fleming's left-hand rule, we find that the resulting movement is upwards, at right angles to the magnetic field.

(2)   **Looking at wire B.** This is carrying current down, away from us, and the magnetic field is from left to right. Applying Fleming's left-hand rule, we find that the resulting movement is downwards, at right angles to the magnetic field.

The combined effect of these two forces causes the coil and former to twist (clockwise) about the pivot.

This twisting effect is opposed by the spiral springs. The amount of twisting force is directly proportional to the current, and because the magnetic field is radial, with lines of force equally spaced, equal amounts of current will produce equal increases in the twisting force. We can see from this that the graduations on the scale will be equally spaced; i.e. the scale will be linear.

Function of components
The shaped pole pieces, soft-iron cylinder, spiral springs and the former serve certain functions:

(1) The curved pole pieces produce lines of force which are parallel to each other and equally spaced. The soft-iron cylinder changes the parallel magnetic field into a radial field, i.e. one in which the lines of force are always at right angles to the movement of the coil and former.

(2) The spiral springs, as well as returning the pointer to zero after the current is switched off, also lead the current in and out of the coil. It is important that the opposition they produce to the coil movement is proportional to the twisting force to ensure a linear scale. One is wound clockwise and the other anticlockwise to compensate for temperature changes.

(3) The former helps the pointer settle quickly at the correct reading. How it does this will be explained in Chapter 9. It also acts as a frame to support the coil.

The direction of the current must be known, because reversing the current would reverse the movement of the pointer.

8.6.4.2 Electric motor

A rotary electric motor is constructed in a broadly similar way and operates on the same fundamental principle as the moving-coil meter. However, in a simple direct-current electric motor, the spiral springs are replaced by **brushes**, which provide a means for current to enter and leave the coil during its continuous rotation. Furthermore, the coil is wrapped around a freely rotating iron core, forming an assembly known as an **armature**.

Chapter 9

Electromagnetic Induction

Induced emf
Fleming's right-hand rule
Electromagnetic induction in a coil
Laws of electromagnetic induction
Mutual induction
Self-induction
Time constant

9.1 Induced emf

The English physicist Michael Faraday (1791–1867) was convinced that because a current produced a magnetic field, the opposite must also be true; i.e. a magnetic field can produce a current. He eventually proved this and showed that when a conductor is moved through a magnetic field, an emf is induced in the conductor. If the ends of the conductor are joined to form a complete circuit then current will flow.

9.1.1 Experiment to demonstrate electromagnetic induction

The experiment to illustrate this is similar to that for the motor effect; i.e. the movement of the conductor must be across rather than parallel to the magnetic field (Fig. 9.1).

9.1.1.1 Further findings

(1) If the direction of movement or field is reversed, the direction of the induced emf is also reversed.
(2) The magnitude of the induced emf is proportional to the speed of movement and strength of the magnetic field.
(3) The effect is the same if the magnet is moved and the conductor remains stationary.
(4) No emf is induced unless there is movement between the conductor and the magnet.

9.1.2 Fleming's right-hand rule

The rule which tells us the direction of the induced emf is **Fleming's right-hand rule**, which states that 'if the first three fingers of the right hand are extended at right angles to each other so that the thumb indicates the direction of movement and the first finger indicates the direction of the magnetic field, then the second

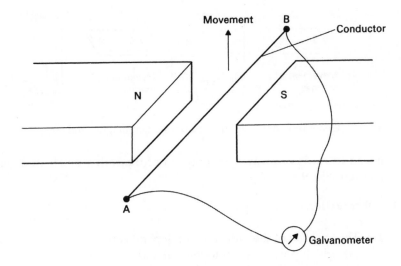

Fig. 9.1 Production of an emf by movement of a conductor through a magnetic field.

finger indicates the direction of the induced emf' (Fig. 9.2).

> Thumb = **movement**
> First finger = **field**
> Second finger = **emf**

The direction of the induced emf will be the same as the direction of the conventional current if the circuit is complete. Thus, in Fig. 9.1, if the conductor is moved upwards, the current will flow from A to B.

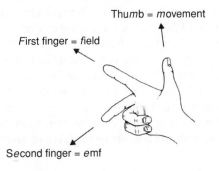

Fig. 9.2 Fleming's right-hand rule.

9.1.3 *Electromagnetic induction in a coil*

The emf induced in a straight conductor is too small to be of any practical value, but its value can be increased by winding the wire into a coil. If the coil is connected to a very sensitive milliammeter (galvanometer) and a bar magnet is

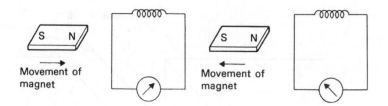

Fig. 9.3   Generation of an emf using a permanent magnet and coil.

moved towards or away from one end of the coil, a much stronger current is detected (Fig. 9.3).

9.1.3.1   Observations

(1) The *direction* of the induced emf depends on
    (a) which pole is nearer to the coil and
    (b) whether the pole is moving towards or away from the coil.
(2) The *magnitude* of the induced emf depends on
    (a) the speed of movement,
    (b) the strength of the magnet,
    (c) the number of turns on the coil and
    (d) the distance of the magnet from the coil.
(3) An emf is induced only when there is relative movement between the magnet and the coil, i.e. a change in magnetic flux linkage.

9.2   Opposition to the flow of current

Let us refer back to our straight conductor: the current that we are inducing in our conductor must also be producing its own magnetic field! As we already know, this field will produce a force on the conductor.

    Can we work out in which direction this force will be? Will it oppose the movement we are putting in, or will it add to it? In Fig. 9.1 if we move the conductor upwards, from Fleming's right-hand rule we can conclude that the current will flow from A to B. By applying Fleming's left-hand rule to find the effect of this induced current, we find that the direction of force is downwards; i.e. there is an opposing force trying to prevent the movement of the conductor.

    All these observations lead us to the **laws of electromagnetic induction**.

9.3   Laws of electromagnetic induction

    Law 1. If a conductor experiences a change of magnetic flux linkage, an emf is induced across the conductor.
    Law 2. The induced emf is proportional to the rate of change of flux linkage (cutting of lines of force).
    Law 3. Lenz's law: The induced emf is in such a direction as to oppose the movement producing it.

Discussion. From Law 2 it follows that the induced emf (E) is given by

$$E \propto -\frac{dN}{dt}$$

where N is the magnetic flux linkage and t is time. The negative sign indicates that the direction of induced emf is such as to *oppose* the changes in magnetic flux (Law 3). The term dN/dt is the rate of change of magnetic flux.

From this proportional relationship, we obtain

$$E = -\frac{dN}{dt} \times \text{constant}$$

If SI units are employed, the constant of proportionality is 1, and the expression becomes simply

$$E = -\frac{dN}{dt}$$

E is then expressed in volts, N in webers and t in seconds. Thus when a conductor experiences a rate of change of magnetic flux linkage of 1 Wb s^{-1}, an emf of 1 V is induced across it; i.e.

$$1 \text{ V} = 1 \text{ Wb s}^{-1}$$

and

$$1 \text{ Wb} = 1 \text{ V s}$$

An application of Lenz's law is found in the moving coil meter. We said that the coil was wound on an aluminium former, so that when the coil moves so does the former. Current is therefore induced to flow in the former when the coil moves, and from Lenz's law we know that the direction of this induced current is such as to oppose the motion causing it.

The effect of this is to reduce the oscillations of the pointer enabling quick accurate readings to be taken. Since current is induced only in the former when the coil is moving, there is no effect on the pointer once it has stopped at its final reading. This effect is called **electromagnetic damping** or **eddy-current damping**.

9.4 Mutual induction

The production of an induced emf does not depend on the use of a permanent magnet. A magnetic field from *any* source will have the same effect, provided that the magnetic flux linked with the conductor can be made to vary.

Consider the arrangement shown in Fig. 9.4. The diagram shows two coils, P and S, wound on a soft-iron core. Coil P is known as the **primary coil** and coil S is the **secondary coil**. If a changing magnetic field is generated by passing a varying current (I_p) through coil P, there will be a changing flux linkage with coil S. This will result in an induced emf E_s across coil S. This phenomenon is known as **mutual induction**.

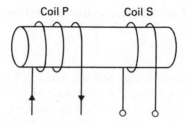

Fig. 9.4 Two coils wound on a soft-iron core.

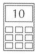

The rate of change of flux linkage, dN/dt, depends on the rate of change of current, dI/dt. Thus, the induced emf (E_s) is given by

$$E_s \propto \frac{dI_p}{dt}$$

and

$$E_s = M\frac{dI_p}{dt}$$

where the constant of proportionality (M) is known as **mutual inductance**.

9.4.1 *Mutual inductance and the henry*

The SI unit of mutual inductance is the **henry** (H). A system has a mutual inductance of 1 H if a rate of change of current of 1 A s^{-1} in coil P induces an emf of 1 V across coil S; i.e. if $E_s = 1$ V when dI_p/d$t = 1$ A s^{-1} then $M = 1$ H.

Electrical transformers and heart pacemakers are important applications of the principle of mutual induction.

9.4.2 *Primary and secondary circuits*

That part of the circuit across which the input voltage is applied and which carries the current I_p is known as the **primary circuit** (and hence includes P, the primary coil).

That part of the circuit across which an induced emf (the output voltage, E_s) appears is known as the **secondary circuit** (and hence includes S, the secondary coil).

9.4.3 *Further observations*

(1) The direction of the induced emf is seen to depend on whether the magnetic field is rising or falling and also on the direction of the current in the primary circuit.

(2) The maximum value of the induced emf will be increased if the two windings are placed closer together, the maximum possible being if the two windings are wound on top of each other (Fig. 9.5).

(3) The value of the induced emf is increased by inserting a soft-iron core into the coils.

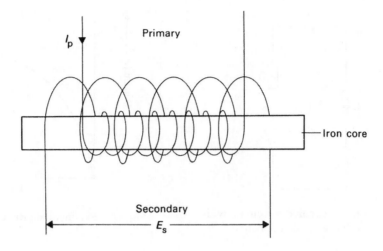

I_p

Primary

Iron core

Secondary

E_s

Fig. 9.5   Primary and secondary coils wound on top of each other on an iron core.

(4)   The value of the induced emf can be increased by increasing the number of turns on the secondary winding. (The magnetic field will cut more turns of wire.)

9.5   Self-induction

We have seen that an emf will be induced in a conductor which is situated in a changing magnetic field. Examining again Section 9.4 and Fig. 9.4 we can see that not only is the secondary coil (S) situated in a changing magnetic field, but so too is the primary coil (P). It is experiencing the changing magnetic flux that the varying current I_p produced. Thus an emf (E_p) is induced across coil P. This phenomenon, known as **self-induction**, occurs irrespective of whether there is a secondary coil present.

Lenz's law (and common sense) tells us that the induced emf *opposes* the changes in the current producing it. Thus, if the primary-coil current (I_p) is increasing (or rising), the induced emf (E_p) will tend to oppose the increase and is known as **back emf**. Similarly, if the primary-coil current is decreasing (or falling), the induced emf (E_p) will oppose the decrease and try to maintain the primary current (I_p). E_p is then known as **forward emf**.

The value of self-induced emf can be calculated from

$$E_p \propto \frac{dI_p}{dt} \text{ (rate of change of primary current)}$$

and

$$E_p = -\frac{L dI_p}{dt}$$

where L is known as the **self-inductance** of the coil and its core. As before, the negative sign indicates that the induced emf is in opposition to the change in I_p. Note that the term *self-inductance* is often shortened to just *inductance*.

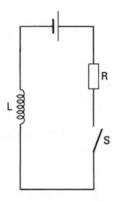

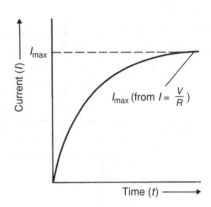

Fig. 9.6   An 'RL' circuit (i.e. a circuit with resistive and inductive components).

Fig. 9.7   Exponential growth of current.

The SI unit of self-inductance is the **henry**. A coil has a self-inductance of 1 H if a rate of change of primary current of 1 A s^{-1} self-induces an emf of 1 V; i.e. if $E_p = 1\text{ V}$ and $dI_p/dt = 1\text{ A s}^{-1}$, then $L = 1\text{ H}$.

9.5.1 The effects of self-inductance

In practice, we find that the self-induced emf *slows down* the rise or fall of the primary current (I_p) and so it takes longer to reach its final value.

9.5.1.1 Rise of current

In the case of the simple inductive circuit shown in Fig. 9.6, after switching *on*, the current rises to a final value of I_F determined by Ohm's law:

$$I_F = \frac{V}{R}$$

The rise in current is a form of exponential growth shown graphically in Fig. 9.7. If I_t is the value of current after time t, then

$$I_t = I_F(1 - e^{-t/T})$$

where T is the **time constant** of the circuit. Note the similarities between this expression and that encountered previously in relation to the charging of capacitors (Section 7.11.2.2).

9.5.1.2 Fall in current

A similar, but reverse, effect occurs when current in the inductive circuit is switched *off*. The current then falls in the manner shown in Fig. 9.8. In this case, the value of current after time t is given by

$$I_t = I_0\, e^{-t/T}$$

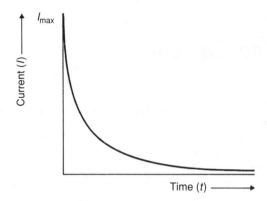

Fig. 9.8 Exponential decay of current.

where I_0 is the initial value of steady current (determined by $I_0 = V/R$). Note the similarities between this expression and that encountered previously in relation to the discharging of capacitors (Section 7.11.3.3).

9.5.1.3 Time constant

The time constant (T) of an inductive circuit is defined in a similar way to that for a capacitive circuit. It represents the time taken for the current to rise (or fall) by 63.2% (see Section 7.11.2, Worked Example 5). Its value in a circuit having inductance (L) and resistance (R) is given by

$$T = \frac{L}{R}$$

Thus, the larger the value of inductance, the longer the current will take to reach its final steady value. The presence of a soft-iron core in the inductor increases its inductance (and therefore the time constant) considerably.

However, the inductance of a circuit has *no* effect on the final steady value of current, because there can be no induced emf unless the value of current is changing. In the case of current growth, the final steady value (I_F is determined only by the values of V and R; i.e. $I_F = V/R$). In the case of current *fall*, the final value of current is zero.

9.5.1.4 Arcing

Rapid switching of the supply current in an inductive circuit leads to a large value of self-induced emf because the rate of change of current (and hence flux linkage) is great. The high voltages so generated may produce *arcing* across switch contacts, possibly causing premature failure of the switch.

Chapter 10
Alternating Current

10.1   Introduction to alternating current

So far we have talked about electric currents which flow in one direction only, i.e. **direct current** (d.c.), and a battery has been the source of current. While batteries are adequate for our experiments so far, and for operating portable devices such as personal hi-fis, they could not supply the needs of the whole country for purposes such as cooking and heating.

Therefore, most of our electricity is produced in electricity-generating stations, using the principle of electromagnetic induction. The simplest and most efficient type of generator is called an **alternator**. This produces a current which changes in direction (alternates) 100 times per second. This type of current is known as **alternating current** (a.c.).

Alternating current is used throughout the world for domestic and industrial purposes, offering important advantages over direct current.

10.1.1   Advantages of alternating current

(1)   It is easier and cheaper to produce than direct current.
(2)   The value of the voltage of alternating current can be changed easily, using a device known as a transformer. Transformers work on alternating current only.

10.2   Generation of alternating current

To summarise what we said in Section 9.1, 'when there is relative movement between a conductor and a magnetic field, so that the conductor experiences a change in magnetic flux linkage, an emf will be induced in the conductor'.

This effect is apparent when either (a) the conductor moves and the magnet is stationary, (b) the magnet moves and the conductor is stationary or (c) the conductor and the magnet are stationary and the strength of the magnetic field varies.

All these methods are used in different types of electrical equipments, but we will examine an example of (b), the rotation of a magnet with respect to a stationary coil. This principle is illustrated diagrammatically in Fig. 10.1, which shows a coil situated close to a rotating permanent magnet.

As the magnet rotates, a varying emf will be induced across the ends of the coil. Assuming that the magnet rotates at a constant speed, the induced emf will be at

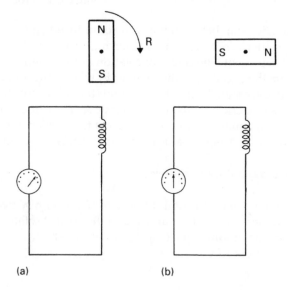

Fig. 10.1   The principle of electromagnetic induction demonstrated with a rotating permanent magnet.

a maximum when the magnetic lines of force cut the coil windings at right angles, as in Fig. 10.1a (see also the Biot–Savart law, Section 8.6.4.1). The induced emf will be zero when the magnetic field is parallel to the coil windings, as in Fig. 10.1b.

10.2.1   *Instantaneous value of induced emf*

The induced emf varies in both magnitude and direction. Its magnitude varies with the rate of change of flux linkage. Its direction varies according to which magnetic pole is approaching the coil. Thus, the instantaneous value of induced emf is directly proportional to the sine of the angle (θ) through which the magnet rotates (see Fig. 10.2).

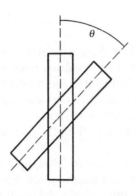

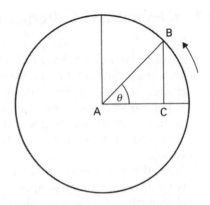

Fig. 10.2   The instantaneous value of induced emf is directly proportional to the sine of the angle (θ) through which the magnet rotates.

Fig. 10.3   A rotating vector showing the relationship between the angle of rotation (θ) and the instantaneous value of induced emf (BC).

The relationship between the value of induced emf and the angular position of the magnet can be found by referring to the vector diagram (Fig. 10.3) in which A represents the centre of rotation of the magnet and the horizontal axis represents the position of the magnet in which zero induced emf is produced, i.e. where the magnetic flux linkage with the coil is not changing. The line AB is the radius of a circle whose centre lies at A. The direction of AB represents the position of the magnet after it has turned through an angle θ. The length of AB represents the *maximum* value of emf that can be induced.

10.2.1.1   Sinusoidal nature of induced emf

The instantaneous value of induced emf (E) is represented by the length of the line BC. It increases as the magnet (and the vector) rotates until $\theta = 90°$, when it reaches its maximum value (E_{Max}), represented by the length of AB.

In the triangle ABC,

$$\sin \theta = \frac{BC}{AB}$$

so

$$BC = AB \sin \theta$$

But since BC $= E$ and AB $= E_{MAX}$, we can deduce that:

$$E = E_{MAX} \sin \theta$$

and that the instantaneous value of induced emf is *directly proportional* to the sine of the angle of rotation of the magnet.

When $\theta = 0°$, then sin $\theta = 0$, so $E = 0$.
When $\theta = 90°$, then sin $\theta = 1$, so $E = E_{MAX}$.
When $\theta = 180°$, then sin $\theta = 0$, so $E = 0$.
When $\theta = 270°$, then sin $\theta = -1$, so $E = -E_{MAX}$.

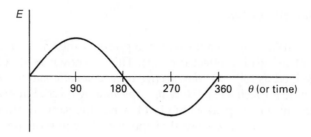

Fig. 10.4 Graphical representation of induced emf (sine wave).

The cycle then repeats itself. Note that for angles between 180° and 360° (0°), E takes on *negative* values, meaning that the polarity of the induced emf is reversed.

Thus, the instantaneous value of induced emf can be represented as a **sine wave** (Fig. 10.4), in which E can be plotted either against the angular rotation (θ), or against time (t). The value of E_{MAX} depends on both the strength of the magnetic field, which interacts with the coil windings, and the rotational speed of the magnet. E_{MAX} is usually known as the **peak value** of emf.

Figure 10.4 represents one complete rotation of the magnet, i.e. 360°. This is known as one cycle. Because the magnet continues to rotate at a constant speed, we can talk about the number of cycles per second. This is known as the **frequency** of the current.

In Britain and Europe, mains electricity is generated at 50 cycles per second (sometimes called 50 hertz, where 1 cycle per second = 1 hertz).

10.3   Peak and effective values of alternating current

When we considered direct current, it was easy to measure the value of potential difference and current because they did not vary with time; i.e. they had constant values. This is, however, not the case with alternating current.

10.3.1   *Peak values*

These are the maximum positive or negative values of voltage or current (see Fig. 10.4).

It is useful to know peak values (a) if we need to calculate the maximum photon energy and/or minimum wavelength of X-rays produced by an X-ray tube operating at a certain kilovoltage (Section 16.1.2.3), and (b) for determining the insulation requirements around a conductor.

10.3.2   *Average values*

Average values are less useful than peak values, the arithmetic average value being zero, because positive and negative values on the graph are equal.

10.3.3   *Effective values*

This is an 'average' value which represents the *effect* of the current, e.g. in terms of its heating effect (power). This is known as its **effective value** and it is defined as follows: '*the effective value of an alternating current is the value of direct current which will produce the same heating effect*'. For example, an alternating current whose peak value is 14 A has the same heating effect as a direct current of 10 A, so we say that the *effective* value of the alternating current is 10 A.

10.3.4   *Relationship between peak and effective values*

For a sinusoidally varying emf (E), peak value = effective value × $\sqrt{2}$ (where $\sqrt{2}$ is approximately 1.4).

$$\text{Effective value} = \frac{\text{peak value}}{\sqrt{2}}$$

or

$$\text{Effective value} = \text{peak value} \times 0.7$$

Effective values are often known as **RMS** values. (This stands for **root mean square** and it indicates the mathematical way in which the effective value is derived.)

Hence, for a sinusoidally alternating emf (E):

$$E_{\text{PEAK}} = E_{\text{RMS}} \times \sqrt{2}$$

and

$$E_{\text{RMS}} = E_{\text{PEAK}} \times \frac{1}{\sqrt{2}}$$

Similarly, for a sinusoidally alternating current (I):

$$I_{\text{PEAK}} = I_{\text{RMS}} \times \sqrt{2}$$

and

$$I_{\text{RMS}} = I_{\text{PEAK}} \times \frac{1}{\sqrt{2}}$$

Worked examples
(1)   The mains voltage is 230 V_{RMS}. Calculate its peak value.

$$\begin{aligned} \text{Peak} &= \text{RMS} \times 1.4 \\ &= 230 \times 1.4 \\ &= 322 \text{ V} \end{aligned}$$

(2) An alternating current whose peak value is 8 A flows through a resistance of 5 Ω. Calculate the power.

$$\text{Power} = I^2 R$$
$$= \frac{8}{\sqrt{2}} \times \frac{8}{\sqrt{2}} \times 5$$
$$= \frac{64}{2} \times 5 \quad (\text{remember } \sqrt{2} \times \sqrt{2} = 2)$$
$$= 160 \text{ W}$$

Note that in this example it is essential to convert peak values of current to RMS because peak values represent the value of current at one moment in time only, whereas RMS values represent the effective value of the current over a complete cycle.

10.4 Practical alternators

10.4.1 *Rotor*

Although we have described the generation of alternating current using a rotating permanent magnet, in practice, the permanent magnet is likely to be replaced by a rotating electromagnet, known as the **rotor**, which is supplied with direct current from a separate generator called an **exciter**.

10.4.2 *Stator*

We have illustrated a stationary coil or **stator**, comprising only a few turns of wire. In practice, the stator would consist of many hundreds of turns of wire wound onto a high-permeability ferromagnetic core which improves magnetic flux linkage, thereby increasing the efficiency of the alternator.

10.4.3 *Polyphase design*

The alternator we have described used only a single stator winding to generate an alternating supply. This is known as a **single-phase alternator**. In practice, however, extra stator coils are present, which provide additional a.c. outputs, known as a **polyphase** design. The additional coils are spaced symmetrically around the rotor. Figure 10.5 shows the most common arrangement, using *three* stator coils spaced 120° apart. Each coil generates its own a.c. cycle, but because of the positions of the coils in relation to the rotor, the peak values of emf will occur at different moments of time. Because the coils are spaced 120° apart, the resultant sinusoidal outputs will be displaced or out of phase by 120° (Fig. 10.6). This design is known as a **three-phase alternator**.

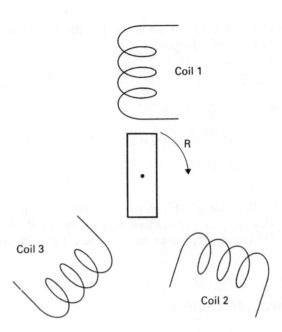

Fig. 10.5 Diagrammatic representation of the arrangement of stator coils around the rotor (R) of an a.c. generator.

10.4.3.1 Star connection

For the purpose of distributing the electrical output of a three-phase alternator, one terminal from each coil is connected to earth, forming a common **neutral** connection. The other three terminals are kept separate and are known as **line conductors** or **lines** (Fig. 10.7). This arrangement reduces the number of conductors required to transmit power and is known as **star connection**.

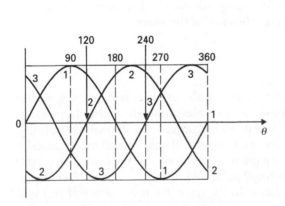

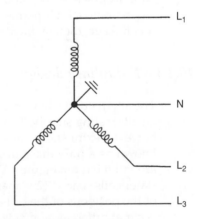

Fig. 10.6 The output from a three-phase generator, showing three sinusoidal outputs out of phase with each other by 120°.

Fig. 10.7 Diagrammatic representation of star-connected stator coils of a three-phase generator, showing the three lines (L_1, L_2 and L_3) and the earthed neutral conductor (N).

10.5   Mains electricity generation and distribution

In the UK, electrical power is generated at approximately 25 kV$_{RMS}$. It is stepped up to 275 or 400 kV$_{RMS}$ for transmission across the countryside and then subsequently stepped back down in stages to 230 V$_{RMS}$ (known as **phase voltage**) for domestic use. Phase voltage is obtained by taking the output from a line conductor and the neutral conductor. Industrial consumers often prefer a 398-V$_{RMS}$ supply known as **line voltage**. This is obtained by taking the output from two of the line conductors.

Heavy-duty electrical equipment, including some X-ray units, is designed to operate from the full **three-phase supply** to reduce power losses in transmission (see Section 10.8).

10.6   Characteristics of alternating current circuits

By definition, the emf and current from an a.c. supply are always changing. We have seen (in Section 9.5) that in a circuit which possesses inductance, changing the value of current produces an induced emf which inhibits the rise and fall of current. Additionally, the charging and discharging of any capacitance in the circuit will also affect the electrical characteristics of the circuit.

Thus in a.c. circuits, resistance is not the only property of the circuit which influences the flow of current. Inductance and capacitance are also important.

10.6.1   *Impedance and reactance*

The *total* current-limiting effect of resistance, inductance and capacitance in a circuit is known as the **impedance** (Z) of the circuit. It is defined as the ratio of RMS voltage to RMS current; i.e.

$$Z = \frac{V_{RMS}}{I_{RMS}}$$

Note the similarity between this and the Ohm's law relationship (Section 7.4.3).

The current-limiting effect of inductance (L) is known as **inductive reactance** (X_L), and the current-limiting effect of capacitance (C_L) is known as **capacitive reactance** (X_C). The SI unit of impedance and both types of reactance is the **ohm** (Ω).

To find out more about the nature of impedance, we shall examine the effects of resistance, inductive reactance and capacitive reactance in more detail.

10.6.1.1   **Resistive a.c. circuits**

Consider a simple a.c. circuit which contains only ohmic resistance (Fig. 10.8). The voltage and current in this circuit are *in phase:* both voltage and current reach their peak values at the same time, and reach their zero values at the same time.

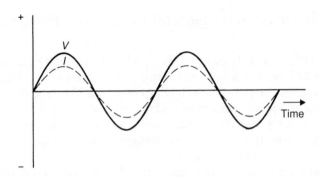

Fig. 10.8   Current (I) and voltage (V) in phase in an a.c. circuit containing only ohmic resistance.

Net power dissipation in resistive circuits
The instantaneous power (P) dissipated in the resistor is given by

$$P = V \times I$$

where V and I are instantaneous values of voltage and current. During the first half-cycle, both V and I are positive; thus, the value of P is positive also. During the second half-cycle, both V and I are negative, so the value of their product (P) is again positive.

The *net* power dissipation (P_T) over a number of complete cycles in a resistive circuit is given by

$$P_T = V_{RMS} \times I_{RMS}$$

10.6.1.2   Capacitive a.c. circuits

Consider a simple a.c. circuit containing only capacitance. When d.c. is supplied to a capacitor, the charge builds on each plate until it reaches a point where no further current flows in the circuit (Section 7.11.1). In effect, the capacitor now has infinitely high resistance. In an a.c. circuit, however, the situation is quite different. The capacitor is being alternately charged and discharged as the supply voltage reverses. The capacitor is therefore being charged and discharged every half-cycle. The value of current flowing at any given time depends on the rate of change of applied voltage at that moment. Because the rate of change of applied voltage is greatest as the voltage passes through zero, it is at these moments that the current will reach its peak values. Thus, the current and voltage in the circuit are *out of phase* (Fig. 10.9). If the circuit contains pure capacitance only, the current will lead the voltage by one-quarter of a cycle (90°). This is shown in a vector diagram (Fig. 10.10).

Capacitive reactance
Capacitive reactance (X_C) is determined by the value of capacitance (C) and the frequency (f) of the supply voltage.

$$X_C = \frac{1}{2\pi f C}$$

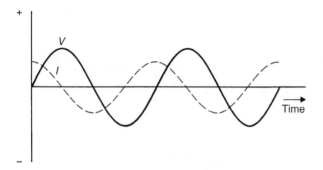

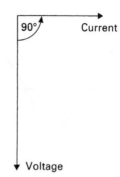

Fig. 10.9　Current (I) leading the voltage (V) by 90° in an a.c. circuit containing only pure capacitance.

Fig. 10.10　Vector diagram showing the current leading the voltage by 90°.

Note that for direct current, f is zero and X_C is infinitely large; i.e. d.c. is unable to pass through a capacitor.

Net power and power factor in capacitive circuits
The net power dissipation (P_T) over a number of complete cycles in a capacitive circuit can be calculated from

$$P_T = V_{RMS} \times I_{RMS} \times \cos \phi$$

where ϕ (the Greek letter 'phi') is the **phase angle** between current and voltage.

The term $\cos\phi$ is known as the **power factor**. In a purely capacitive circuit, $\phi = 90°$ and $\cos 90° = 0$, so *net* power is zero. Closer analysis shows that during every other half-cycle, the circuit draws power *from* the supply, but during the remaining half-cycles the circuit feeds power *into* the supply. There is *no* net transfer of power over a complete cycle.

Note that in a purely resistive circuit, $\phi = 0$, so $\cos \phi = 1$. Thus, $P_T = V_{RMS} \times I_{RMS} \times 1$, which agrees with the conclusion reached in Section 10.6.1.1.

10.6.1.3　Inductive a.c. circuits

Consider a simple circuit containing only inductance. When direct current is supplied to an inductor, the current is initially opposed by the back emf induced across it. Once a steady current is established, however, a perfect inductor offers no resistance to the flow of current. In an a.c. circuit, the situation is again very different because the direction and magnitude of current flow through the inductor are constantly changing. This generates a perpetually changing magnetic flux linkage which induces an emf. The effect of the induced emf is to oppose changes in the current, preventing it from remaining in phase with the supply voltage. The current and voltage are therefore *out of phase*, with the voltage *leading* the current (Fig. 10.11). In a purely inductive circuit, the voltage leads the current by one-quarter of a cycle (90°), as shown in the vector diagram (Fig. 10.12).

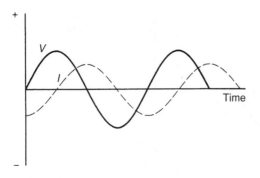

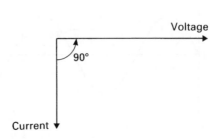

Fig. 10.11   Voltage (V) leading the current (I) by 90° in an a.c. circuit containing only pure inductance.

Fig. 10.12   Vector diagram showing the voltage leading the current by 90°.

Inductive reactance
Inductive reactance (X_L) is determined by the inductance (L) and the frequency (f) of the supply:

$$X_L = 2\pi fL$$

Note that for direct current, f is zero and X_L is zero; i.e. a pure inductance offers no opposition to the flow of steady current.

Net power and power factor in inductive circuits
The net power dissipation (P_T) in an inductive circuit is given by

$$P_T = V_{RMS} \times I_{RMS} \times \cos \phi$$

where ϕ is again the phase angle between current and voltage, and $\cos \phi$ is the power factor. In a purely inductive circuit the phase angle is 90°; thus, the power factor is zero and the net power consumed over a number of cycles is zero. However, at any particular instant power may be entering or leaving the system. These characteristics underpin the operation of transformers (Section 10.7).

10.6.1.4   Resistor–capacitor and resistor–inductor circuits

In practice, circuits always contain some resistance as well as capacitance or inductance (Fig. 10.13). The total impedance (Z) of such circuits is given by:

$$Z = \sqrt{(R^2 + X^2)}$$

where X is total reactance. Thus, in a resistive–capacitive circuit (Fig. 10.13a):

$$Z = \sqrt{[R^2 + (1/2\pi fC)^2]}$$

and in a resistive–inductive circuit (Fig. 10.13b):

$$Z = \sqrt{[R^2 + (2\pi fL)^2]}$$

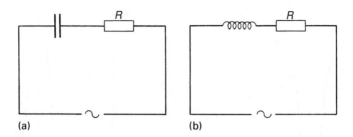

Fig. 10.13   (a) Resistor–capacitor and (b) resistor–inductor circuits.

The effect of resistance is to *reduce* the phase angle (ϕ) between voltage and current to less than 90°. The power factor (cos ϕ) is then no longer zero and the circuit has a *positive* net power consumption.

10.6.2   Resonant circuits

If both inductance *and* capacitance are present in an a.c. circuit, a phenomenon known as **resonance** occurs. Inductors (or **chokes**) and capacitors can be connected either in series or in parallel.

10.6.2.1   Series-resonant circuits (Fig. 10.14)

The *total* reactance (X) of an inductor and capacitor in series is given by:

$$X = X_L + X_C$$

(Compare this with the formula for resistors in series derived in Section 7.5.1.) Therefore,

$$X = 2\pi f L - 1/(2\pi \ fC)$$

This is zero (and the impedance is at a minimum) when:

$$2\pi f L = \frac{1}{2\pi f C}$$

i.e. when

$$f = \frac{1}{2\pi \sqrt{(LC)}}$$

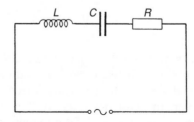

Fig. 10.14   A series-resonant circuit.

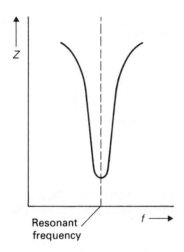

Fig. 10.15 Graph of impedance (Z) against frequency (f) for a series-resonant (accepter) circuit. Note the very low impedance at resonant frequency.

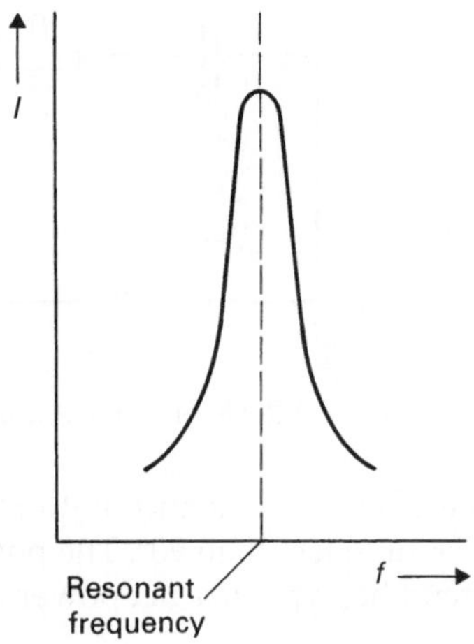

Fig. 10.16 Graph of current (I) against frequency (f) for an accepter circuit, showing the current peaking at resonant frequency.

At this frequency, known as **resonant frequency**, the impedance of the circuit is determined only by R. At any other frequency, above or below resonant frequency, impedance will increase (Fig. 10.15).

Consider the current flow through such a circuit (Fig. 10.16). Resonant circuits of this type are known as **acceptor circuits** and can be used to suppress currents at all frequencies other than resonant frequency. This is the principle of the **tuning circuits** employed in radio and television receivers. The value of the resonant frequency of such a circuit can be changed by altering the value of L and/or C, e.g. by using a **variable choke** or a **variable capacitor**.

10.6.2.2   Parallel-resonant circuits (Fig. 10.17)

The total reactance (X) of an inductor and capacitor in parallel is given by:

$$\frac{1}{X} = \frac{1}{X_L} + \frac{1}{X_C}$$

(compare this with the formula for resistors in parallel derived in Section 7.5.2) from which:

$$X = \frac{X_L X_C}{X_L + X_C}$$

When $X_L + X_C$ is zero (i.e. at resonant frequency), the combined reactance is infinite and current flow is blocked. Such a circuit is called a **rejecter circuit** and its characteristic is that it will transmit *any* current except one whose frequency coincides with resonant frequency (Figs. 10.18 and 10.19). One application of a rejecter circuit is to act as a selective **filter** to remove a specific frequency from a multiple frequency signal.

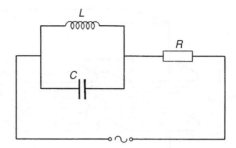

Fig. 10.17   A parallel-resonant circuit.

The resonant frequency of rejector circuits is again given by:

$$f = \frac{1}{2\pi\sqrt{(LC)}}$$

and can be varied by altering the value of L and/or C.

10.7   Transformers

In Section 9.4, we showed how electrical energy could be transferred from one circuit to another by means of a link of changing magnetic flux; the phenomenon was called **mutual induction**. A transformer is an electrical machine which is a direct application of the principle of mutual induction.

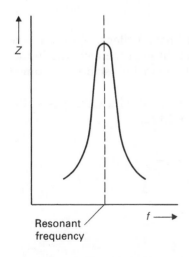

Fig. 10.18   Graph showing impedance (Z) against frequency (f) for a parallel-resonant (rejecter) circuit. Note the very high impedance at resonant frequency.

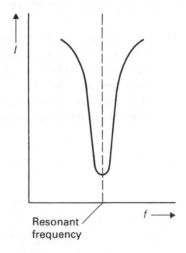

Fig. 10.19   Graph of current (I) against frequency (f) for a rejecter circuit, showing the suppression of current at resonant frequency.

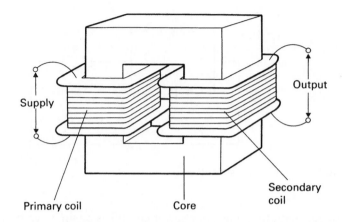

Fig. 10.20   Diagrammatic representation of the construction of a simple transformer.

10.7.1   Basic construction (Fig. 10.20)

The transformer consists of two coils, electrically insulated from one another:

- A **primary coil** – defined as the coil to which the supply is connected
- A **secondary coil** – defined as the coil from which the output is taken

The magnetic field generated by the primary coil is passed to the secondary coil through a **ferromagnetic core**. The circuit symbol for a transformer is shown in Fig. 10.21.

10.7.2   Principle of operation

(1)   The application of an alternating emf (primary voltage, V_P) across the primary coil drives a primary current (I_P) through the coil. The inductance of the coil causes I_P to lag V_P by 90° if minimal resistance is assumed (see Section 10.6.1.3).

(2)   The primary current (I_P) sets up a magnetic field which changes as the instantaneous value of current changes (Fig. 10.22).

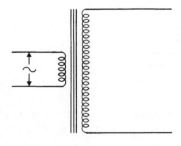

Fig. 10.21   Circuit symbol for a transformer.

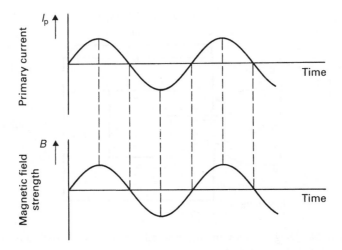

Fig. 10.22   Changes in primary current (I_P) and magnetic field strength (B) in a transformer.

(3)   The core passes the changing magnetic field through the secondary coil.
(4)   The secondary coil experiences the changing magnetic flux linkage and an emf (V_S) is induced in this coil by mutual induction (Fig. 10.23).
(5)   A sinusoidally changing voltage appears across the secondary coil (as long as the core does not saturate).

10.7.2.1   Voltage per turn

In the primary coil, each individual turn of wire has a specific voltage across it; e.g. if V_P is 230 V_{RMS} and the primary winding has 1150 turns, then the voltage

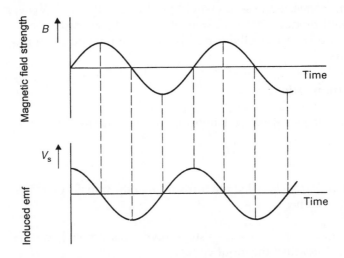

Fig. 10.23   Changes in magnetic field strength (B) and induced emf (V_s) in the secondary coil of a transformer.

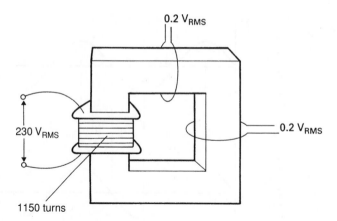

Fig. 10.24 Diagram showing the emf induced across two separate secondary turns wound on a transformer core.

across each single turn is

$$\frac{230}{1150} = 0.2 \, V_{RMS}$$

i.e. the **voltage per turn** is 0.2. In a perfect (**ideal**) transformer, this would lead to a changing magnetic field capable of inducing 0.2 V_{RMS} on any *other* turn of wire wrapped around the same core (Fig. 10.24). The voltage per turn is thus the same for both primary and secondary windings:

$$\frac{V_P}{N_P} = \frac{V_S}{N_S}$$

Thus, a secondary coil of only *one* turn would generate 0.2 V_{RMS}; *two* such turns connected in series would produce $2 \times 0.2 = 0.4 \, V_{RMS}$; *two hundred* turns would produce $200 \times 0.2 = 40 \, V_{RMS}$. In other words, we can select any voltage we wish from the transformer by employing an appropriate number of turns.

10.7.2.2 Turns ratio

The voltage-per-turn relationship may be rewritten as:

$$\frac{V_S}{V_P} = \frac{N_S}{N_P}$$

where N_S/N_P is called the **turns ratio** of the transformer. The value of the turns ratio may be:

- *Less than 1* – known as a **step-down transformer**, because the output voltage is *lower* than the input voltage
- *More than 1* – known as a **step-up transformer**, because the output voltage is *higher* than the input voltage

More rarely the turns ratio may be:

- *Equal to 1* (i.e. $N_S = N_P$) – known as a **one-to-one transformer**

10.7.3 The effect of load

Experiment shows that the presence or absence of a secondary coil makes *no difference* to the current and voltage in the primary coil *as long as the secondary coil is on open circuit* or **off-load**, i.e. as long as no secondary current flows. Under *off-load* conditions, the transformer behaves as a pure inductance and consumes no net power: its power factor is zero (see Section 10.6.1.3). If the secondary coil is **on-load**; i.e. if it is connected across a load such as a resistor or an X-ray tube, then a secondary current (I_S) flows.

As the current flows through the secondary coil it generates a changing magnetic field. This opposes (weakens) the magnetic field set up by the primary coil. The effect of this is to reduce the self-induced emf generated in the primary coil and it no longer neutralises the applied voltage. The result is that a current (I_P) is able to flow in the primary coil. Thus if the transformer is *off-load*, no primary current flows, but when it is *on-load*, primary current does flow.

Note that a more rigorous explanation results from realising that the effect of secondary current is to reduce the *phase difference* between primary voltage and current. This increases the power factor from its zero value (off-load) to a positive value (on-load), which, in turn, increases the net power consumption above zero.

In fact, the power output from an ideal transformer exactly matches the power it draws from the supply:

Power out (from secondary) = power in (to primary)

10.7.4 Power losses in transformers

Not *all* the power absorbed from the supply by the primary coil of a transformer is available for use across the secondary coil. There is some wastage, due largely to shortcomings in the windings (known as **copper losses**) and in the core (known as **iron losses**).

10.7.4.1 Copper losses

Even though made of an excellent electrical conductor such as copper, transformer windings have measurable resistance (R). When a current (I) flows through the windings, heat is generated at the rate of I^2R watts (Section 7.10.3). For example, a doubling of the current flow would generate four times the heat. This wasted power, known as **copper loss**, can be reduced by minimising the resistance of the windings, e.g. by using wires as thick as practicable.

10.7.4.2 Iron losses

Iron losses arise from deficiencies in the ferromagnetic core of the transformer. They can be traced to three sources:

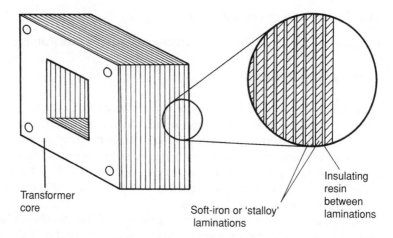

Transformer
core

Soft-iron or 'stalloy'
laminations

Insulating
resin
between
laminations

Fig. 10.25   Construction of a transformer core showing its laminations.

(1)   **Magnetic leakage.** The transformer core may not pass all the magnetic flux from primary to secondary coil and magnetic leakage is said to occur. Good core design practically eliminates losses due to magnetic leakage.

(2)   **Hysteresis losses.** Due to the effect of hysteresis (see Section 8.4.3.1), the magnetisation of the core lags slightly behind the magnetising current and a finite amount of energy is required to rotate the magnetic domains in the core. Choice of core material with high relative permeability reduces these hysteresis losses.

(3)   **Eddy-current losses.** The changing magnetic field induces currents to flow in the core material itself. (It is an electrical conductor.) These **eddy currents** have a heating effect on the core, representing a waste of energy. The magnitude of the eddy currents can be greatly reduced by interrupting their conducting pathways through the core with insulated **laminations** (Fig. 10.25). Some small high-frequency transformers employ a high-resistance **ceramic core** to limit eddy-current losses.

10.7.4.3   Mains hum

The alternating magnetic fields present in transformers may set up mechanical vibrations which lead to the emission of sound waves at the frequency of the electrical supply (e.g. 50 Hz in the UK). This gives rise to the familiar humming or buzzing sound produced by many transformers. A small amount of energy is lost in generating these sound waves. Vibration is minimised by securing together the core laminations with bolts or rivets and with resin. The windings are also set in insulating resin to prevent vibration.

10.7.5   *Transformer efficiency*

The **efficiency** of a transformer (indeed, of *any* machine) is the ratio of its usable power output (P_{OUT}) to the power input (P_{IN}) that it draws from the supply.

Efficiency is often expressed as a percentage:

$$\text{Percentage efficiency} = \frac{P_{\text{OUT}}}{P_{\text{IN}}} \times 100$$

Overall, transformers are extremely efficient machines (98% or better with large transformers). However, when running at very high power levels, even a 2% loss is significant. For example, an X-ray high-tension transformer may run at over 100 kW during an exposure. A 2% power loss is then 2 kW, which represents a considerable amount of potentially damaging heat. Thus, transformers may incorporate a cooling system in their design. Air or mineral oil is commonly used as a coolant.

10.7.6   *Voltage regulation*

The resistance of transformer windings leads to a lower voltage appearing across the secondary coil when it is *on-load* than when it is *off-load*. The difference between the off-load and on-load voltages is called the **voltage drop** (V_{DROP}):

$$V_{\text{DROP}} = V_{\text{OFF-LOAD}} - V_{\text{ON-LOAD}}$$

Its value depends on the resistance (R) of the secondary coil and on the magnitude of current (I_S) drawn from the secondary:

$$V_{\text{DROP}} = I_S \times R$$

This effect is similar to the voltage drop in a battery on-load, due to its internal resistance (Section 7.8).

The voltage drop in transformers is often expressed as a fraction or a percentage of the off-load voltage ($V_{\text{OFF-LOAD}}$). This quantity is known as the **voltage regulation** of the transformer:

$$\text{Percentage regulation} = \frac{V_{\text{DROP}}}{V_{\text{OFF-LOAD}}} \times 100$$

Because its value for a given transformer varies with the current drawn, the current must be specified when regulation is quoted; e.g. 'Regulation is 5% at 800 mA'.

10.7.7   *Transformer rating*

To protect transformers from damage, manufacturers specify maximum safe operating conditions known as the **rating** of the transformer. There are two major aspects to consider: **power rating** and **voltage rating**.

10.7.7.1   **Power rating**

Observing the specified power rating prevents the transformer being damaged by overheating. Transformers can produce very high power output for a short time without overheating. The limit to their output under these conditions is known as the **instantaneous** or **surge rating**. Its value primarily depends on the **heat capacity** of the transformer (Section 2.3.2). However, for prolonged operation the transformer output must be drastically reduced to within its **continuous rating**, which depends on the rate at which the transformer can dissipate heat and therefore on the efficiency of its cooling system.

The power rating of a large transformer is often quoted in **kilovolt amps** or **kVA**. This is the product of the RMS values of voltage and current. It is quoted in kilovolt amps rather than kilowatts to indicate that the effect of the power factor has not been taken into account (Section 10.6.1.2).

10.7.7.2 Voltage rating

The electrical insulation employed in a transformer is designed to withstand voltages up to a specified maximum or peak value. Manufacturers therefore indicate the maximum voltage to which the transformer should be subjected. A safety margin is built in, but if the transformer suffers excessive voltage (an **overvoltage**), its electrical insulation may break down, arcing may occur and the transformer may be damaged beyond repair.

10.7.8 Applications of transformers

In X-ray equipment, step-up transformers are used to provide the high voltage required across the X-ray tube. Step-down transformers are used to reduce the mains voltage to supply ancillary and control circuits. Step-down transformers are also used in everyday life, e.g. to supply power to mobile phone chargers and laptop computers.

10.8   Transmission of power (National Grid)

We now have a simple way of not only generating alternating current but also changing the value of its voltage. We have the choice of transmitting this power from the generating stations to people's homes, hospitals, industries, etc., either at high voltages and low currents, or at low voltages and high currents. Let us try to discover which would be the best.

Fig. 10.26 shows electrical power from the generating station being transmitted down the cables of the National Grid system.

If we look at just one conductor (e.g. A → B), from Ohm's law we know that there will be a drop in voltage between its ends and that this drop in voltage will be proportional to the current flowing through it; i.e. the larger the current, the larger the voltage drop.

Another way of looking at this question is to remember that the heat produced is proportional to the square of the current ($H \propto I^2$). Therefore by making the current as small as possible, we will reduce the power losses due to the production of heat.

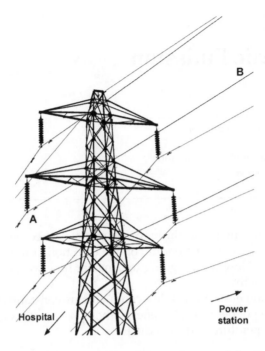

Fig. 10.26   Transmission of power. (Adapted from photograph by Gary Houston.)

For these two reasons it is therefore more economical to transmit power at *high voltages* and *low currents*. (In practice, power is transmitted through the National Grid system at a variety of voltages, e.g. 400 KV, 275 kV and 132 kV.)

Chapter 11

Thermionic Emission

Principle of thermionic emission
   Work function
Thermionic emission in a vacuum tube
   Vacuum diode valve
   Triode valve

When a current flows through a conductor, free electrons move along the wire, their direction depending on the direction of the potential difference (see Chapter 7). Now we are going to consider how we can release electrons completely from the wire.

Atoms and electrons inside a conductor are constantly vibrating. The amount of vibration depends on the energy they possess. This energy in turn depends on the temperature of the conductor.

11.1 Principle of thermionic emission

At room temperature, conduction electrons can move freely within a wire because of attraction between neighbouring atoms, but are unable to leave the *surface* of the material because of the combined effect of all the other atoms tending to pull them back. As the temperature of the conductor increases, the kinetic energy of the electrons increases until a point is reached when a few electrons have sufficient energy to overcome the binding forces of the atoms and then escape from the surface of the material. This process is known as **thermionic emission**. Tungsten, a material commonly used, exhibits thermionic emission at about 2000°C.

Figure 11.1 shows no emission of electrons until 2000°C is reached. Thereafter small increases in temperature produce large increases in electron emission. If the temperature of the material is further increased, eventually a point will be reached where some of the *atoms* may acquire enough energy to escape the surface of the material. This process is known as evaporation.

11.1.1 Work function

The minimum energy needed to release a free electron from the surface of a material is known as the **work function**. Work function (W) is usually expressed in electronvolts (eV). Table 11.1 shows examples of the values of work function for materials with low work functions.

Note that thermionic emission is not the *only* method of releasing electrons from the surface of a material. In some cases, a similar effect can be produced

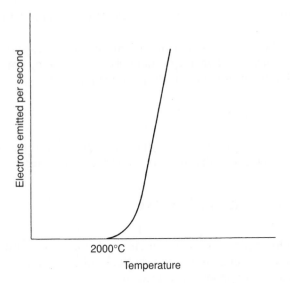

Fig. 11.1   Graph of thermionic emission against temperature (tungsten wire).

Table 11.1   Examples of materials having low work functions

Material	Work function (eV)
Caesium	1.9
Sodium	2.0
Tungsten	4.5
Copper	4.7

by bombarding the material with electromagnetic radiation (see photoelectric effect; Sections 14.5.4 and 15.4.1).

11.2   Thermionic emission in a vacuum tube

Thermionic emission will occur more readily if the pressure of air around the material is removed, e.g. if the conductor is sealed in an evacuated glass bulb or vacuum tube. Let us look at what would happen under these conditions.

The most practical way of heating a conductor is to pass a current through it. Assuming the conductor is a thin **filament** of tungsten, as its temperature approaches 2000°C electrons will start to be emitted from the surface. Because all the electrons possess a negative charge, they will tend to repel each other and form a cloud around the filament.

Because the conductor has emitted electrons, it will tend to acquire a positive charge and will therefore attract some of the electron cloud back to itself. Thus electrons are being emitted from and returning to the surface of the filament (imagine them on elastic bands). Another effect of this negatively charged cloud of electrons is to repel further electrons which are trying to escape from the filament.

Thus when a filament reaches its emission temperature, a state of equilibrium is soon achieved, where the number of electrons being emitted from the filament is equal to the number of electrons returning to it.

11.2.1   Space charge

The cloud of electrons around the filament is known as **space charge**, and its tendency to limit further electron emission is the **space charge effect**.

11.3   The vacuum diode valve

Let us add another conductor or **electrode** into our vacuum tube. We now have a simple valve called a vacuum diode. Its circuit symbol is shown in Fig. 11.2.
The valve comprises the following:

(1)   Filament or **cathode** (negatively charged electrode)
(2)   **Anode** (positively charged electrode)
(3)   Glass envelope
(4)   Vacuum

11.3.1   Rectifying properties of a vacuum diode

Let us connect the valve into a simple circuit.

The circuit in Fig. 11.3 comprises a battery, switch, ammeter, diode valve, high-tension d.c. source and a battery to heat the filament (filament heating current = I_f).

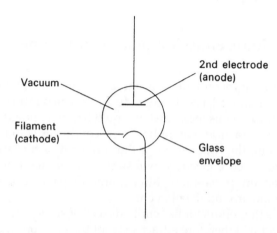

Fig. 11.2   Circuit symbol representing a thermionic vacuum diode valve.

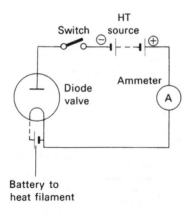

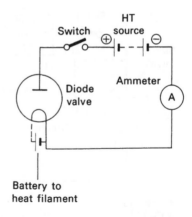

Fig. 11.3 Diode valve in circuit with anode negative.

Fig. 11.4 Diode valve in circuit with anode positive.

As the temperature of the filament rises, the space charge effect is established. If the switch is now closed, the anode will be made negative with respect to the cathode. Because the anode is unheated, it will not emit electrons, and no current will flow through the circuit.

What happens if we reverse the polarity of the battery? The anode is now positive with respect to the cathode (Fig. 11.4). Thus, electrons will be attracted across the valve from the filament reducing the space charge effect. This reduction in the space charge allows further electrons to be emitted; i.e. an **anode current** (I_a) will flow through the circuit.

What we have, in effect, is a device which acts as a *conductor* of current in one direction, but an *insulator* to current trying to flow in the opposite direction. When used in this way, the valve is acting as a **rectifier**.

11.3.2 *Vacuum diode characteristics*

An X-ray tube is an example of a modified diode valve. It is therefore important to study the characteristics of the vacuum diode valve in some depth.

Consider the circuit shown in Fig. 11.5. Suppose that the variable resistor is adjusted so that the filament emits a moderate number of electrons per second and we start with the anode potential (V_a) at zero and gradually increase it.

(1) Initially, no anode current (I_a) will flow, because there is no potential difference across the valve to attract the space charge away.
(2) As the anode potential rises, the anode current also rises, slowly at first and then more rapidly until a point is reached where further increases in V_a do not produce any increase in I_a. This is because all available electrons emitted from the filament are being attracted across to the anode.

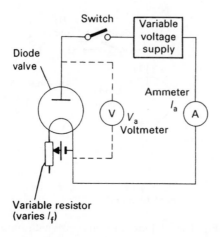

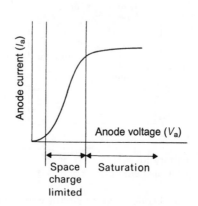

Fig. 11.5 Experiment to demonstrate diode characteristics. I_f = filament heating current; V_a = anode voltage (voltage across valve); I_a = anode current (current through valve).

Fig. 11.6 Graph of anode voltage against anode current (fixed filament temperature).

This situation is shown graphically in Fig. 11.6.

(1) **Space charge limited.** This is where *some*, but not all, of the electrons from the space charge are drawn across to the anode. In this region increases in V_a produce increases in I_a.

(2) **Saturation.** *All* electrons which are emitted from the filament are drawn across the valve.

In the saturation region, increases in V_s *do not* produce increases in I_a. This is the condition under which X-ray tubes operate so that increases in kV *do not* produce increases in mA.

In the saturated portion of the graph, increases in I_a can only be obtained by increasing the filament temperature. This is done by raising the filament heating current (I_f).

Look at what happens to the graph when the filament temperature is increased (Fig. 11.7). We see that at temperature T_2 (higher than T_1) saturation is again reached, but saturation current is higher. Raising the temperature again to T_3 gives a further rise in saturation current. This important graph is known as the **characteristic curve** for a vacuum diode valve.

11.3.3 *Uses of vacuum diodes*

Before the development of solid-state diodes (Section 13.1), vacuum diode valves were used to provide rectification in X-ray equipment. The only example of a vacuum diode used in modern X-ray equipment is the X-ray tube itself, which is a modified form of vacuum diode. We shall examine the X-ray tube more closely in Chapter 12.

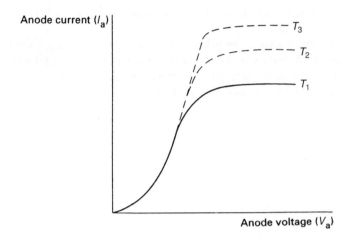

Fig. 11.7　Effect of varying filament temperature.

11.4　Triode valve

The vacuum triode has a third electrode, known as a grid (Fig. 11.8). The grid is constructed in the form of a wire mesh. This is situated in close proximity to the cathode, and by applying a negative bias to the grid the resistance of the valve can be altered or the valve can be used as an electronic switch. This offers the advantage of very rapid switching because there are no moving parts (except electrons).

These characteristics of the vacuum triode valve can be applied in X-ray equipment:

- **Grid-controlled X-ray tubes.** These tubes are modified vacuum triodes. The switching action of the grid can be used to facilitate very rapid exposure switching, as required, for example, in angiocardiography. The ability to vary the resistance of the X-ray tube, and therefore vary the voltage drop across

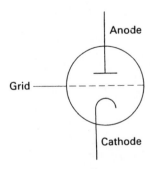

Fig. 11.8　Vacuum triode.

it, can be used to limit the output of low-energy ('soft') X-radiation in dental X-ray equipment.

- **Variable-focus X-ray tubes.** By isolating the focusing hood from the filament and applying a variable negative bias to it, focusing of the electron stream can be adjusted, thereby altering the dimensions of the focal spot and therefore the size of the source of X-rays (see Section 12.6).

Chapter 12

X-Ray Tubes

Construction of simple X-ray tubes
   Design features of a stationary-anode tube
   Design features of a rotating-anode tube
   Rotating-anode induction motor
Modern materials and X-ray tube design
   Tube envelopes
   Anode disc
   Rotor bearings
   Mammography tubes
Line focus principle
   Focal spot size
   Anode heel effect
   Biangular tubes
X-ray tube shield
Cooling of X-ray tubes

12.1 Requirements for producing X-rays

In Section 11.3.2 we said that an X-ray tube was a special type of diode valve. To meet the requirements of producing X-rays, some modifications have been made, particularly to the size and shape of the anode and cathode.

To produce X-rays we need to make fast-moving electrons suffer sudden and violent changes of direction (Section 16.1.1.1). The electrons are accelerated across to the positive anode which they hit at high speed. As they interact with atoms in the anode, some of their energy is converted into X-rays. Details of these interactions are discussed in Chapter 16.

Approximately 99% of the energy released by these electrons appears as heat; it is clear that heat is going to be a major consideration in the design of the anode. Another problem, particularly in diagnostic work, is the size of the source of X-rays known as the **focus** or **focal spot**. For example, imagine two sources of X-rays: (a) a small point source and (b) a larger finite source (Fig. 12.1). In example (a), a sharp shadow is cast. Contrast this with example (b), where the shadow is no longer sharp; the edges of the image are seen to be spread out, not clearly defined as in (a). This unsharpness is known as the **penumbra effect**.

To overcome this problem we ideally need a point source of X-rays, but this presents us with two additional problems. Firstly, if all the electrons strike one point on the anode, the heat produced at this point would cause the anode to melt. Secondly, how can we get all the electrons to arrive at one point, remembering

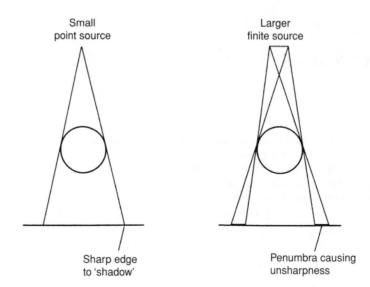

Small
point source

Larger
finite source

Sharp edge
to 'shadow'

Penumbra causing
unsharpness

Fig. 12.1   Effect of small and large focal spots.

that they are all negatively charged, so will tend to repel each other as they travel from the cathode to the anode and therefore spread out?

To see how these problems are overcome, let us examine the construction of stationary- and rotating-anode X-ray tubes.

12.2   X-ray tube – principles of construction

For many years, the basic design and materials used in the construction of X-ray tubes remained relatively unchanged. However, over the last 25 years advances in technology have led to the introduction of new materials and modifications to the traditional design of the X-ray tube. Because the physical principles underlying the operation of the X-ray tube have not changed, we will use the simpler traditional model to explain these principles. Later in this chapter we shall consider the impact of new materials on the design and operation of the tube.

There are two fundamental approaches to the design of X-ray tubes, depending on whether the anode is stationary or rotating.

12.3   Stationary-anode X-ray tube

The stationary-anode X-ray tube has few applications in modern radiography equipment. However, its small size and weight can be an advantage in specialised applications, such as intra-oral and orthopantomographic dental radiography, where only a low X-ray output is required.

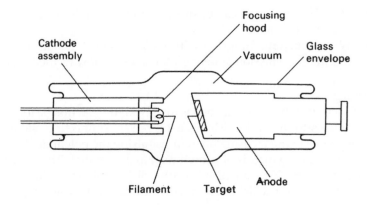

Fig. 12.2   Stationary-anode X-ray tube (diagrammatic).

12.3.1   *Design features of the stationary-anode X-ray tube* (Fig. 12.2)

12.3.1.1   Glass envelope

This is made of borosilicate glass (pyrex) to withstand the high temperatures. It also acts as an electrical insulator between the negative cathode and the positive anode. It contains the vacuum and supports the electrodes.

12.3.1.2   Vacuum

All the air is excluded from within the glass envelope. This prevents oxidation of the electrodes and acts as an electrical insulator. It also ensures that thermionic electrons moving across the tube do not collide with any gas atoms which would be ionised and reduce the kinetic energy of the thermionic electrons.

12.3.1.3   Cathode

The cathode consists of a coiled filament of tungsten wire enclosed in a **focusing hood** or **focusing cup**.

Filament
The function of the filament is to release a supply of electrons into the vacuum by thermionic emission. The filament is coiled in order to provide a large surface area for electron emission while confining the emission to a small volume of space. Tungsten is chosen as the filament material for the following reasons:

(1)   **Melting point.** It has a high melting point (3387°C).
(2)   **Vapour pressure** (pressure at which a substance no longer evaporates). It has a low vapour pressure of about 5000 kPa, which means that when hot, it releases less vapour into the vacuum than do other materials.

(3) **Ductility.** Tungsten can be drawn (stretched) into the fine wire needed to form the filament.

(4) **Work function.** Tungsten with its low work function of 4.5 eV exhibits thermionic emission at temperatures well below its melting point.

Focusing hood

The function of the focusing hood is to prevent the electron beam from diverging as it crosses to the anode. This is achieved by connecting one of the filament supply wires to the focusing hood, thus raising the potential of the hood to that of the filament, which is at a high negative potential. The edges of the hood produce an electric field which is responsible for this focusing effect. Figure 5.8 illustrates the electric field between the cathode and the anode of an X-ray tube.

12.3.1.4   Anode

The main bulk of the anode is made of copper because copper is a good conductor of heat (high thermal conductivity). The thermal conductivity of copper is about 400 W m^{-1} K^{-1}, compared with 174 W m^{-1} K^{-1} for tungsten. The anode has a large mass and heat capacity to allow it to absorb more heat. Other characteristics of copper, particularly its low melting point and low proton number, make it a bad choice as a source of X-rays. A tungsten block known as the **target** is therefore inset into the surface of the anode and the electrons are focused onto this.

Tungsten is chosen as the target material for the following reasons:

(1) High proton number ($Z = 74$) (efficient at producing X-rays)
(2) Reasonable thermal conductivity (174 W m^{-1} K^{-1}) (It helps to conduct heat away from the target to the mass of the anode.)
(3) High melting point (3387°C)
(4) Low vapour pressure (about 5000 kPa)
(5) Easily machined to give a smooth surface

12.4   The rotating-anode X-ray tube

The rotating-anode X-ray tube is the design chosen for the vast majority of applications. It is based on the same basic principle as the stationary-anode tube, but certain modifications have been made, particularly to the anode assembly to help overcome the limitations imposed by having a very small area on which the heat produced at the target is concentrated.

12.4.1   *Design features of a basic rotating-anode X-ray tube* (Fig. 12.3)

12.4.1.1   Glass envelope and vacuum

Rotating-anode tubes tend to be larger than stationary-anode tubes, but in general the structure and function of the glass envelope and vacuum remain the

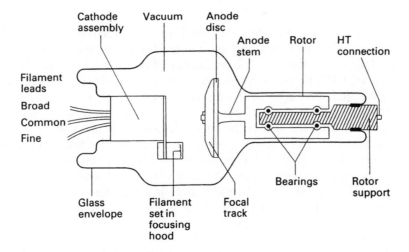

Fig. 12.3 Rotating-anode X-ray tube insert (diagrammatic).

same. In modern tubes, the glass envelope has been replaced by one made of a combination of glass and metal, or ceramic and metal (see Section 12.5.1).

12.4.1.2 Cathode

The cathode assembly is offset from the long axis of the X-ray tube to face the target track near the periphery of the anode disc. It is usual to incorporate two filaments, one larger than the other, set side by side into the cathode assembly, giving the radiographer a choice of a fine or a broad focal spot. The filaments are supplied by three leads, one to the fine focus filament, one to the broad, and a common lead, which is also connected to the focusing hood.

12.4.1.3 Anode

The anode assembly is a very complex component because it incorporates an induction motor to enable the anode disc to rotate. It is convenient to look at individual parts of the assembly.

Anode disc
A simple anode disc is made of tungsten and is saucer shaped (with a *concave* rear surface). It can vary in diameter from 90 to 120 mm.

The **target track** (or **focal track**) is near the periphery of the disc to maximise its length. The track itself is usually a mixture of 90% tungsten and 10% **rhenium**. The presence of rhenium reduces the **crazing** effect caused by thermal stresses. Because its proton number ($Z = 75$) is close to that of tungsten ($Z = 74$), rhenium has little effect on the X-ray output. Details of the materials found in modern **compound anode** designs are given in Section 12.5.2.

Anode stem

The anode stem connects the anode disc to the rotor. It is made of **molybdenum**, a hard white metal with proton number 42 and a melting point 2620°C. The stem is designed to minimise the conduction of heat from the anode disc to the rotor bearings. It is therefore constructed with a relatively small diameter, giving it a small area of cross section (see Section 2.4.1.1). The worked example following Section 2.4.1.1 in Chapter 2 demonstrates how effectively the anode stem protects the rotor from the heat of the anode disc. It is interesting to note that although molybdenum has a lower thermal conductivity than that of tungsten at room temperature (137 Wm^{-1}, compared with 174 Wm^{-1}), this difference reduces at higher temperatures. At the typical operating temperatures of the anode stem, the difference in thermal conductivity is no longer a significant factor in the choice of molybdenum for the anode stem.

Rotor

The copper rotor forms the moving part of the **induction motor** which drives the rotation of the anode disc (see Section 12.4.2). The high electrical conductivity of copper encourages strong currents to be induced in the rotor by the stator windings situated outside the glass envelope. This enhances the efficiency of the induction motor. The surface of the rotor is blackened to improve the dissipation of heat by the emission of **infrared radiation** (see Section 2.4.3.1).

Rotor support

The rotor support is made of steel to take the weight of the anode assembly. The positive high-tension connection is made to the end of the rotor support outside the glass envelope.

Bearings

The bearings are made of steel ball races. They are coated with lead or silver to act as a lubricant. Oil and grease are prohibited because they would vaporise and destroy the vacuum. The bearings also transmit the high tension to the rotor and anode disc.

12.4.2   *Rotating-anode induction motor*

12.4.2.1   Principle of operation

A rotating magnetic field is produced by the stator windings which are wound onto a laminated ferromagnetic core surrounding the anode end of the glass envelope. As the magnetic field rotates, the stationary rotor experiences a continually changing magnetic field. The resulting changes in magnetic flux linkage induce an emf in the rotor. The induced emf causes an induced current to flow in the rotor, creating its own magnetic field. The polarity of this magnetic field *opposes* that of the stator field (Lenz's law; Section 9.3). Consequently, the force of attraction between the two magnetic fields causes the rotor to turn, as it follows the rotating stator field.

The rotating stator field is generated by two pairs of windings, A_1A_2 and B_1B_2, spaced at right angles to each other around the rotor (Fig. 12.4). The windings

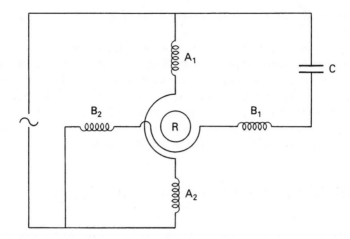

Fig. 12.4   Diagram of an induction motor circuit designed to produce a rotating magnetic field. The circuit includes a phase-shifting capacitor (C), stator windings (A₁, A₂, B₁, B₂) and rotor (R).

are supplied with alternating current. A capacitor (C) is connected in series with one pair of windings (B₁B₂). Let us consider the current flow in each pair of windings:

- **Windings A₁A₂** (*no* capacitor) – The inductive nature of this circuit causes the current flowing through windings A₁A₂ to *lag behind* the voltage supply (Section 10.6.1.3). If appropriate values of inductance and resistance are chosen for this circuit, the current can be made to lag the voltage by 45°.
- **Windings B₁B₂** (*with* capacitor) – The capacitive nature of this circuit causes the current through windings B₁B₂ to *lead* the voltage supply (Section 10.6.1.2). If an appropriate value of capacitance is chosen for this circuit, the current can be made to lead the voltage by 45°.

The two different circuit characteristics produce a phase difference of 90° between the currents in the two pairs of stator windings. The effect of this phase difference is, for example, to make the north magnetic pole of the windings move in sequence from A₁ to B₁ to A₂ to B₂ and then back to A₁. The cycle is then repeated. The result is a magnetic field which rotates at a speed matching the frequency of the alternating current supply.

Note that in practice, the laminated stator core has more than four poles. The stator windings are shared between 16 or more pole pieces in order to provide a broader magnetic field, which envelops the entire circumference of the rotor.

12.4.2.2   Speed of rotation

If the arrangement described in Section 12.4.2.1 is connected to an a.c. supply at mains frequency (50 Hz in the UK and Europe), the stator field rotates at 50 revolutions per second, or 3000 revolutions per minute (rpm). In fact, the rotor turns at slightly less than the speed of the stator field because of the effects of friction in the rotor bearings.

Speeds around 3000 rpm are too slow for the short (*millisecond*) X-ray exposure times used in current practice. If a higher rotation speed is employed, the focal track is longer, enabling the heat generated at the focus to be spread over a larger area. The rotor and anode disc in a modern **high-speed X-ray tube** are therefore driven at speeds approaching 9000 rpm (150 Hz) or 12 000 rpm (200 Hz). These high rotation speeds are achieved by increasing the frequency of the stator supply with frequency-multiplying circuits.

12.5   Modern materials and X-ray tube design

Two of the most significant developments in X-ray tube construction arise from the use of materials other than glass for the tube envelope and the introduction of **compound anode** discs.

12.5.1   X-ray tube envelopes

Glass is far from an ideal material for the X-ray tube envelope because it is susceptible to the effects of tungsten vapour. Although tungsten has a low vapour pressure, some tungsten vapour is released into the vacuum from both the filament and the anode target. The tungsten vapour condenses on the relatively cool glass envelope and eventually forms a thin, electrically conducting coating on the inside of the glass. In time, this can lead to arcing and possibly loss of the vacuum due to puncture of the glass. The increasingly common use of high X-ray currents, requiring higher filament temperatures which release more tungsten vapour, exacerbates this problem. Glass is also susceptible to damage from electron bombardment.

To eliminate these problems, **metal envelopes** have been developed. These offer many advantages because they can tolerate electron bombardment without damage, the deposition of tungsten is no longer a problem and a low-attenuation **beryllium window** can be incorporated into the envelope to transmit the X-ray beam with reduced inherent filtration (Section 17.3.2).

An obvious potential problem with metal envelopes is that metal is an electrical conductor and would short-circuit the anode and cathode potentials of the X-ray tube. This difficulty is overcome by incorporating ceramic or glass insulating sections at the ends of the tube, where the anode and cathode are attached. The envelope is then known as a **metal-ceramic** or **metal-glass** design.

Metal-envelope X-ray tubes are more robust, have a longer working life and provide a higher X-ray output than tubes with a glass envelope.

12.5.2   Anode disc

Modern X-ray tube anodes are discus shaped (with a *convex* back surface) and use a combination of materials producing a **compound anode** design.

12.5.2.1 Molybdenum anodes

The anode disc in most modern rotating-anode X-ray tubes is made from solid molybdenum onto which a thin tungsten–rhenium focal track is coated. The specific heat capacity of molybdenum (250 J kg^{-1} K^{-1}) is greater than that of tungsten (130 J kg^{-1} K^{-1}). A molybdenum anode disc is therefore a more effective **heat sink** than a tungsten anode disc of the same mass. This means that a given X-ray exposure produces a lower temperature rise in a molybdenum anode than it would in a tungsten anode (Section 2.3.4). Molybdenum also has a lower density than that of tungsten ($10\,200$ kg m^{-3} compared with $19\,250$ kg m^{-3}), meaning that a molybdenum anode has only about half the mass of a tungsten anode with the same dimensions.

12.5.2.2 Stress-relieved anode

Some high-output, heavy-duty X-ray tubes have radial slots cut into the anode disc to reduce the stresses caused by repeated cycles of heating and cooling.

12.5.2.3 Carbon backing

Heavy-duty X-ray tubes may incorporate a thick layer of graphite (carbon) attached to the back of the anode disc. This increases considerably the heat capacity of the anode while adding little to its mass.

12.5.3 Spiral bearings (also known as liquid bearings)

At least one manufacturer produces rotating-anode X-ray tubes with **spiral groove** rotor bearings. These use liquid metal alloys as a lubricant and provide a virtually silent and friction-free bearing. The bearings are claimed to have excellent electrical and thermal conductivity and permit the development of anodes which rotate continuously during the daily operation of the X-ray tube.

12.5.4 Specialised mammography tubes

X-ray tubes used for mammography have special requirements. In particular, they must produce a high output of near-monochromatic, low-energy X-radiation. This is achieved by using a molybdenum target, which emits **characteristic radiation** at 17 and 19 keV, together with a molybdenum filter, which removes most of the unwanted radiation from the beam (Section 17.3.2.1).

Mammography tubes may suffer problems associated with the presence of a **space charge**, the result of operating at low kilovoltages and high tube currents. To help overcome these problems, mammography tubes may operate two filaments simultaneously and may employ a reduced cathode–anode spacing.

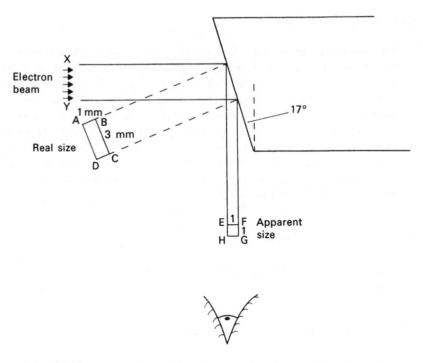

Fig. 12.5 Principle of line focus.

12.6 Principle of line focus

You will notice that in both the stationary- and rotating-anode X-ray tube the target is at an angle of about 17°. The reasons for this are most important. If we look back to our ideal situation, namely, (a) a large area over which to spread the heat and (b) a small area to give a point source of X-rays, some compromise must be reached.

The principle of line focus is illustrated in Fig. 12.5. XY represents a parallel beam of electrons 1 mm wide, arriving at the target. It hits a rectangle 1 mm × 3 mm. This *real* area is represented by ABCD.

If we now look up at the source of X-rays from the viewpoint of the patient, the area appears to be much smaller than the real area because of the effect of the 17° angle. In fact, the area producing X-rays appears to be 1 mm × 1 mm. This is known as the **apparent** (or **effective**) focal spot size. This effect is known as the **principle of line focus**.

12.6.1 *Calculating the apparent focal spot size*

The size of the apparent focal spot can be calculated using simple trigonometry. In Fig. 12.6, RST is a right-angle triangle, in which RT represents the *real* side dimension of the rectangle on which the electron beam strikes the target (3 mm in our example), θ represents the target angle (17° in the example) and ST represents

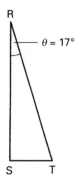

$\theta = 17°$

Fig. 12.6 The triangle used in the calculation of the apparent focal spot size (ST) of an X-ray tube with target angle θ. The real focal spot size is represented by RT.

the dimension of the *apparent* focal spot. Then

$$\sin \theta = \frac{ST}{RT}$$

so

$$ST = RT \sin \theta$$

i.e.

Apparent focus $=$ real focus $\times$ sin (target angle)

In our example, $\theta = 17°$ and RT $= 3$ mm. Consulting the sine function on an electronic calculator shows that sin $17° = 0.2924 \approx 0.3$. Thus,

Apparent focus $= 3 \times 0.3$

$$\approx 0.9 \text{ mm}$$

12.6.2   *Demonstration of the line focus principle*

You can demonstrate this principle for yourself by drawing a rectangle, say, 3 cm $\times$ 1 cm, on a piece of card and colouring the area. This represents the area of the target that the electrons strike. Now look first at the card from the direction that the electrons would approach, holding the card at an angle of roughly 17°, and then turn the card and look at it from the position of the patient (Fig. 12.7).

In the first case a large area is seen, and in the second a much smaller area. These represent the real and apparent focal spot sizes.

12.6.3   *Effects of choosing small apparent focal spot sizes*

From what we said in Section 12.1 about unsharpness being caused by the penumbra effect, it would seem sensible to use the smallest possible apparent focal spot for all examinations. However, it should be realised that choosing a very small apparent focal spot size means that the real area will also be reduced in size, thus reducing the area on the target over which the heat is spread.

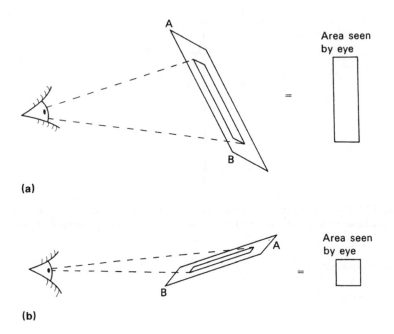

Fig. 12.7   Illustration of the principle of line focus: (a) looking at anode from direction of electron beam and (b) looking at anode from direction of film.

Most modern X-ray tubes have anode angles between $10°$ and $13°$, and employ focal spot sizes of 0.6 and 1.3 mm. Smaller and variable focal spot sizes are available for specialised applications.

12.6.4   Effects of choosing small target angles

There are two important effects associated with the choice of target angle: size of apparent focal spot and area covered by X-ray beam.

12.6.4.1   Size of apparent focal spot

For a given apparent focal spot size (e.g. 1.2 mm), the real area covered by the electron beam is larger for a small target angle. Compare the height of the electron beams a_1 and a_2 in Fig. 12.8, each producing the same apparent focal spot size.

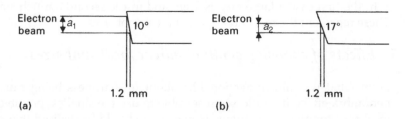

Fig. 12.8   Effect of target angle on focal spot size: (a) small target angle – 1.2 mm apparent focal spot; (b) large target angle – 1.2 mm apparent focal spot.

The precise effect on the *real* dimensions of the focal spot can be calculated using the relationship derived in Section 12.6.1:

Apparent focal spot size = real focal spot size × sin (target angle)

Thus,

$$\text{Real focal spot size} = \frac{\text{apparent focal spot size}}{\text{sin(target angle)}}$$

In the example shown in Fig. 12.8a:

$$\text{Real focus} = \frac{1.2}{\sin 10°}$$

$$= \frac{1.2}{0.17} \text{ mm}$$

$$= 6.9 \text{ mm}$$

In the example shown in Fig. 12.8b:

$$\text{Real focus} = \frac{1.2}{\sin 17°} \text{ mm}$$

$$= \frac{1.2}{0.29} \text{mm}$$

$$= 4.1 \text{ mm}$$

This represents a 40% reduction in the surface area over which the heat must be spread.

12.6.4.2 Area covered by X-ray beam

As can be seen from Fig. 12.9, the extent of the X-ray beam is limited by the angle of the face of the target. (X-rays will not pass easily through tungsten or copper.) This means that it is not possible to cover large X-ray films at short focus-film distances, with a target angle of 10°. (It is for this reason that radiotherapy tubes use target angles of 35° in order to cover large areas of the patient at short distances.)

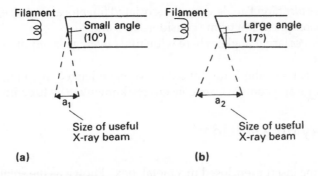

Fig. 12.9 Effect of target angle on the size of an X-ray beam.

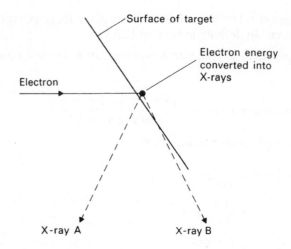

Fig. 12.10   Anode heel effect.

12.6.4.3   Anode heel effect

Close examination of the X-rays emitted from the target shows that because they are produced below its surface, they have to pass through some tungsten before they can escape from the tube.

Compare the two rays A and B shown in Fig. 12.10. A has to pass through only a small amount of tungsten, whereas B has to pass through a much greater thickness before escaping from the tube. This greater thickness of tungsten causes more of the X-ray beam to be absorbed towards the anode end of the tube. This means that the strength of the X-ray beam varies from A to B, being stronger at A. This is known as the **anode heel effect**.

12.6.4.4   Biangular X-ray tubes

A **biangular** X-ray tube design uses an anode which has two different target angles on the same anode disc. This arrangement offers, in the same X-ray tube, the advantages of both:

- a *smaller* target angle with its associated finer focal spot size, where geometric unsharpness is a prime consideration, and
- a *larger* target angle, where wide film coverage is required.

The parts of the X-ray tube that we have looked at so far, namely the glass envelope and contents, are collectively known as the **tube insert**.

12.7   X-ray tube shield

The tube insert is enclosed in a metal 'box', known as the shield (Fig. 12.11). It is designed to perform four functions: radiation protection, electrical protection, thermal protection and physical protection.

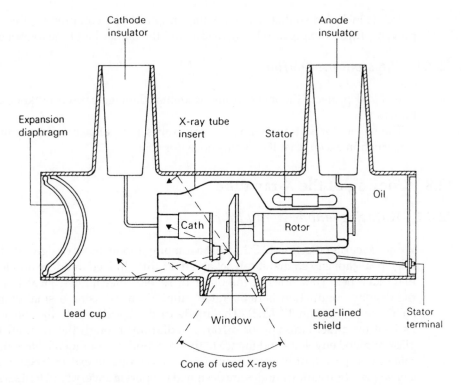

Fig. 12.11 Rotating-anode X-ray tube insert and housing. (Figure reproduced courtesy of IGE Medical Systems Ltd.)

12.7.1 Radiation protection

The steel casing is lined with lead to prevent radiation emerging in all directions. A perspex port is provided to allow the X-ray beam to escape in the useful direction only. It is convex upwards to reduce filtration of the X-ray beam by the oil.

12.7.2 Electrical protection

To prevent patients and staff coming into contact with high voltages, the shield is earthed. Where high-tension cables enter the shield, insulated sockets are used. The shield is filled with pure mineral oil, which acts as an electrical insulator, preventing sparking across the insert or from the insert to the shield.

12.7.3 Thermal protection

Because the anode reaches very high temperatures, the oil also acts as a cooling medium (see below).

To enable the oil to expand when it gets hot, an expansion diaphragm is included in the shield. This allows the oil to expand and contract as its temperature changes, without letting any air enter the insert. In some types of equipment a switch is included so that when the diaphragm is fully compressed, the switch prevents further exposures being made until the oil has had time to cool down.

12.7.4   *Physical protection*

The shield protects the insert from accidental damage caused by knocks and bumps.

The shield for stationary-anode X-ray tubes is smaller but very similar in construction except that it contains no stator coils.

12.8   Cooling of the X-ray tube

12.8.1   *Rotating-anode X-ray tubes*

We noted earlier (Section 12.5.2.1) that a rotating-anode disc is designed to have a large heat capacity so that it can act as a **heat sink**. Indeed, modern anode discs may have heat capacities of the order of several megajoules. Heat loss from the disc by conduction is deliberately minimised by using a small-diameter anode stem (Section 12.4.1.3). The anode disc must dissipate the majority of its heat by direct emission of **infrared radiation** through the vacuum to the glass or metal envelope and thence to the surrounding cooling oil. Note that the rate of dissipation of heat by radiation is *temperature dependent* (Section 2.4.3). Consequently, rotating anodes are designed to operate at very high temperatures (white hot) in order to maximise heat dissipation by radiation.

Heat passes through the oil by **convection** to the tube shield and is then **conducted** through the shield. Finally, **convection** currents in the surrounding air remove the heat from the tube shield.

Many modern X-ray tubes employ **positive cooling**. This can be achieved by fitting air circulation fans to the tube shield. In some high-output, heavy-duty metal-ceramic tubes, direct cooling of the anode disc and bearings is achieved by circulating cooling oil into the rear of the disc itself. The oil then dissipates its heat by passing through an external heat exchanger. A similar method is employed in radiotherapy X-ray tubes.

12.8.2   *Stationary-anode X-ray tubes*

In contrast to rotating-anode tubes, stationary-anode tubes are designed to maximise heat dissipation from the target by **conduction** through the anode. The anode itself is a large-diameter copper block. Its large area of cross section, combined with the high thermal conductivity of copper (395 W m^{-1} K^{-1}), provides ideal conditions for heat conduction to occur. The majority of the heat is therefore conducted along the anode and directly into the cooling oil.

Chapter 13

Solid-State Devices

Much of the rapid advance in technology over the last 30 years has been due to the application of semiconductor materials. The development of silicon chips the size of a fingernail, which can contain many millions of electronic components, has enabled a new generation of electronic equipment to be produced, ranging from personal computers to mobile telephones.

In this chapter, we shall look at some of the simpler solid-state devices, which find many applications in the rectification, switching and control systems of X-ray equipment. The term **solid state** is used here to distinguish semiconductor-based components from their earlier vacuum-valve predecessors.

To understand how solid-state devices work it is first necessary to explore the properties of semiconductors.

13.1 Properties of semiconductors

Semiconductors, as the name suggests, have resistance values somewhere between conductors and insulators. Examples of common semiconductors are silicon, selenium and germanium.

The nature of semiconducting materials was introduced in terms of electron energy levels in Section 6.1.1.2. We noted that in semiconductors, there is only a narrow forbidden energy gap between the top of the valance band and the bottom of the conduction band. This means that at room temperature, some electrons from the valence band are able to acquire sufficient energy to transfer from the valence band into the conduction band and therefore be available for electrical conduction.

13.1.1   The structure of semiconductors

To understand the properties of semiconductors it is necessary to look first at their atomic structure, in particular their outermost electron shells, or valence shells.

In semiconductors, we find that neighbouring atoms share their valence electrons. For example, silicon has four valence electrons of its own, but it requires eight to complete its valence shell. To overcome this, each atom shares electrons with four of its neighbours, thus satisfying its need for eight electrons (Fig. 13.1). This sharing of electrons is known as **covalent bonding** (Section 4.4.2).

13.1.1.1   Pure semiconductors

You might imagine from the structure of silicon that it would be a perfect insulator, because all the electrons are linked to neighbouring atoms, there being no free electrons to permit a flow of current. This, however, is not the whole truth, as we shall see.

At normal room temperatures, or if we supply energy to the semiconductor material, e.g. heat, light or electrical energy, a few of the covalent bonds become broken and an electron can acquire sufficient energy to make the transition to the conduction band, leaving a 'hole' behind. The hole is filled by another electron from the valence band of a neighbouring atom, which, in turn, leaves another hole and so on.

Thus, we can imagine electrons and holes continuously wandering about within the material until an electron drops back from the conduction band to fill the hole. Because electrons are negative charges, we can consider holes as being positive charges. This will be a useful concept later on.

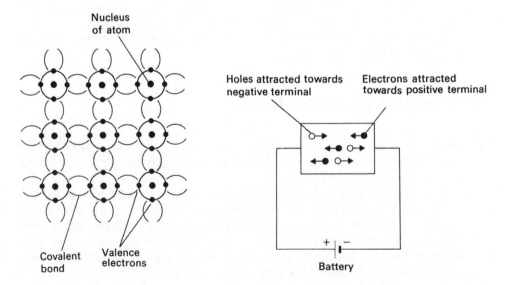

Fig. 13.1   Silicon crystal.   Fig. 13.2   Conduction in semiconductors.

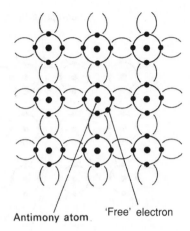

Antimony atom   'Free' electron

Fig. 13.3   N-type semiconductor material.

Imagine now the effect of applying a potential difference (PD) to the semiconductor (Fig 13.2).

Intrinsic conduction
As expected, the electrons move towards the positive potential and the holes towards the negative; i.e. we have a small flow of current. In a pure semiconductor there is one free electron and one hole per 1000 million atoms. This current which occurs in pure semiconductors is known as **intrinsic conduction** and is too small to be of significance in this section.

13.1.1.2   N-type semiconductors

The number of conduction electrons in a semiconductor can be altered by adding atoms of other materials.

If we add a very small amount of an impurity, such as antimony to silicon (e.g. 1 ppm), we find that a change in the structure of the crystal occurs (see Fig. 13.3). Silicon has four valence electrons, whereas antimony has five. Four of the valence electrons of the antimony atom form covalent bonds with the silicon atoms, leaving the fifth valence electron 'free'. We have therefore increased the conductivity of the silicon (i.e. decreased its resistance) by the introduction of antimony.

By adding impurities which have *five* valence electrons (such as antimony) we produce an **n-type semiconductor**. Conduction which occurs as a result of added impurities is called **extrinsic conduction**.

N.B. Although n-type semiconductors contain free electrons, they are still electrically neutral, because they have the same number of electrons as protons.

13.1.1.3   P-type semiconductors

Just as the number of electrons in a semiconductor can be increased by adding impurities, so can the number of holes.

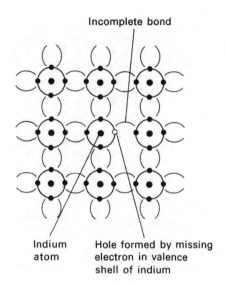

Fig. 13.4   P-type semiconductor.

If we add a very small amount of an impurity, such as indium to silicon, we again notice a change in the structure of the crystal (see Fig. 13.4). Silicon atoms have four valence electrons and indium atoms have three. The three valence electrons of indium form covalent bonds, leaving a hole where the fourth should be. We have therefore increased the conductivity of the silicon by the introduction of a hole, which is free to move and combine with other electrons.

By adding impurities such as indium, whose atoms have three valence electrons, we produce a **p-type semiconductor**.

N.B. Once again this material is still electrically neutral. Remember also that electrons and holes are wandering around continuously in the materials.

13.1.2   Conduction in P- and N-type semiconductors

Let us look at what happens when a battery is connected across an n-type semiconductor (Fig. 13.5). Free electrons flow out of the semiconductor to the positive terminal of the battery and electrons from the negative terminal flow into the semiconductor to take their place; i.e. a current flows.

In the case of p-type semiconductors (Fig. 13.6), current again flows through the circuit. This time we can imagine holes flowing out of the semiconductor material towards the negative terminal of the battery.

Conclusions
In n-type semiconductors, current flow is due to electrons. *Electrons* are therefore known as **majority carriers**. In p-type semiconductors, current flow is due to holes; i.e. *holes* are majority carriers.

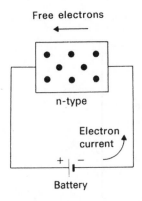

Free electrons

n-type

Electron
current

Battery

Fig. 13.5 Conduction in n-type semiconductors.

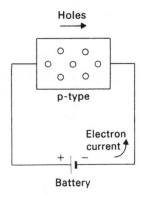

Holes

p-type

Electron
current

Battery

Fig. 13.6 Conduction in p-type semiconductors.

13.1.3   P–N junction

When a p-type and an n-type semiconductor are joined together, an interesting effect is noticed (Fig. 13.7). Some of the free electrons from the n-type wander across the junction into the p-type, and similarly some of the holes from the p-type wander across the junction into the n-type. The electrons that have wandered into the p-type combine with some of the holes and form negative ions. Similarly, some of the holes which have wandered across into the n-type combine with some of the free electrons and form positive ions; i.e. the previously neutral p- and n-type materials become charged (Fig. 13.7).

This movement of electrons and holes continues until a charge builds up on either side of the junction, which then repels any further electrons or holes from crossing the junction. We can consider this charge barrier as being an imaginary battery (Fig. 13.8). The region in the vicinity of the junction where there are now

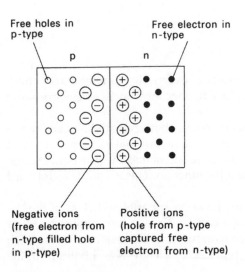

Free holes in
p-type

Free electron in
n-type

p   n

Negative ions
(free electron from
n-type filled hole
in p-type)

Positive ions
(hole from p-type
captured free
electron from n-type)

Fig. 13.7   P–N junction.

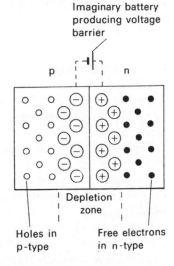

Imaginary battery
producing voltage
barrier

p   n

Depletion
zone

Holes in
p-type

Free electrons
in n-type

Fig. 13.8   P–N junction showing voltage barrier and depletion zone.

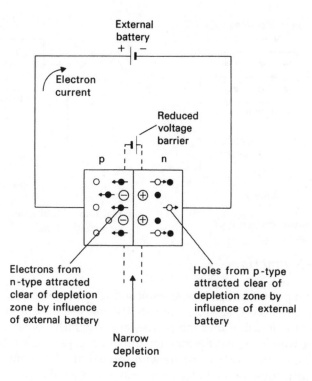

Fig. 13.9   Conduction in a p–n junction.

no free electrons or holes is known as the **depletion zone** or **depletion layer**. It acts as an almost perfect insulator.

13.1.3.1   Forward biasing

To permit a continuous flow of current we must overcome this imaginary battery or voltage barrier, because it is preventing further movement of electrons and holes.

This can be achieved by connecting an external battery with its negative terminal to the n-type semiconductor and its positive terminal to the p-type; i.e. it is connected to *overcome* the voltage barrier set up across the junction, leaving only a very small depletion zone around the junction. This is known as **forward bias** (Fig. 13.9).

Most of the charges now crossing the junction are attracted clear of the depletion zone by the effect of the external battery. Thus, a continuous stream of electrons is able to flow through the semiconductors. Electrons and holes which move through the semiconductor are replaced by electrons and holes from the battery.

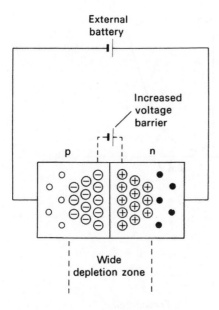

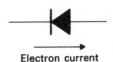

Fig. 13.10   Reverse bias of a p–n junction.

Fig. 13.11   Circuit symbol for a solid-state rectifier.

13.1.3.2   Reverse biasing

Now let us consider what happens when the external battery is connected the other way round, i.e. with the positive terminal to the n-type semiconductor and the negative terminal to the p-type. This time the external battery is connected in such a way as to reinforce the voltage barrier, making the depletion zone wider and therefore preventing any flow of electrons or holes across the barrier. Therefore, no current can flow through the semiconductors. This is known as **reverse bias** (Fig. 13.10).

Conclusion
When the p-type material is positive and the n-type negative, the semiconductor conducts. When the p-type material is negative and the n-type positive, the semiconductor does not conduct.

We have a device which will allow current to flow through it in one direction only. It can therefore be used as a rectifier, and it is known as a **solid-state rectifier** or **junction diode**. The circuit symbol is shown in Fig. 13.11. Junction diodes have replaced vacuum diodes to provide rectification in X-ray equipment.

13.1.3.3   Variation of current through a junction diode

Figure 13.12 shows the characteristic way in which the current flowing through a silicon junction diode varies with the applied PD.

If an increasing *forward-biased* PD is applied, a point is soon reached (at approximately 0.6 V) where the potential barrier at the depletion zone is overcome

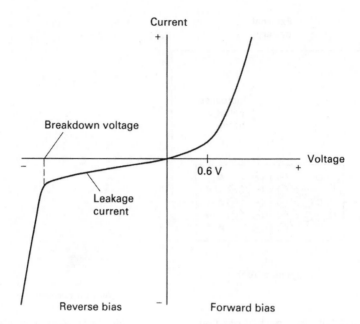

Fig. 13.12 Graph of the current flowing through a junction diode plotted against the voltage applied across it.

and the diode conducts. Once this point is reached, the resistance of the diode decreases as the PD increases.

If an increasing *reverse-biased* PD is applied, the depletion layer widens and the resistance of the diode is very high, permitting only a small **leakage current** to flow. If the reverse-biased PD continues to increase, a point is eventually reached where the barrier breaks down and a large inverse current flows. The reverse-biased PD at which this occurs is known as **breakdown voltage**.

13.1.4 Other types of diodes

13.1.4.1 Light-emitting diodes

X-ray equipment uses **light-emitting diodes** (LEDs). LEDs are made from compounds which emit light when they are forward biased. The light is emitted as a result of the combination of electrons and holes. The wavelength (and therefore colour) of the light depends on the precise combination of materials used.

13.1.4.2 Photodiodes

These diodes are normally held in a reverse-biased state. When one of the surfaces of a photodiode is exposed to light, electrons are able to absorb sufficient energy from the light to jump from the forbidden gap into the conduction band, changing the diode from a non-conducting state to a conducting state.

13.2   Rectification in X-ray equipment

We mentioned earlier that an X-ray tube is a modified form of vacuum diode valve. It therefore has similar rectifying properties to a vacuum diode valve (Section 11.3.1). If the alternating output of an X-ray high-tension transformer is connected directly across an X-ray tube, the tube will *conduct* current (and therefore generate X-rays) during the half-cycles when the anode is positive. However, it will *block* the flow of current (and produce no X-rays) during the inverse half-cycles when the anode is negative. This simple circuit arrangement, known as **self-rectification**, was used for many years in portable and dental X-ray equipment.

However, X-ray tubes work most efficiently when the PD applied across them is unidirectional. This is because it is normal during the operation of an X-ray tube for the anode temperature to reach a level where thermionic emission can occur (Section 12.8.1). Under these circumstances, *if a reverse* potential is applied across the tube, electrons emitted from the hot anode could be attracted across the tube and bombard the delicate filament, eventually destroying it.

By connecting four rectifiers in a **full-wave** or **bridge circuit**, it is possible to re-route the output of the high-tension transformer and thereby make use of *both* half-cycles of the alternating high tension. This **full-wave rectified** type of generator was used for many years in general-purpose and high-power mobile X-ray equipment. The design has now been superseded by medium-frequency and high-frequency generators, but a four-rectifier bridge circuit still forms a key element in such equipment. For this reason, we shall now describe the principle of the bridge circuit used to provide full-wave rectification.

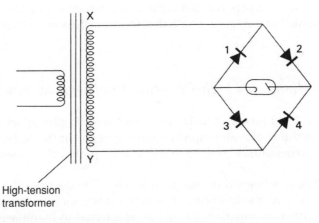

High-tension
transformer

Fig. 13.13   Full-wave rectified circuit.

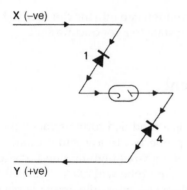
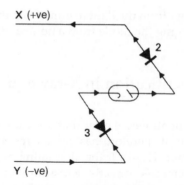

Fig. 13.14 Electron flow during the first half-cycle. Arrows indicate direction of electron flow.

Fig. 13.15 Electron flow during the second half-cycle. Arrows indicate direction of electron flow.

13.2.1   Full-wave rectification circuit

Figure 13.13 shows a bridge circuit connected between the high-tension transformer and the X-ray tube. X and Y are the output leads from the high-tension transformer providing alternating voltage.

Let us first look at what happens when X is negative and Y is positive (Fig. 13.14). Electrons move from X to 1 to X-ray tube to 4 to Y (attracted by positively charged Y). You will notice that the electrons can only pass through the X-ray tube; other routes are blocked by rectifiers 2 and 3.

Now let us look at the next half-cycle when X is positive and Y is negative (Fig. 13.15). Electrons move from Y to 3 to X-ray tube to 2 to X (attracted by positively charged X); i.e. electrons pass through the X-ray tube in the same direction during the second half-cycle.

If we now look at graphs of voltage and current in different parts of the circuit, we see that current flows through the X-ray tube during every half-cycle (Fig 13.16).

If we now incorporate the voltage and current across the X-ray tube into one graph, we can compare it with that for the self-rectified circuit (Fig 13.17).

13.2.2   Medium- and high-frequency (multi-pulse) generators

As we stated earlier, modern X-ray high-tension generators are described as either medium- or high-frequency generators and are sometimes known as **multipulse generators**. Figure 13.18 shows a simplified block diagram of such a generator.

While it is beyond the scope of this book to describe the detailed operation of this circuit, the following section illustrates some of the principles involved. For further information, the reader is referred to manufacturers' literature or specialised texts on X-ray equipment.

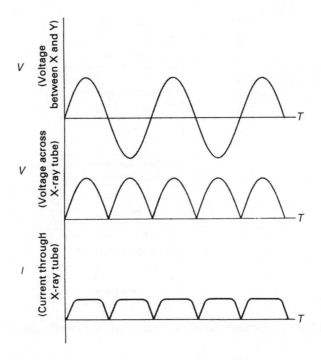

Fig. 13.16 Voltage and current graphs at points in the full-wave circuit.

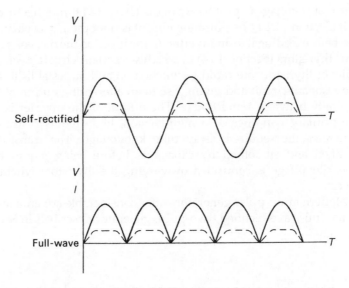

Fig. 13.17 Comparison of voltage and current graphs in self- and full-wave rectification. Solid line = voltage; dotted line = current.

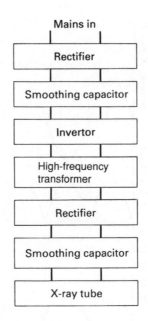

Fig. 13.18 A diagrammatic illustration of a modern multi-pulse X-ray circuit.

13.2.2.1 Principle of operation

The mains voltage (e.g. at 50 Hz in the UK) is fed through a **bridge rectifier** circuit (Section 13.2.1). Its pulsating output is smoothed by capacitors to a constant d.c. before feeding it to an **inverter**. In the inverter, the d.c. voltage is fed through four **thyristors** (Section 13.4) to a **series-resonant circuit** (Section 10.6.2.1). The pairs of thyristors are rapidly switched on and off, establishing oscillations in the resonant circuit and giving rise to an alternating output at high frequency, typically between 4 and 8 kHz. The output of the inverter is used to supply the primary windings of a high-tension, high-frequency transformer which generates the required X-ray tube kilovoltage. The transformer output is rectified and smoothed by capacitors before being fed to the X-ray tube. The kilovoltage is controlled by varying the thyristor switching rates in the inverter.

Modern multi-pulse generators offer considerable advantages over the traditional full-wave rectified, two-pulse generator described in Section 13.2.1. For example:

- The tube kilovoltage is selected electronically and with no appreciable delay, guaranteeing a virtually constant d.c. supply across the X-ray tube.
- High-frequency generators are smaller than other designs. A modern multi-pulse generator may have only one-quarter the weight of its predecessors.

13.3   Transistors

Solid-state semiconductor devices have virtually replaced all thermionic vacuum components in modern electrical equipment. The transistor was invented in 1948 and found one of its first commercial applications in portable radios. The technology of incorporating many thousands of miniature electrical components, such as transistors, resistors and capacitors, into a single silicon chip is known as **large-scale integration** and subsequently, **very large scale integration (VLSI)**. Such **integrated circuits** have been discussed briefly in Section 6.3.3.

Transistors consist of three semiconductor materials sandwiched together. They enable a small current to control the flow of a larger current and have many applications, including switching and amplification.

13.3.1   Construction of transistors

There are two types of transistors known as an **n–p–n type** or a **p–n–p type**, depending on the precise arrangement of semiconducting layers (see Fig. 13.19). The three layers are known as the **collector**, the **base** and the **emitter**. The emitter and the collector are made of the same type of semiconductor (n-type in an n–p–n transistor and p-type in a p–n–p transistor). However, the emitter contains thousands of times more doping impurities than does the collector. Although in Fig. 13.19, the base appears to be the same thickness as the collector and emitter, in practice it is much thinner. An electrical connection is provided to each layer.

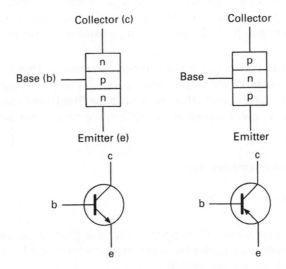

Fig. 13.19   N–P–N (left) and p–n–p (right) transistors and their circuit symbols. In each case, the arrow indicates the direction of conventional current flow.

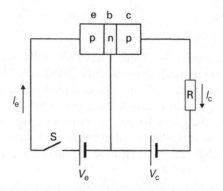

Fig. 13.20   A p–n–p transistor in a common-base circuit.

13.3.2   *Principle of operation of a p–n–p transistor*

13.3.2.1   Common-base circuit

Referring to Fig. 13.20:

- When the switch (S) is open, no current flows in the emitter–base circuit. In this state, very little current flows in the base–collector circuit because the base–collector junction is reverse biased.
- When the switch is closed, the emitter–base junction is forward biased and holes will cross the emitter–base junction. Most of the holes will travel through the base (which is very thin) and provided the potential (V_c) on the collector is sufficient, they will be attracted through the collector, giving an increased collector current (I_c). The remaining holes combine with electrons in the base, constituting a small base current (I_b).

In practice, V_c may be significantly greater than V_e. This means that considerable power may be dissipated in the resistor (R) compared with the power supplied to the emitter circuit. In this **common-base circuit** configuration, the transistor is acting as a **power amplifier**. An alternative circuit arrangement is the common-emitter circuit.

13.3.2.2   Common-emitter circuit

Referring to Fig. 13.21:

- When the switch (S) is open, no current flows in the emitter–base circuit. In this state, little current flows through the transistor because the collector–base junction is reverse biased.
- When the switch is closed, the emitter–base junction is forward biased and holes cross the junction. Many of these holes travel through the base and are attracted by the potential on the collector. The larger the current (I_b) in the

emitter–base circuit, the more holes are available and the larger the current (I_c) through the resistor.

In practice, the collector current (I_c) is much greater than the base current (I_b); thus, the transistor is acting as a **current amplifier**.

Current gain
The current gain (β) of a transistor is given by:

$$\beta = \frac{\text{collector current}}{\text{base current}}$$

$$= \frac{I_c}{I_b}$$

The value of current gain is constant for a given transistor but varies for different types of transistors. A typical value is around 100, with a collector current of 100 mA being associated with a base current of 1 mA.

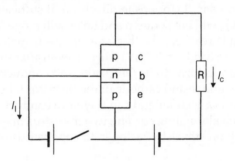

Fig. 13.21   A p–n–p transistor in a common-emitter circuit.

13.3.3   N–P–N transistors

The operation of an n–p–n transistor can be explained in a similar way to the p–n–p type, except that the majority carriers are electrons. Because electrons move faster than holes, n–p–n transistors operate more quickly than p–n–p transistors and are therefore employed where response speeds are critical, e.g. in computer circuits.

13.4   Thyristors

The thyristor, or **silicon-controlled rectifier**, is a four-layer (n–p–n–p) solid-state device, which is used for switching larger currents than a transistor can handle. It has two large terminals (the **anode** and the **cathode**) which connect to the main circuit and a smaller third terminal called the **gate**.

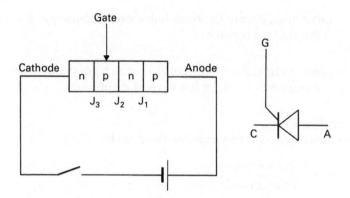

Fig. 13.22   A thyristor and its circuit symbol (right).

In the thyristor shown in Fig. 13.22, junctions J_1 and J_3 are forward biased, and junction J_2 is reverse biased. Thus, little current will flow through the main circuit, and the thyristor is in its *OFF* state.

If a positive voltage pulse is applied to the gate terminal, holes will flow across J_3 (and electrons in the opposite direction). If sufficient current flows across J_3, the barrier at J_2 will break down and holes will move from N to P across J_2. Once this situation is reached, the thyristor has been switched into its *ON* state and will continue to conduct the main current even after the gate voltage is removed.

The thyristor returns to its *OFF* state, and conduction ceases, only when the PD across the anode and cathode of the thyristor falls to zero.

A thyristor is a rectifier and can therefore conduct current only in one direction. To switch alternating current, two thyristors may be connected in **opposed parallel**, with one thyristor facing in the opposite direction to the other.

Chapter 14

Electromagnetic Radiation

Having studied the constructional aspects of the X-ray tube and its electrical supplies we shall now concentrate on the radiation it produces. X-radiation is one example from a whole range of radiations known as electromagnetic radiations. Other examples include visible light, ultraviolet and infrared rays, radio waves and gamma rays. While there are important differences between these examples of electromagnetic radiation, there are also similarities between them. For example, they all:

- Travel through a vacuum
- Travel at the same speed (the speed of light)
- Result from changes in the motion of electric charges

14.1   The origin of electromagnetic radiation

We saw in Section 3.4 that an electric charge (such as an electron or an atomic nucleus) exerts an influence on other electric charges in its neighbourhood; it is accompanied by an electric field. Furthermore, in Section 8.6 we observed that *moving* electric charges are accompanied by a *magnetic* field. When charges accelerate, i.e. experience a change in their motion (an increase or decrease in speed, or a change in direction), disturbances are set up in these electric and magnetic fields. The disturbances, known as **electromagnetic radiation**, travel outwards from the charges at the speed of light (about $300\,000$ km s^{-1}, or 3×10^8 m s^{-1}). The nature of the electromagnetic radiation produced, whether X-rays, visible light, radio waves, etc., depends on the particular way in which the electric charges are disturbed, but in all cases electromagnetic radiation conveys energy away from the disturbed electric charges. If any matter happens to lie in the path of electromagnetic radiation, it may absorb part of this energy and thereby be affected in some way.

14.2   Modelling the behaviour of electromagnetic radiation

How can we explain the behaviour of electromagnetic radiation? As with other fundamental physical problems, we need to find a conceptual model which will help us to understand its behaviour. In fact, *two* quite different, but complementary, models are necessary to explain the range of observed behaviour of electromagnetic radiation. However, we should not be alarmed or surprised by this. After all, it is not a new experience: in Section 4.5.4, we discussed the need for two models to explain the behaviour of matter. According to which particular aspects of behaviour we wish to explain, we may model electromagnetic radiation either as a continuous wave phenomenon (**wave theory**) or as a stream of individual packets of energy (**quantum theory**). We shall explore each model in turn, including the circumstances in which it is applied.

14.3   Wave theory of electromagnetic radiation

The electromagnetic disturbances created when charges accelerate can be visualised as continuous waves. What are the properties of these waves? A useful, and widely quoted, analogy is to imagine an object floating on perfectly calm water. When the object is moved, disturbances are produced in the water, which cause surface waves to be generated, carrying the disturbances outwards and away from the source (Fig. 14.1). Other objects floating nearby would experience these surface waves and be disturbed by them. We may infer that to produce this effect, the surface waves must be carrying energy. Electromagnetic waves also carry energy.

Notice that the water surface moves up and down. It does not flow in the direction of the wave even though we may sometimes gain such an impression, e.g. when observing waves breaking on a seashore.

14.3.1   *Graphical representation of waves*

The surface waves on water are illustrated in the form of graphs in Figs. 14.2 and 14.3. Figure 14.2 is a graph representing the contour of the water surface

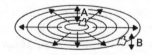

Fig. 14.1   Two bottles floating on still water. Disturbances to bottle A are passed on to bottle B by surface waves on the water; i.e. energy is transmitted from A to B.

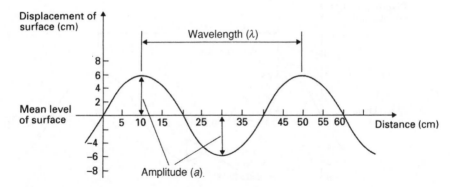

Fig. 14.2   A graph of displacement against distance for surface waves on water. The diagram represents a frozen moment in time, a sort of 'snapshot' of the contours of the water surface. In the example shown, the amplitude (*a*) of the wave is 6 cm and its wavelength (λ) is 40 cm.

'frozen' at an instant of time. The vertical axis shows the vertical displacement of the surface above and below its mean (undisturbed) level. The horizontal axis of the graph depicts distance measured in the direction of travel of the surface waves. Both axes are therefore scaled in units of distance. Three characteristic wave features can be identified on this graph:

- The **amplitude** (*a*) of the wave – the maximum amount by which the surface is raised above (or depressed below) its mean level
- The **wavelength** – the distance between corresponding points on two adjacent waves (The Greek letter lambda (λ) is normally used to represent wavelength.)
- The **general shape** of the wave – which is recognisable as a **sine wave** (see also Section 10.2.1.1)

Note that this graph gives no indication of how fast the wave is travelling across the surface of the water.

Figure 14.3 is a graph showing how the level of the water surface at one particular point varies with time as it oscillates up and down. As before, the vertical axis shows the *displacement* of the water surface above or below its mean level. However, the horizontal axis represents the passage of time. Unlike Fig. 14.2, therefore, the axes of this graph are scaled in *different* units because they represent quite different quantities (time and distance). The wave characteristics identified on this graph are:

- The **amplitude** (*a*) of the wave – the maximum amount by which the surface is raised above (or depressed below) its mean position
- The **period** (*T*) of the wave – the time taken for the surface to undergo one complete cycle of oscillation
- The **general shape** of the wave – again a **sine wave**

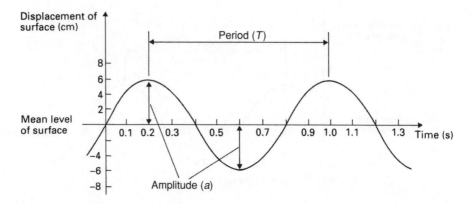

Fig. 14.3   A graph of displacement against time for surface waves on water. The graph shows how the level of one particular point on the water surface varies with the passage of time. The sinusoidal pattern indicates that the surface is undergoing repeating cycles of rising and falling. In the example shown, the wave amplitude (a) is 6 cm, while the period (T) of the wave is 0.8 s. The wave frequency (f) is $1/T = 1/0.8 = 1.25$ Hz (see Section 14.3.2.4). **N.B.** Although at first sight this graph appears very similar to Fig. 14.2, the two graphs provide different information about the wave motion because their horizontal axes are fundamentally different. In order to interpret wave diagrams correctly, we must always take care to check whether the horizontal axis of the graph represents distance or whether it represents time.

Again, we cannot tell from this graph alone how fast the surface wave was travelling, but as we shall see in Section 14.3.2.6, by combining information from both graphs it is possible to deduce the speed of the wave.

14.3.2   *Wave characteristics applied to electromagnetic radiation*

We have defined a number of wave characteristics as they relate to surface waves on water, but to apply them to electromagnetic waves we must first identify what is oscillating: in other words, what is represented by the vertical axes of the graphs when they are used to describe electromagnetic waves.

The quantity which varies with time is the electric (and magnetic) **field strength**. Figure 14.4 illustrates the magnitudes of these electric and magnetic fields frozen in time, at different points on a line drawn outwards from the source of the radiation. Notice that the electric and magnetic fields are perpendicular to each other. In fact, an oscillating electric field *always* generates a perpendicular oscillating magnetic field. Similarly, an oscillating magnetic field *always* produces a perpendicular oscillating electric field (by **electromagnetic induction** – see Section 9.1). It is the *combination* of these two mutually dependent oscillating fields which we call an electromagnetic wave.

Notice that as well as being mutually perpendicular, the oscillations of both fields are at right angles to the direction of travel of the electromagnetic wave. A wave motion whose oscillation is at right angles to its direction of travel is called a **transverse wave**. Electromagnetic waves are therefore transverse waves.

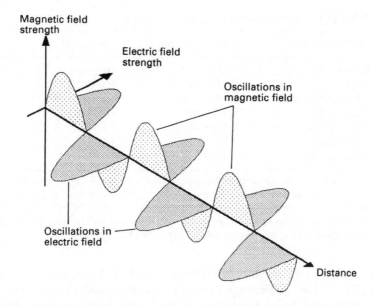

Fig. 14.4   A diagrammatic 'snapshot in time' of electromagnetic waves. The diagram is an attempt to show in three dimensions how the magnetic field strength and the electric field strength vary at different distances, measured along the direction of travel of the wave. As with Figs 14.2 and 14.3, a similar diagram could have been drawn to show how the field strengths at a fixed point vary with the passage of time. The distance axis would then be replaced by a time axis. Note that the decision to show the magnetic field as vertical is a purely arbitrary one; any direction could have been selected. However, whatever direction is chosen for the magnetic field, the electric field and the direction of travel are always mutually perpendicular to it.

14.3.2.1   Amplitude (*a*)

The amplitude of an electromagnetic wave at a particular point in space is the maximum electric (or magnetic) field strength experienced at that point. The amplitude of electromagnetic waves is important in determining the *energy flow* they represent. The controlled variation (or *modulation*) of the amplitude of electromagnetic waves can be used as a means of transmitting a message or **signal**. Radio wave communication using this technique is known as **amplitude modulation** (AM) transmission, but it is more susceptible to interference and signal corruption than the alternative technique known as **frequency modulation** (FM). For most types of electromagnetic radiations, however, we are far more likely to express energy flow in terms of the **intensity** than amplitude (see Section 14.3.3).

14.3.2.2   Wavelength (λ)

Wavelength is the distance between corresponding points on two successive waves. The wavelength of electromagnetic waves covers a tremendous range of values, from as little as 10^{-16} m (for high-energy gamma rays) to over 10^{4} m

Table 14.1 Types of electromagnetic radiations[a,b]

Type of radiation	Wavelength (m)	Period (s)	Frequency (Hz)
Gamma rays	10^{-16}–10^{-9}	10^{-24}–10^{-16}	10^{24}–10^{16}
X-rays	10^{-12}–10^{-7}	10^{-20}–10^{-16}	10^{20}–10^{16}
Ultraviolet rays	10^{-8}–10^{-6}	10^{-17}–10^{-15}	10^{17}–10^{15}
Visible light	10^{-6}–10^{-5}	10^{-15}–10^{-14}	10^{15}–10^{14}
Infrared rays	10^{-5}–10^{-3}	10^{-14}–10^{-11}	10^{14}–10^{11}
Microwaves	10^{-4}–10^{-2}	10^{-12}–10^{-10}	10^{12}–10^{10}
Radio waves	10^{-3}–10^{4}	10^{-11}–10^{-4}	10^{11}–10^{4}

[a] Radiations are listed in order of increasing wavelength and period, and decreasing frequency.
[b] Note the overlaps between the range of values quoted for radiations placed next to each other in the list; e.g. the range of wavelengths for gamma rays overlaps with that for X-rays. In such cases, the radiations are distinguished by the different processes which produce them. Note also that the figures quoted are approximate orders of magnitude only.

(for long-wave radio transmissions). Each different form of electromagnetic radiation has a *different* wavelength, as illustrated in Table 14.1. Visible-light wavelengths lie in the middle of the range, between about 400 and 700 nm ($1\,\text{nm} = 10^{-9}$ m).

14.3.2.3 Period (*T*)

The period (T) of an electromagnetic wave is the time taken for the electromagnetic field to undergo one complete cycle of oscillation. For electromagnetic radiation, the rate of oscillation is extremely rapid, giving a period whose value varies from about 10^{-24} s (for high-energy gamma rays) to 10^{-4} s (for long-wave radio). Each different form of electromagnetic radiation has a *different* period (Table 14.1).

14.3.2.4 Frequency (*f*)

The frequency (f) of an electromagnetic wave is the number of oscillations of the electromagnetic field per unit time. If we know the time occupied by *one* oscillation (i.e. the period T), we can determine how many oscillations occur in one unit of time (i.e. the frequency f). In fact, the frequency of a wave is given by:

$$f = \frac{1}{T}$$

T has very low values for electromagnetic waves, so the frequency must be very great, varying from about 10^4 Hz (for long-wave radio) to 10^{24} Hz (for high-energy gamma rays). Again, each different form of electromagnetic radiation has a *different* frequency (Table 14.1).

14.3.2.5 Speed (*c*)

All electromagnetic radiations travel at the same speed (c) in a vacuum. The value of c, commonly known as the **speed of light**, is $299\,792\,458\ \text{m s}^{-1}$, usually quoted

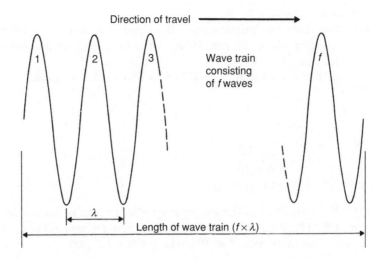

Fig. 14.5   The relationship between wavelength (λ), wave frequency (f) and wave speed (c). Suppose a continuous electromagnetic wave system is passing from left to right. If the frequency of the wave system is f, then f waves must (by definition) be passing a given fixed point in unit time (e.g. 1 s). The diagram shows a wave train containing f consecutive waves selected from the continuous wave system. This wave train will therefore take unit time to pass by. Because its total length is $f \times \lambda$, it must be travelling a distance $f\lambda$ in unit time. However, as we saw in Section 1.2, distance travelled per unit time is speed (c). Therefore, $c = f\lambda$. This fundamental relationship is true not only for electromagnetic waves but for *all* regular wave systems.

as 3×10^8 m s^{-1} (about 186 000 miles per second). For most purposes, the travel time of electromagnetic waves on earth is so small as to seem instantaneous. Only when very large distances are involved does the delay due to the travel time of electromagnetic waves become noticeable. For example, when conducting an interview via a communications satellite link, a television presenter may find the delay (about 0.5 s) long enough to disrupt the flow of conversation. Astronauts and astronomers have to contend with much longer delay times.

14.3.2.6   Relationship between speed, wavelength and frequency (Fig. 14.5)

If f is the frequency of a wave, f waves will pass a given point in unit time. If each wave has a length λ, the total length of f waves will be $f \times \lambda$. It follows that a collection of waves (a **wave train**) of total length $f\lambda$ will pass the given point in unit time. The speed of the waves (c) must therefore be given by:

$$c = f\lambda$$

This relationship holds for *all* forms of wave motion, including electromagnetic waves, surface waves on water and sound waves (Section 22.1.4), but for electromagnetic waves the value of c is constant, so the relationship is of special significance. It means that if we know the wavelength of electromagnetic radiation, we can always work out its frequency, and if we know its frequency, we can always work out its wavelength.

Worked examples

(1) The infrared emission from the solid-state laser in a laser imager has a wavelength of 850 nm. What is the frequency of this emission? ($c = 3 \times 10^8$ m s^{-1})

The wavelength, $\lambda = 850$ nm $= 850 \times 10^{-9}$ m. Using

$$c = f\lambda$$
$$f = \frac{c}{\lambda}$$
$$= \frac{3 \times 10^8}{850 \times 10^{-9}}$$
$$= 3.5 \times 10^{14} \text{ Hz}$$

(2) The frequency of the long-wave radio transmissions of BBC Radio 4 UK is 198 kHz. What is the wavelength of these radio signals? ($c = 3 \times 10^8$ m s^{-1})

The frequency, $f = 198$ kHz $= 198 \times 10^3$ Hz.

Using

$$c = f\lambda$$
$$\lambda = \frac{c}{f}$$
$$= \frac{3 \times 10^8}{198 \times 10^3}$$
$$= 1510 \text{ m}$$

The wavelength is just over 1.5 km.

14.3.3   Radiation intensity

As we have seen, electromagnetic waves convey energy. It is often important to quantify this energy flow or **energy flux**, e.g. when investigating the biological effects of exposure to ionising radiation. The concept known as **intensity** is one way of quantifying energy flux. The intensity of an electromagnetic wave system is the rate of energy flow through unit area, measured at right angles to the direction in which the waves are travelling.

Figure 14.6 illustrates this concept. It shows a parallel beam of electromagnetic waves falling on an imaginary flat surface placed perpendicular to the direction of the radiation. The radiation is said to be **normal** to the surface, where the term *normal* means 'at right angles to'. The intensity of the radiation is numerically equal to the quantity of energy falling in unit time through a 'window' of unit area in the surface.

Suppose the rate of energy flow through an area A is dE/dt (literally, the rate of change of energy with time). Then the intensity of the beam (I) is given by:

$$I = \frac{1}{A} \times \frac{dE}{dt}$$

In SI units, A is measured in square metres (m^2) and dE/dt in joules per second (J s^{-1}) or watts (W), so the SI unit of intensity is the watt per square metre (W m^{-2}).

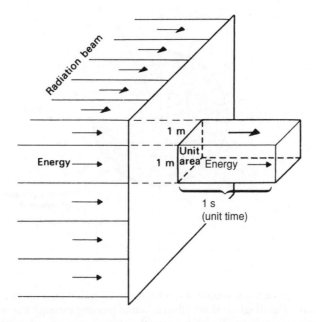

Fig. 14.6   A diagram illustrating the concept of radiation intensity. The intensity of a beam of radiation is the amount of energy flowing per unit time per unit area measured at right angles to the direction of the beam. In SI units, intensity is expressed in watts per square metre (W m^{-2}).

The concept of intensity can be applied to *other* types of energy flow, as well as to electromagnetic waves; e.g. in diagnostic imaging, it is used to express the energy flux of **ultrasound** beams. Table 14.2 gives typical values of intensity for a variety of different applications.

Table 14.2   Typical examples of energy flux intensity for a variety of different applications

Application	Intensity (W m^{-2})
Light from a neodymium glass laser (1)	10^{16}
Total electromagnetic radiation arriving at the earth's surface from the sun (2)	1000
Total electromagnetic radiation arriving from a 100-W lamp at a distance of 1 m	8
Radio waves detected by a domestic satellite TV dish (3)	4×10^{-12}
Dimmest light detectable by the human eye (4)	10^{-14}
Radio waves arriving on earth from distant galaxies (5)	10^{-15}
Diagnostic ultrasound beam (6)	1000
Sound from an exploding firework 100 m away (1)	2
Quietest sound detectable by the human ear (7)	10^{-13}

Sources: (1) Cutnell & Johnson (2007); (2) Halliday et al. (2001); (3) Wilson (1993); (4) Microsoft (2005); (5) Kraus & Marhefka (2002); (6) Blackwell (1988); (7) Sternheim & Kane (1991).

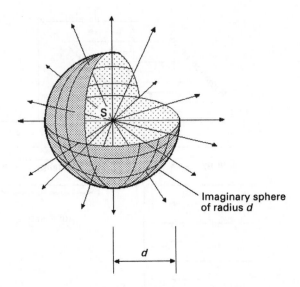

Fig. 14.7   S is a point source of electromagnetic radiation, emitting equally in all directions. The diagram shows the radiation passing through the surface of an imaginary sphere of radius d. Because the surface area of such a sphere is $4\pi d^2$, we can deduce that the intensity of radiation conforms to an inverse square relationship (see Section 14.3.5). Note that part of the sphere has been cut away to reveal the source more clearly.

14.3.4   Rectilinear propagation of radiation

Electromagnetic waves travel in straight lines; i.e. they exhibit rectilinear propagation. They may deviate when passing through a junction between one medium and another; e.g. light is bent (refracted) on passing from air to glass, as in an optical lens. Refraction is *not* apparent with X- and gamma rays, and for most practical purposes we may assume that these radiations travel in straight lines without deviation.

Because electromagnetic waves travel in straight lines, it follows that if they are generated from a point source (S in Fig. 14.7) they will diverge, causing a reduction in the intensity of the radiation as the distance from the source is increased. In other words, as we move further from a source of radiation, its effects become weaker. The precise way in which this reduction in intensity occurs is defined in the inverse square law, which we first described in Section 3.3.2 in relation to electric field strength. The inverse square law follows directly from the fact that radiation travels in straight lines.

14.3.5   Inverse square law for radiation

If we assume that a point source S is radiating its energy equally in all directions at a constant rate dE/dt, we can determine the intensity of the radiation at any distance from the source. At a distance d from the source, the radiation will be spread over the inner surface of an imaginary sphere of radius d (Fig. 14.7). The surface area of such a sphere is $A = 4\pi d^2$. However, in Section 14.3.3, we showed that radiation intensity (I) is given by:

$$I = \frac{1}{A}\frac{dE}{dt}$$

so

$$I = \frac{1}{4\pi d^2}\frac{dE}{dt}$$

Of the terms on the right-hand side of this equation, only the distance d is a variable. (The term 4π is constant, and we defined dE/dt as being a constant rate of production of energy.) We can therefore conclude that:

$$I \propto \frac{I}{d^2}$$

In other words, *the intensity of electromagnetic radiation is inversely proportional to the square of the distance from its source*. This is a clear statement of an **inverse square law** linking radiation intensity with distance. However, in order to arrive at this conclusion, we made a number of assumptions (either explicitly or by implication) which do not always reflect reality.

14.3.5.1 Conditions demanded by the inverse square law

- *The source of radiation is a point source*. The term **point source** means that the source is infinitely small. Even if it were desirable, we can never achieve a point source in practice. However, as long as the dimensions of the source are very small compared with the distance (d) at which we are considering intensity, the inverse square law provides a close approximation to the truth. For example, the effective size of the X-ray source in a diagnostic X-ray tube is about 1 mm square. This is about one-thousandth of the distance of the X-ray film from the source, and therefore approximates to a point source for the purposes of intensity calculations (but see Section 12.1 for image unsharpness considerations).
- *The radiation travels in straight lines*. This is a correct assumption if the radiation travels only through a vacuum, but if the radiation interacts with any obstacle in its path, its direction may be modified, e.g. due to **reflection**, **refraction**, **diffraction** or **scattering**. The precise natures of the radiation and of the obstacle determine which, if any, of these processes is of practical significance (see Section 17.2.5).
- *The radiation is emitted equally in all directions*. This is certainly *not* true of the output from an X-ray tube! However, if the energy distribution is uniform *over the area being investigated* (e.g. the 24 cm × 30 cm area of an exposed film) then intensity calculations may still be valid.
- *The energy is radiated at a constant rate*. In some instances, this may well be true. In other cases it is not, e.g. the output from an X-ray tube supplied by a single-phase, two-pulse, high-tension generator is far from being constant (Section 13.2.1). However, the *average* X-ray output over a number of wave cycles is likely to be constant and the *mean* intensity of radiation may obey the inverse square law.

- *No radiation energy is lost on its way from the source to the point of measurement.* It was assumed implicitly that in Fig. 14.7 *all* the energy leaving the source arrived at the inner surface of the sphere. In other words, nothing impeded the radiation. If the radiation passed only through a vacuum, this assumption would be correct. In practice, this is rarely the case. For example, a diagnostic X-ray beam must pass through various **filters** (see Section 17.3.2) as it leaves an X-ray tube, and it passes through the patient's tissues before it reaches the film. The radiation interacts with such obstacles, imparting energy to them. Consequently, radiation intensity reduces with distance not only because of its divergent nature (from which the inverse-square-law relationship was derived), but because its energy has been depleted through interactions with matter.

14.3.5.2   The inverse square law in practice

The conclusion we must draw from the above discussion is that discretion must be used in applying the inverse square law to practical problems. Before the inverse square law can be applied with any confidence, each of the assumptions implicit in the law must be considered in the light of the conditions ruling at the time. We must ask ourselves four questions:

- Is the distance very much greater than the size of the radiation source?
- Does the radiation have an unimpeded path to follow?
- Is the beam of radiation uniformly distributed over the area we are considering?
- Is the radiation being emitted at a steady rate?

Only if we can answer *yes* to each question should we expect inverse-square-law calculations to produce accurate predictions.

Worked example
It is recommended that to prevent film fogging, a darkroom safelight containing a 25-W lamp should be placed no closer than 1.2 m to the bench worktop (Ball & Price, 1995). Use the inverse square law to estimate a suitable lamp wattage if the safelight has to be positioned only 1 m above the worktop. Assume that light output is proportional to lamp wattage.

We assume that to avoid film fogging, the intensity (I) of the light falling on the worktop must be maintained at the same level (or less) after repositioning the safelight. Because

$$I \propto \frac{1}{d^2}$$

$$I = \frac{1}{d^2} \times k$$

 where k is a constant of proportionality. Initially, the intensity (I_1) of light on the worktop provided by the 25-W lamp is:

$$I_1 = \frac{1}{d_1^2} \times k$$

where d_1 is the initial height of the lamp above the worktop. Therefore:

$$I_1 = \frac{k}{1.2^2}$$
$$= 0.69 \times k$$

After repositioning the safelight, the intensity (I_2) of light on the worktop provided by the same 25-W lamp would be:

$$I_2 = \frac{1}{d_2^2} \times k$$

where d_2 is the *new* height of the lamp above the worktop. Hence:

$$I_2 = \frac{k}{1^2}$$
$$= 1 \times k$$

So, the intensity would increase by the ratio 1:0.69 if we continued to use a 25-W lamp. We therefore need a lamp which is 0.69 times the previous wattage to bring the intensity of light on the worktop back to its former level:

$$0.69 \times 25 = 17.25 \text{ W}$$

Of course, we cannot *actually* purchase a 17.25-W lamp, but common sense tells us that a 15-W lamp would suffice because it is close to the required wattage, and being slightly less powerful, we can be sure it would not fog any of our films.

Note: It is very doubtful whether the conditions described in this problem approximate to those demanded by the inverse square law. For example, the size of an actual safelight source is *not* negligible compared with its distance above the worktop because a typical safelight has an emitting area whose side length is only about one-quarter to one-fifth of this distance.

14.4   Radiation – continuous or grainy?

In Section 14.3 we compared electromagnetic waves with surface waves on water. Let us now consider this analogy further.

When examined from a distance the surface waves on water appear perfectly continuous. However, we understand from our knowledge of the structure of matter that in fact water is a 'grainy' substance because it consists of vast numbers of individual molecules. If we were able to examine the water surface closely enough, we would be able to distinguish the individual particles from which it is formed and we would see that the surface is *not* continuous.

Of course, if our interest is in the effects of surface waves on structures similar in size to the waves, the particulate nature of water is largely irrelevant, but if our interest is on a microscopic or molecular level, then the movements of the individual molecules of water become paramount. In other words, our choice of explanation depends on the nature of the interactions we are investigating. Each explanation is valid as long as it is applied in the appropriate circumstances.

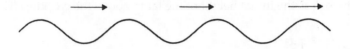

Fig. 14.8   Radiation as a continuous wave.

There are many examples of this 'smooth-versus-grainy' approach to understanding. For instance, it can be applied to the image on a radiograph. Examined at normal viewing distance, the radiographic image demonstrates varying shades of grey, representing the different body tissues. Examined with a powerful magnifying lens, the image is seen to consist of large numbers of individual black particles (of silver) and the anatomical significance of the image is lost: we cannot see the wood for the trees.

Electromagnetic radiation may also be considered as being both *smooth* (i.e. wave-like) and *grainy* (i.e. particle-like). Electromagnetic radiation has a **dual nature**.

14.5   Quantum theory of electromagnetic radiation

Until now we have concentrated on the smooth, continuous, wave nature of radiation (Fig. 14.8). For many purposes this is an entirely adequate explanation. However, when we wish to examine how radiation interacts at an atomic or even subatomic level, as we shall in the case of X- and gamma rays, the wave theory is inappropriate and we need to consider the *grainy* nature of the radiation.

14.5.1   *Quanta*

In the 1890s, the scientist Max Planck proposed that energy can only be transferred in discrete amounts known as **quanta**. (*Quanta* is the plural form of the word *quantum*.) Planck's hypothesis was later confirmed experimentally. Quanta are to energy what elementary particles such as protons and electrons are to matter, but they represent amounts of *energy* which cannot be further subdivided. One quantum may represent a different amount of energy from another, but each individual quantum is a discrete entity which cannot be split into smaller parts.

The study of the nature and consequences of this **quantisation** of energy forms the basis of the **quantum theory**, which has had a fundamental effect on the way we perceive electromagnetic radiation and on physical science generally.

Quantum theory has a reputation for being totally incomprehensible and obscure. Certainly, some of the associated mathematics can be intimidating, but in essence, there is no mystery about the underlying concept of quantisation and it has many parallels outside the realm of physics. For example, an everyday action such as handling money in the form of loose cash is quantised. It is possible to transfer cash only in amounts which are multiples or combinations of the available currency notes and coinage. For example, UK coinage comprises tokens, representing the values 1 p (i.e. one penny), 2 p, 5 p, 10 p, 20 p, 50 p

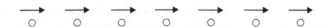

Fig. 14.9 Radiation as a stream of photons.

and £1 (100 p). These are the quanta of British coinage. Notice that like energy quanta, although coins represent a range of different money values, individually they cannot be divided into smaller amounts: cutting a 10 p coin in half does not produce two 5 p coins! When major organisations are dealing with large-scale financial transactions, running perhaps into millions of pounds, the quantisation of the money system seems irrelevant. It is only when dealing with much smaller amounts that the quantum nature of money becomes significant. This, too, has close parallels with the quantisation of energy, as we saw in Section 14.4.

14.5.2 Photons

Quantum theory tells us that when energy is transferred by electromagnetic radiation, it cannot be transferred in the continuous fashion which wave theory implies. Instead, we conceive each individual quantum of energy being carried by a 'particle' of radiation known as a **photon**. Electromagnetic radiation can therefore be visualised as a stream of photons travelling at the speed of light (Fig. 14.9).

Photons have no mass or electric charge, but consist only of pure energy. They have some of the properties of particles (e.g. they may rebound or be scattered if they collide with particles such as electrons). Photons are indivisible; they cannot be split into smaller units.

14.5.3 Photon energy and Planck's law

We saw in the previous section that photons of electromagnetic radiation carry energy. However, we gave no indication of the *amount* of energy involved, except perhaps to imply that it was small rather than large. Max Planck considered this problem when he proposed the quantum nature of radiation. He deduced that the energy of a photon (known as **photon energy**, E) depends only on the frequency (f) of the electromagnetic waves associated with it. He defined a simple mathematical relationship between these two quantities:

$$E \propto f$$

and

$$E = hf$$

where h is a constant of proportionality. Further work by Einstein and others confirmed Planck's ideas. The relationship $E = hf$ is now known as **Planck's law**, while the constant h, known as **Planck's constant**, has the value 6.626×10^{-34} J s (joule seconds).

Planck's law provides a welcome link between the *wave nature* of electromagnetic radiation (characterised by its frequency) and the *particle nature* of electromagnetic radiation (characterised by its photons). If we know the wave characteristics of a particular form of electromagnetic radiation, then we can predict the energy of its photons. Conversely, if we know the photon energy of the radiation, we can predict its wave characteristics. Let us illustrate this by working through three examples.

Worked examples

(1) Calculate the photon energy of 100-MHz radio waves used for FM radio transmission. Assume Planck's constant $h = 6.6 \times 10^{-34}$ J s.

Because we have values for Planck's constant and frequency ($f = 100$ MHz $= 100 \times 10^6$ Hz), we can apply Planck's law directly:

$$E = hf$$
$$= 6.6 \times 10^{-34} \times 100 \times 10^6$$
$$= 6.6 \times 10^{26} \text{ J}$$

Thus, each photon of the 100-MHz radio waves carries only 6.6×10^{-26} J of energy. Note that because the energy of a photon is *always* a very small fraction of a joule, it is usual to express photon energy in **electronvolts** (eV) rather than joules (1 eV $= 1.6 \times 10^{-9}$ J). The energy of the radio waves then becomes 4.1×10^{-7} eV, which is still a very small figure.

(2) Gamma rays emitted by a source used in radionuclide imaging have a photon energy of 140 keV. What is the wavelength of this particular gamma radiation? Assume that $h = 6.6 \times 10^{-34}$ J s and $c = 3.0 \times 10^8$ m s^{-1}.

The value of photon energy (E) must first be converted into joules; i.e.

$$E = 140 \text{ keV} = 140 \times 10^3 \text{ eV}$$
$$= 140 \times 10^3 \times 1.6 \times 10^{-19} \text{ J}$$
$$= 2.24 \times 10^{-14} \text{ J}$$

This problem is further complicated by the fact that we wish to find the wavelength (λ) rather than the frequency (f) of the gamma rays. However, we know from the relationship $c = f\lambda$, discussed in Section 14.3.2.6, that $f = c/\lambda$, so Planck's law can be expressed in the alternative form:

$$E = h\frac{c}{\lambda}$$

from which

$$\lambda = \frac{hc}{E}$$
$$= \frac{6.6 \times 10^{-34} \times 3.0 \times 10^8}{2.24 \times 10^{-14}}$$
$$= 8.8 \times 10^{-12} \text{ m}$$

The wavelength of 140-keV gamma rays is 8.8×10^{-12} m (8.8×10^{-3} nm), which (reassuringly) falls neatly within the range of gamma-ray wavelengths quoted in Table 14.1.

(3) Visible-light wavelength extends from about 400 nm (blue-violet) to 700 nm (red). Compare the energies carried by photons of blue-violet and red light. Assume $h = 6.6 \times 10^{-34}$ J s and $c = 3.0 \times 10^8$ m s^{-1}.

Because we are not given the frequencies of blue-violet and red light, we must again use Planck's law expressed in the form:

$$E = h\frac{c}{\lambda}$$

Then for blue-violet light, where $\lambda = 400$ nm $= 400 \times 10^{-9}$ m:

$$E = \frac{6.6 \times 10^{-34} \times 3.0 \times 10^8}{400 \times 10^{-9}}$$
$$= 4.9 \times 10^{-19} \text{ J} \quad \text{(or 3 eV)}$$

while for red light, where $\lambda = 700$ nm $= 700 \times 10^{-9}$ m:

$$E = \frac{6.6 \times 10^{-34} \times 3.0 \times 10^8}{700 \times 10^{-9}}$$
$$= 2.8 \times 10^{-19} \text{ J} \quad \text{(or 1.7 eV)}$$

Hence, a red-light photon carries appreciably *less* energy than a blue-violet-light photon.

14.5.4   *Radiation quanta and the photoelectric effect*

The photon energy difference between red light and blue-violet light demonstrated above had consequences which were crucial to the early development of quantum theory. In the 1890s, it was discovered that when certain metals are exposed to light, electrons are released from the surface of the metal, a phenomenon known as the **photoelectric effect** (see also Section 15.4.1). However, there were problems in using the wave theory of radiation to explain some aspects of the photoelectric effect. For example, while exposure of a certain metal to blue-violet light produces a photoelectric effect, exposure of the same material to *red* light does not, no matter how intense the light source. This result could not be explained by wave theory. Einstein showed later that it is not the *cumulative* effect of radiation energy on the electrons which causes the photoelectric effect, but the interaction between individual electrons and single 'particles' (i.e. photons) of light. A photon of blue-violet light has sufficient energy to release an electron, whereas a photon of red light does not. This provided confirmation of the quantum nature of electromagnetic radiation.

14.6   Electromagnetic spectrum

Electromagnetic radiation can be produced by various means, resulting in different values of frequency, wavelength and photon energy. Radiations also differ in the methods required to detect them. The complete range of electromagnetic radiations set out in order of frequency, wavelength or photon energy is called the **electromagnetic spectrum** and is illustrated in Table 14.3. Radio waves are at one end of the spectrum, having low photon energy, while at the other end gamma rays are very energetic. Visible-light rays have medium photon energy, while X-rays lie towards the high-energy end of the spectrum. Table 14.3 also

Table 14.3   The electromagnetic spectrum[a–c]

Type of radiation	Photon energy (eV)	Method of Production	Method of detection
Gamma rays	10^9–10	Radioactive decay	Scintillation in gamma camera, ionisation chamber, photographic film
X-rays	10^5–10	Electron interactions in target of X-ray tube	Ionisation chamber, photographic film, fluorescence
Ultraviolet rays	100–3	Electron transitions in carbon arc or mercury vapour lamp	Fluorescence, photographic film, photoelectric cell
Visible light		Fluorescence, incandescence, lasers	Photographic film, the eye, photomultiplier tube
Blue-violet	3		
Green	2.2		
Red	1.7		
Infrared rays	1.7–10^{-4}	Atomic transitions, molecular vibrations	Infrared film, thermopile, sensation of heat
Microwaves	10^{-3}–10^{-5}	Klystrons, magnetrons	Heating effect, crystal detectors
Radio waves	10^{-4}–10^{-11}	Oscillating electric currents in conductor	Tuned circuit in radio receiver

[a] Radiations are listed in order of decreasing photon energy (expressed in eV).
[b] Apart from visible light, only approximate photon energy values are given.
[c] The table provides some examples of how each type of radiation is produced and how it is detected. The processes which are most relevant to diagnostic imaging will be covered in later sections of the book.

indicates how the various forms of electromagnetic radiations are produced and how they may be detected.

14.7   Spectral emission curves

The electromagnetic radiation emitted from a source often comprises streams of photons carrying different amounts of energy. In wave theory terms, the radiation would be said to consist of a collection of electromagnetic waves having different wavelengths and frequencies. For example, a beam of white light contains photons with energies ranging from 1.7 to 3 eV (and wavelengths from 400 to 700 nm). It is useful, in such cases, to be able to investigate the composition of the beam of radiation by studying the contribution made to the beam as a whole by the different photon energies (or different wavelengths) present. When a radiation beam is investigated, the results are often presented in the form of a **spectral emission curve** (or **spectrum**), which is a graph of the intensity of radiation plotted either against wavelength or against photon energy.

This approach is similar to one that might be used to explore the distribution of intelligence in a group of students. A spread of intelligence quotient (IQ) values would be encountered, and the frequency with which each different IQ occurs could be found. A frequency diagram or distribution curve would be a good way of summarising the IQ spectrum. Figure 14.10 shows the sort of result that might be expected.

14.7.1   Relative intensity

On spectral emission curves it is usual to plot intensity as a relative rather than an absolute value. The maximum or peak intensity is assigned the value of 1 (or 100%), and all other intensities are quoted relative to this. Relative intensity has no units, because it is merely a number representing the ratio between two similar quantities. As we saw in Section 14.3.3, absolute intensity is expressed in watts per square metre ($W\ m^{-2}$).

14.7.2   Wavelength spectrum

Figure 14.11 shows the **wavelength spectrum** of the visible and infrared radiation emitted from a heated solid, such as the filament of an electric light bulb. The distribution of wavelengths follows a characteristic pattern with a central peak of intensity, but with intensity tailing off each side of the peak. The position of the central peak indicates the wavelength of the most predominant waves (in this case at 2000 nm), but the beam also contains wavelengths above and below this value. As we move further from the dominant wavelength, the intensity falls, indicating that fewer of these particular waves are present. Notice that the intensity falls to zero at a wavelength of about 550 nm. Such a well-defined **minimum wavelength** is a feature of many beams of electromagnetic radiation, including X-ray beams (see Section 16.1.2.3).

Statisticians might describe the wavelength spectrum in Fig. 14.11 as reminiscent of a **normal distribution**. (The distribution of IQ illustrated in Fig. 14.10 is a normal distribution.) A true normal distribution curve is *symmetrical* about the central peak, but spectral emission curves for beams of radiation are rarely symmetrical.

14.7.3   Photon energy spectrum

Figure 14.12 shows the same radiation beam as in Fig. 14.11, but this time a **photon energy spectrum** is illustrated. It has broadly the same shape as before, with a central peak. This indicates the photon energy of the most plentiful photons (in this case 0.6 eV), but the beam also contains photons with energies above and below this value. The further we move from the predominant photon energy, the fewer the number of photons present. Notice how one aspect of the asymmetry present in Fig. 14.11 has been reversed in Fig. 14.12. The well-defined **minimum wavelength** (550 nm) on the wavelength spectrum has been replaced by a well-defined **maximum energy** (about 2.2 eV) on the photon energy spectrum. This is because the short-wavelength parts of a wavelength spectrum correspond to the high-photon-energy parts of a photon energy spectrum. (From Planck's

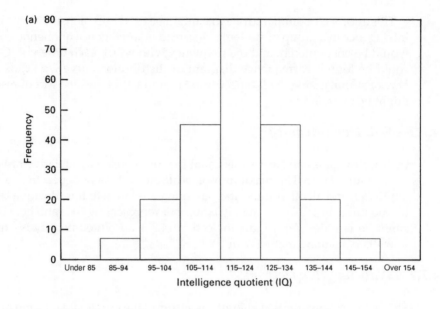

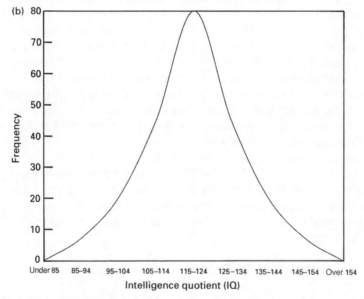

Fig. 14.10 The bar chart (a) is a frequency diagram showing the distribution of intelligence quotient (IQ) in an imaginary group of 224 students. The frequency axis represents the number of students whose IQs lie within each band. The central peak shows that more students have IQs in the 115–124 band than in any other. Seven students have IQs over 144, which would probably qualify them to become members of Mensa! (b) The same distribution pattern is shown as a smooth curve. Its overall shape, which is typical of a normal distribution, bears some resemblance to the shape of the spectral emission curve shown in Fig. 14.11.

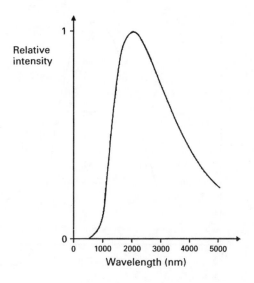

Fig. 14.11 The wavelength spectrum of the radiation emitted by a solid heated to a temperature of 1400 K. Although most of the energy is radiated in the infrared part of the spectrum, a small amount of visible light is also emitted at wavelengths between about 550 nm (green light) and 700 nm (red light). The solid is therefore almost 'white hot'.

law, short-wavelength, high-frequency radiation has a *high* photon energy, while long-wavelength, low-frequency radiation has a *low* photon energy.)

The vast range of photon energy values sometimes present in a radiation beam may be difficult to accommodate satisfactorily on the horizontal axis of

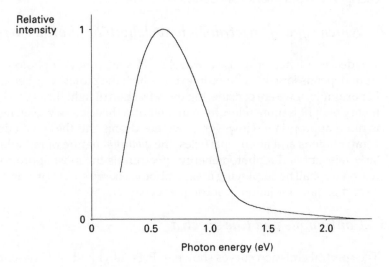

Fig. 14.12 The photon energy spectrum of radiation emitted by a solid at 1400 K. A small amount of visible light is radiated (with photon energies between about 1.7 and 2.2 eV).

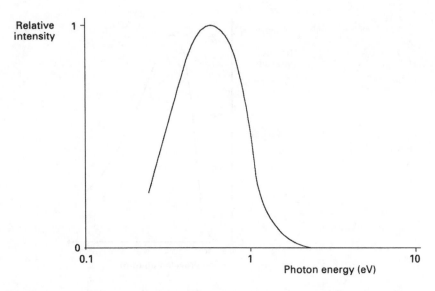

Fig. 14.13 The same photon energy spectrum as shown in Fig. 14.12, but with a logarithmic scale of photon energy. Notice how the high-energy end of the scale has been compressed. Note also that we have chosen to commence the energy scale at 0.1 eV. (It not possible to show zero on a logarithmic scale.)

the spectral emission curve. To overcome this problem, the linear scale may be replaced by a *logarithmic* scale. This has the effect of expanding the lower end of the photon energy range while compressing the upper end. The use of a logarithmic scale modifies the shape of the curve, and care must be taken when interpreting such graphs. Figure 14.13 shows a logarithmic version of the photon energy spectrum previously described in Fig. 14.12.

14.7.4   *Which type of spectrum – wavelength or photon energy?*

The decision whether to use a wavelength spectrum or a photon energy spectrum depends largely on the context in which the radiation is being considered. For example, if we are considering the refraction of light through a lens, the *wave* theory of light is more relevant than quantum theory, so a wavelength spectrum is more appropriate. However, if we are discussing the interactions between X-ray photons and atomic particles, the *quantum* nature of radiation is particularly relevant and a photon energy spectrum is the most appropriate. For this reason we shall be employing mainly photon energy spectra in our discussions of X- and gamma radiation in subsequent chapters.

14.7.5   *Continuous and line spectra*

The spectral emission curves shown in Figs. 14.11 and 14.12 describe a beam of radiation in which many different photon energies are present with no discontinuities such as gaps or sudden peaks. The graph is a smooth curve and is known as a **continuous spectrum**. In some circumstances it is possible to produce a beam

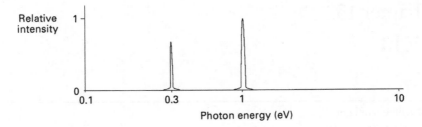

Fig. 14.14   A characteristic (line) spectrum of electromagnetic radiation plotted on a logarithmic scale of photon energy. In this example, the radiation consists of photons having only two specific energy levels (1 eV and about 0.3 eV), both lying in the infrared part of the spectrum.

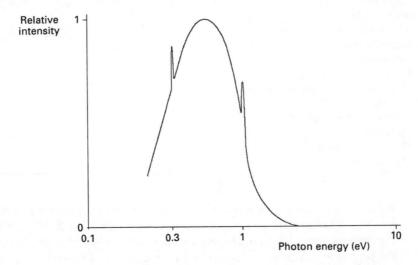

Fig. 14.15   A combined characteristic and continuous spectrum. The radiation whose characteristic spectrum was shown in Fig. 14.14 has been combined with the radiation whose continuous spectrum was shown in Fig. 14.13. Notice how the radiation intensity at 1.0 and 0.3 eV has been increased due to the contribution made by the characteristic radiation. This type of spectrum indicates the presence of two different radiation-producing processes.

containing only a few specific photon energies. The spectral emission curve for this type of beam is shown in Fig. 14.14 and is known as a **line spectrum** or **characteristic spectrum**. Line spectra may also be drawn as wavelength rather than energy graphs. Continuous and line spectra are produced by different processes. In some cases we may get both types of spectra superimposed (Fig. 14.15) because more than one process may be involved in producing the radiation.

Chapter 15
Light

Brightness of light
   Luminous intensity
   Luminous flux
   Intensity
   Illuminance
   Luminance
   Brightness
Colour of light
Production of light
   Incandescence
   Luminescence
   Lasers
   Photon-stimulated luminescence
Photoelectric effect
   External photoelectric effect
   Photoconduction
   Photovoltaic effect
   Photoionisation

Before describing the properties of X- and gamma radiation we shall spend a short time investigating some of the properties of visible light with which we are perhaps more familiar. Hopefully, we will then find it easier to understand the processes which are involved in the production of X-rays.

15.1 Brightness of light

There are a number of terms used to describe the brightness of light. We shall refer to those which may be encountered in the diagnostic imaging sciences. The first two terms relate to measures of the output of a light source.

15.1.1 Luminous intensity

The **luminous intensity** of a light source is a measure of its brightness. Historically, the luminous intensity of a source was measured by comparing it with the light output of a standard candle which (by definition) was said to have an intensity of 1 candle-power. The SI equivalent of the candle-power is the **candela** (cd). Because of difficulties in producing a standard candle of consistent output, the candela is defined by reference to a different source (the light output of a black-body radiator at specified temperature). Nevertheless, a light source whose luminous intensity is 1 cd has roughly the same brightness as that of a candle.

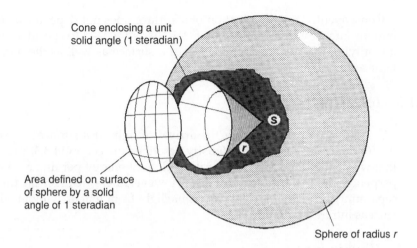

Cone enclosing a unit
solid angle (1 steradian)

Area defined on surface
of sphere by a solid
angle of 1 steradian

Sphere of radius *r*

Fig. 15.1 The concept of a solid angle. The diagram shows a cone, whose apex is at the centre (S) of an imaginary sphere of radius r. The apex of the cone encloses a solid (i.e. three-dimensional) angle, just as the apex of a triangle encloses a plane (i.e. two-dimensional) angle. The solid angle defines an area A on the surface of the sphere. If $A = r^2$, the solid angle is 1 steradian(sr). Because the total surface area of a sphere is $4\pi r^2$, the solid angle enclosed by a complete sphere is 4π sr. (Compare this with two-dimensional geometry, in which a complete circle subtends an angle of 2π radians.) If a 1-cd light source is placed at S, then 1 lm of luminous energy flux will emerge from the cone.

15.1.2 *Luminous flux*

The output of a light source can also be expressed in terms of its **luminous flux**, which is the rate at which it emits visible-light energy over a given solid (i.e. three-dimensional) angle. The SI unit of luminous flux is the **lumen** (lm). One lumen is defined as the flux emitted in a unit solid angle (1 steradian) from a 1-candela point source (see Fig. 15.1); i.e.

1 candela = 1 lumen per steradian

or

$$1 \text{ cd} = 1 \text{ lm sr}^{-1}$$

A 100-W tungsten-filament electric light bulb produces a light output of about 1200 lm, while a 100-W fluorescent tube produces about 5000 lm (Horder, 1971). This shows that fluorescent tubes generate light more efficiently than conventional light bulbs.

As light energy travels outwards from a source it usually loses intensity because it:

- diverges or spreads out (see Section 14.3.5) and/or
- becomes attenuated (weakened) by absorption in the medium through which it is passing.

Consequently, the illumination of a surface does not depend *only* on the luminous intensity of the light source. We therefore need to consider methods of quantifying the level of illumination of a surface as well as the output of the light source.

15.1.3   Intensity

We could attempt to quantify the arrival of light at a surface by referring to the fundamental concept of **intensity** described in Section 14.3.3. You will recall that we defined intensity as the rate of flow of energy per unit area measured perpendicular to the direction of flow. However, there are practical difficulties in separating the energy arriving as visible light from that arriving in other forms such as infrared radiation.

15.1.4   Illuminance

More probably, we would quote the **illuminance**, which is the level of illumination expressed in lumens per square metre ($lm\,m^{-2}$) or in **lux** (lx), where $1\,lx = 1\,lm\,m^{-2}$. This is the method preferred by architects and lighting engineers to specify suitable lighting levels for different activities. For example, a desktop lighting level of 500 lx may be perfectly adequate for the work undertaken in a radiology manager's office, but on a workbench where hand assembly of miniature electronic circuitry is being undertaken, an illuminance of 2000 lx or higher would be desirable (Oborne, 1995).

15.1.5   Luminance

Although a particular level of light might fall on a surface, its *apparent* brightness may vary because different types of surfaces reflect different amounts and different qualities of light according to their physical nature. For example, a white surface appears brighter than a black surface because it reflects more light. We can specify the amount of light arising or being reflected from a surface by quoting the **luminance**. Luminance is a measure of the light emitted per unit area from a surface (Workman & Cowen, 1994). The SI unit of luminance is the candela per square metre ($cd\,m^{-2}$).

15.1.6   Brightness

Brightness is how we describe our *subjective* impression of the luminance of a surface or a light source. For example, we might judge the luminance of a surface by combining an assessment of the intensity of light received from it, with a knowledge of other factors (such as distance) which influence the intensity of the light received. Generally, we perceive different intensities of light as different brightnesses; e.g. light which is of high intensity appears brighter than light of low intensity. However, external influences complicate the judgement of brightness. Under subdued lighting conditions, the X-ray image on the screen of a television monitor may appear acceptably bright, but in strong daylight the same image would appear much dimmer, even though its luminance has not changed and we are viewing it from the same distance (Ball & Price, 1995).

15.2 Colour of light

Light beams which have different wavelengths, frequencies and photon energies affect the human eye differently and we see them as being of different colours (Ball & Price, 1995). Light of short wavelength (around 400 nm) appears blue or violet, while long-wavelength light (approaching 700 nm) appears red or orange. The complete range of wavelengths in the visible-light region of the electromagnetic spectrum is represented by the range of colours in the rainbow, i.e. red, orange, yellow, green, blue and violet. If, as in sunlight, light waves with all these wavelengths are present in the right proportions, we perceive the mixture as *white* light. White light can also be synthesised by combining lights of as few as three specific wavelengths (representing the **primary colours** red, green and blue). The white parts of the image on a colour television screen are produced by combining red, green and blue light in this way.

Light comprising but a single wavelength or colour is known as **monochromatic light**. The light from the sodium-vapour lamps often used for street lighting is practically monochromatic (see Section 15.3.1.1).

15.3 Production of light

Light may be generated in two main ways, namely, by incandescence and by luminescence.

15.3.1 Incandescence

Incandescence is the emission of visible light from a substance as a direct result of raising its temperature. When a substance is heated, its internal energy increases (Section 2.1). The increase in internal energy causes electrons in the atoms which form the substance to enter higher energy states. Such excited atoms are unstable and the electrons soon return to their former energy levels (see Section 4.3.5.4). As they do so, the electrons give up their surplus energy in the form of photons of electromagnetic radiation, the energies of which represent the energy changes experienced by each individual electron. Depending on the nature of the substance being heated, the spectrum of the radiation emitted may be a **line spectrum**, a **band spectrum** or a **continuous spectrum**.

15.3.1.1 Line spectrum

If the heated substance is a **monatomic gas** such as sodium vapour, whose molecules contain only one atom, the individual atoms are far enough apart for

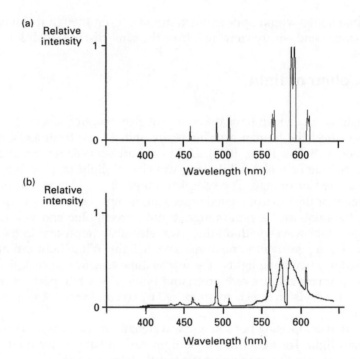

Fig. 15.2   (a) The line spectrum resulting from the emission of light from a heated monatomic gas or vapour (in this case sodium). The most dominant emission from incandescent sodium vapour is at wavelengths of 589.0 and 589.6 nm (yellow), represented by a double peak on the diagram. Emissions at the other wavelengths shown (467, 497, 515, 568 and 616 nm) are far less intense. Sodium incandescence can be demonstrated by sprinkling common salt (sodium chloride) onto the flame of a gas cooker. The sodium vapour released causes the flame to glow with a characteristic bright-yellow light. (b) The spectrum of light emitted from the type of high-pressure sodium-vapour lamp used for street lighting. Many of the sodium characteristic lines can be identified, but the emission is complicated by other elements such as neon which are present. (Adapted from Cayless & Marsden, 1997.)

their electron energy states not to be influenced by neighbouring atoms. As we saw in Section 4.3.5, all atoms of a specific element have the same characteristic set of electron energy states, so when the excited atoms of the monatomic gas return to their ground state, the energies of the photons emitted reflect these particular energy changes. On a wavelength spectrum, each specific photon energy is represented by radiation of a specific wavelength. The result is a *line* spectrum such as that for a sodium-vapour lamp shown in Fig. 15.2. The precise combination of photon energies or wavelengths present is a unique characteristic of the element concerned.

15.3.1.2   Band spectrum

If the heated substance is a gas or vapour whose molecules contain *more* than one atom, the resulting electromagnetic radiation produces **band spectra** comprising

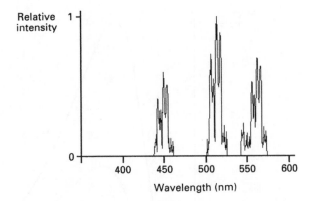

Fig. 15.3   An example of band spectra produced by a gas or vapour whose molecules contain more than one atom. Each cluster of lines is known as a band. The spacing of the bands depends on the molecular structure of the material concerned.

separate groups of lines known as bands (Fig. 15.3). In this case, the atoms within each molecule are close enough to each other to influence the permitted electron energy states. What in an isolated atom was a single discrete energy level now becomes a cluster of energy levels or an **energy band** (Section 6.1.1). The precise combination of energies or wavelengths in a band spectrum is characteristic of the molecules concerned.

15.3.1.3   Continuous spectrum

If the heated substance is a solid or liquid, the atoms are so close together that a nearly infinite number of permitted electron energy levels are created, giving rise to a continuous range of possible electron energy changes. Consequently, the resulting radiation produces a **continuous spectrum**. However, the continuous spectrum is *not* characteristic of the substance which produces it. Instead, the relative intensities of the various wavelengths are largely determined by the *temperature* of the emitting substance. At all temperatures above 0 K (absolute zero) infrared radiation is emitted.

   If the temperature reaches a high enough level, some of the radiation will be visible light. We say the object is 'red hot', meaning red light is being emitted. As the temperature is increased, the minimum wavelength will get shorter and yellow, green and even blue light will be produced. If all these are present, the eye would perceive the mixture as white light and we would say the object was 'white hot'. Figure 15.4 shows the spectrum of light emitted by a solid at 700, 1000 and 1800 K. We can recognise these as forms of the continuous spectrum showing that at 700 K no visible light is produced, only invisible heat rays (infrared). At 1800 K all the colours of the spectrum are emitted and white light results. At the intermediate temperature (1000 K) some visible light is emitted, as well as infrared rays, and we see the object glowing red. It is the process of incandescence which causes the tungsten filament of a conventional electric light bulb to emit light.

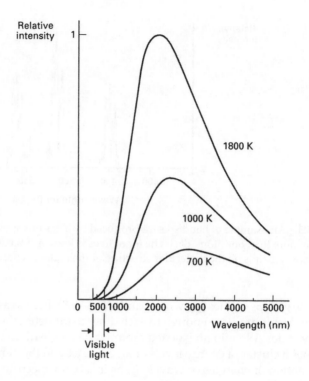

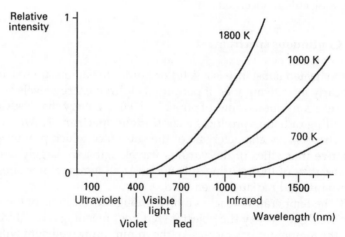

Fig. 15.4 The wavelength spectra of electromagnetic radiation emitted from an incandescent solid: (a) the complete spectrum of radiation from a solid at temperatures of 700, 1000 and 1800 K (approximately 1000, 1300 and 2100°C). The diagram indicates that in all cases, the greater part of the emission is in the infrared region of the spectrum; (b) an enlarged view of the visible part of the same spectra. At 700 K, no visible light is emitted. At 1000 K, some red light is emitted (660–700 nm); the solid is red hot. At 1800 K, light from the red (660 nm), orange (630 nm), yellow (600 nm) and green (550 nm) parts of the spectrum is emitted; the solid now appears 'white' hot.

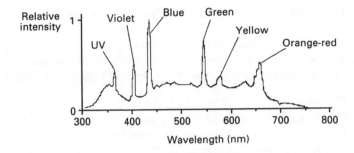

Fig. 15.5   The emission spectrum of a 65-W artificial-daylight fluorescent lamp. Even though the lamp operates at a relatively low temperature, the prominent emissions due to fluorescence in the ultraviolet, violet, blue and green parts of the spectrum give the light its daylight quality and a colour temperature rated at 6500 K. (Adapted from Cayless & Marsden, 1997.)

15.3.1.4   Colour temperature

As we have seen, the colour of light emitted by an incandescent solid depends essentially on its temperature. This relationship forms the basis of the quantity known as **colour temperature**, which provides a convenient means of describing the *quality* of light from a particular source. The colour temperature of a light source is the kelvin temperature to which a black-body radiator (see Section 2.4.3.1) must be raised for it to emit light of a similar quality to the source. For example, average daylight has a colour temperature of 6500 K because a black body at a temperature of 6500 K would emit light of the same quality. It is no coincidence that the surface of the sun, which is the source of our daylight, is at a temperature approaching 6500 K. Although it is based on the phenomenon of incandescence, the concept of colour temperature can be applied even if the source is emitting light by a different process. Thus, the light emitted by the *artificial-daylight* fluorescent tubes used in X-ray illuminators (viewing boxes) is described as having a colour temperature of 6000 K (Fig. 15.5). Table 15.1 includes examples of the colour temperature of various other light sources.

Table 15.1   Approximate colour temperatures of some common light sources

Light source	Colour temperature (K)
Candle	1930
Electric light bulb	2800
'Warm-white' fluorescent tube	3000
'Daylight' fluorescent tube	4500
Direct sunlight at noon	5400
Electronic flash (camera)	6000
'Tropical daylight' fluorescent tube	6000
Blue sky	12 000–18 000

Source: Horder (1971).

15.3.1.5   Alternative methods of stimulating light emission

Increasing the temperature of a substance is not the only way to promote its electrons to higher energy levels. Other methods of raising the energy level of electrons and therefore stimulating the material to emit light include the following:

- Exposing the material to ultraviolet light
- Exposing the material to ionising radiation, such as X- or gamma rays
- Bombarding it with high-energy particles
- Applying a strong electric field

Stimulating a material in one of these ways may cause it to emit visible light at temperatures *well below* those of incandescent bodies. Such a method of 'cold light' emission is known as **luminescence**.

15.3.2   *Luminescence (cold light emission)*

The term luminescence encompasses phenomena such as phosphorescence, fluorescence, thermoluminescence, scintillation and the stimulated emission of light employed in lasers. In each case the emission of light occurs at temperatures below those required to produce incandescence.

Luminescence in solids is exhibited by the group of crystalline semiconducting materials which are collectively known as **phosphors** even though they do not necessarily contain any traces of the element phosphorus. To explain luminescence we need to apply the **electron band theory** of solids discussed in Chapter 6. Reference to Section 6.1.1 and Fig. 15.6 reminds us of some of the relevant features of semiconductors:

- **Conduction bands.** Any electrons in the conduction band may move freely through the material.

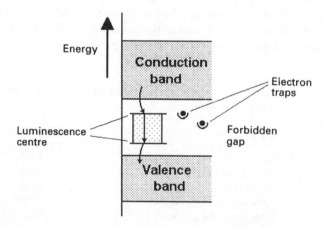

Fig. 15.6   An electron energy band diagram, showing the special features of luminescent phosphors. In the diagram, one electron is returning from conduction band to valence band via a luminescence centre; two other electrons are shown lodged in electron traps in the forbidden gap. See Section 15.3.2 for further explanation.

- **Valence bands.** Electrons in the valence band are bonded to the nucleus of an atom. Electrons removed from the valence band leave behind electron vacancies or **holes**.
- **Forbidden gaps.** In a pure semiconductor, the forbidden gap between the valence and conduction band contains *no* permitted energy levels, so electrons cannot exist in the forbidden gap.
- **The doping process.** Traces of a carefully chosen 'impurity' or **doping agent** are added during the manufacture of the semiconductor. The presence of such an agent, sometimes known as an **activator**, modifies the properties of the semiconductor by introducing permitted energy levels known as **luminescence centres** into the forbidden gap. In certain circumstances, electrons use these centres as 'steps' as they transfer downwards from the conduction band to the valence band.

Additionally, there are:

- **Electron traps.** The crystal structure of a semiconductor is never perfect. Imperfections create extra energy levels known as **electron traps** in the forbidden gap. An electron which settles in an electron trap can escape from it only if it can gain sufficient energy to enable it to jump *upwards* into the conduction band.

Stimulation of a luminescent phosphor by any of the methods listed in Section 15.3.1.5 causes electrons to be lifted from the valence band into the conduction band. They leave behind holes in the valence band. The sequence of events which then follows depends on the particular type of luminescence involved. We shall consider each process in turn.

15.3.2.1 Fluorescence

Fluorescent phosphors have no electron traps but many luminescence centres. Valence electrons raised to the conduction band are able to return immediately via the luminescence centres to fill the holes in the valence bands. As the electrons fall through the luminescence centres they emit their surplus energy in the form of flashes of visible light (Fig. 15.7). The return of the electrons and the subsequent emission of light is practically instantaneous, taking less than 10^{-8} s. The energy (and wavelength) of light emitted depends on the difference in energy across the luminescence centre. It is always less than the energy which originally stimulated the fluorescence. For example, stimulation of a phosphor with ultraviolet light results in the emission of lower energy (longer wavelength) *visible* light. Because the X- or gamma-ray photons used in diagnostic imaging may carry well over 100 000 eV (100 keV) of energy, they are each capable of triggering the release by fluorescence of many hundreds of visible light photons which individually carry only 2 or 3 eV. The absorption of each X- or gamma-ray photon is then marked by a tiny flash of light known as a **scintillation**. Examples of fluorescent phosphors used in diagnostic imaging are thallium-activated **sodium iodide** (in a gamma camera), terbium-activated **gadolinium oxysulphide**

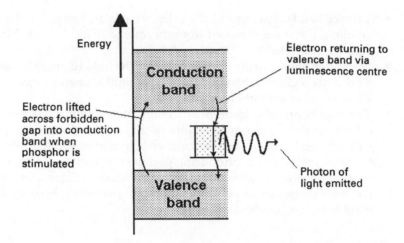

Fig. 15.7   An energy band diagram representing a fluorescent phosphor. After being excited into the conduction band, an electron returns to the valence band via the luminescence centre. The light emitted has a photon energy equal to the energy difference across the luminescence centre. This determines the wavelength and therefore the colour of the fluorescence.

(in intensifying screens) and sodium-activated **caesium iodide** (in an image intensifier).

The spectrum of light emitted by a fluorescent phosphor depends on (and is characteristic of) its crystalline structure. Figure 15.8 shows the spectral emission curves of two fluorescent phosphors commonly used in diagnostic imaging.

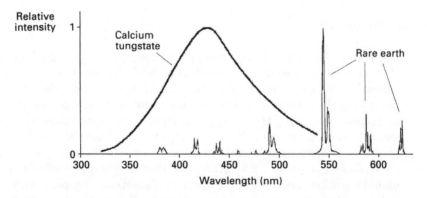

Fig. 15.8   The spectral emission curves of two fluorescent phosphors used in X-ray intensifying screens. The continuous curve is the emission curve of calcium tungstate, which fluoresces mainly in the ultraviolet and blue parts of the spectrum. This type of phosphor is known as a broad-band emitter. The discontinuous emission curve is typical of a 'rare earth' phosphor, such as terbium-activated gadolinium or lanthanum oxysulphide. This emission curve comprises a number of narrow-band spectra, with peak emission occurring near 550 nm in the green part of the spectrum. (Data adapted from Lawrence, 1977.)

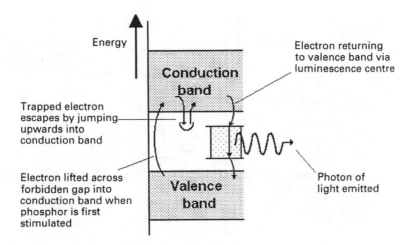

Fig. 15.9   An energy band diagram representing a phosphorescent phosphor. After being excited into the conduction band, an electron becomes lodged in an electron trap in the upper levels of the forbidden gap. At room temperature, the electron eventually acquires the small injection of energy to lift itself back into the conduction band from where it can return to the valence band via a luminescence centre. Again, the light emitted has a photon energy equal to the energy difference across the luminescence centre.

15.3.2.2   Phosphorescence

This process is caused by the presence of **electron traps** between the conduction and valence bands. When the phosphor is stimulated, and electrons are promoted to the conduction band, the traps interfere with the return of electrons to the valence band. Some of the electrons fall into the traps and then cannot escape downwards to the valence band. They must first acquire enough energy to jump *upwards* back into the conduction band, from where they may try again to transfer down to the valence band via a luminescence centre, emitting photons of light as they do so (Fig. 15.9). As long as the electron traps are close to the conduction band, even at room temperature the 'background' internal energy in a phosphor provides sufficient energy to lift the trapped electrons sooner or later into the conduction band. The acquisition of energy enabling electrons to escape from their traps and produce luminescence is a random process which takes time to accomplish. Unlike fluorescence, the emission of light due to phosphorescence therefore continues for a while after the initial stimulation of the phosphor has ceased. In fact, the emission of light decays **exponentially** with a time constant (see Section 7.11.2.1) which depends partly on the temperature of the phosphor. At a high temperature, a phosphorescent phosphor will initially glow more brightly, but become dim more rapidly, than at a lower temperature.

15.3.2.3   Thermoluminescence

This process is similar in principle to phosphorescence, but the electron traps are situated *well below* the conduction band; at room temperature, background

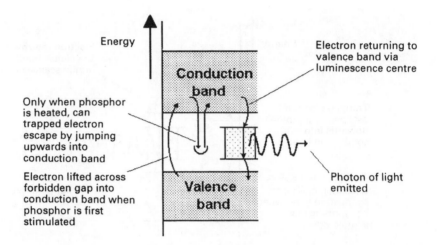

Fig. 15.10   An energy band diagram showing a deep-lying electron trap in a thermoluminescent phosphor. A trapped electron can escape only if it acquires a substantial injection of energy sufficient to lift it from the trap into the conduction band. At room temperature, background internal energy is not great enough to achieve this, and only when the phosphor is oven-heated to around 200°C can the electron escape into the conduction band. It then returns to the valence band via a luminescence centre, emitting a photon of light as it does so.

internal energy in the phosphor is *not* sufficient to raise trapped electrons to the conduction band (Fig. 15.10). However, if the phosphor is actively heated (e.g. to 200°C in an oven), its internal energy is increased; some of the trapped electrons are then able to reach the conduction band and participate in luminescence. Part of the energy absorbed by the phosphor when it was first stimulated is therefore *stored* until the phosphor is heated, when the energy is released as light. This process forms the basis for **thermoluminescent dosimetry**, which we shall describe in Section 19.2.3.

15.3.2.4   Scintillation

Scintillation is a particular form of fluorescence. As we saw in Section 15.3.2.1, stimulation of a fluorescent phosphor with a single high-energy photon of X- or gamma rays can lead to the emission of hundreds of visible light photons. Because all these light photons are emitted simultaneously, a tiny flash of light which may be visible to the naked eye is generated in the phosphor. Exposure of the phosphor to a *stream* of X- or gamma-ray photons results in a series of tiny flashes, each one representing the absorption of a single high-energy photon. The production of such a series of light flashes is known as **scintillation**, and a phosphor used for this purpose is called a **scintillation crystal**. Scintillation in thallium-activated sodium iodide is employed in the gamma camera (see Section 20.6.2.1).

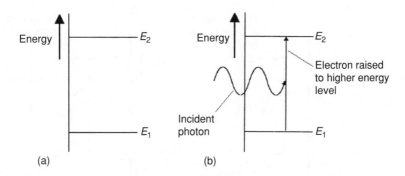

Fig. 15.11   (a) Two electron energy levels E_1 and E_2 in an atom. E_1 is the normal (unexcited) energy level of the atom, while E_2 is a higher (excited) level. (b) The arrival of a light photon, of energy equal to the energy difference $E_2 - E_1$, is very likely to stimulate an electron to rise from its former energy level E_1 to the higher energy level E_2. Such a phenomenon is known as stimulated absorption. Because the energy of the incident photon is totally absorbed in exciting the atom in this way, the photon no longer exists.

15.3.2.5   Stimulated emission of light

Stimulated emission is the mechanism by which **lasers** generate light. Consider an atom which has only two energy levels: an upper level E_2 and a lower level E_1. The atom will normally be in its lower level, but if it is exposed to light whose photon energy is exactly $E_2 - E_1$, it is very likely to absorb a photon and be excited to the upper energy level E_2 (Fig. 15.11). This is known as **stimulated absorption** because the absorption of energy has been stimulated by exposure to light.

Almost immediately (10^{-9}–10^{-8} s later), the excited atom will return to its lower energy state by emitting a photon of light of energy $E_2 - E_1$. This light emission can occur in two ways:

- **Spontaneous emission**
- **Stimulated emission** (where the emission is prompted by an incident photon of light; see Fig. 15.12)

Under normal conditions, spontaneous emission is far more likely to occur than stimulated emission (about 10^{33} times more likely!). To increase the likelihood of stimulated emission occurring, we have to ensure that:

- More atoms are in the excited state than in the unexcited state, a condition known as **population inversion**. An incoming photon is then more likely to interact with an excited atom than a stable atom.
- There is a high density of light photons available to stimulate the emissions.

To create a population inversion, large numbers of atoms are 'pumped' into an excited state by injecting energy into the medium from an external source

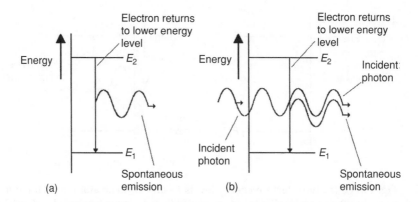

Fig. 15.12 (a) An excited atom spontaneously releasing its excess energy as a photon of light. Because the process is a random one, it is not possible to predict the precise moment when an excited atom will undergo spontaneous emission. Different excited atoms in the same material will release their photons at different times. (b) The arrival of a light photon of energy $E_2 - E_1$ stimulates the excited atom to release a photon and return to its unexcited state. This is known as stimulated emission. The photon released is of precisely the same energy as, and is in phase with, the incident photon. Their effects therefore reinforce each other. The two photons can now stimulate other excited atoms to release their energy and an avalanche effect occurs.

(e.g. optical radiation from a low-pressure xenon flash tube, passage of electric current, or particle collisions created by electrical discharge).

The necessary high density of photons is created by the stimulated emission itself. Each photon emitted is of exactly the right energy to stimulate *more* emissions. Additionally, the photons emitted are made to traverse up to 100 times back and forth through the laser medium by placing reflecting surfaces at each end of the medium. This increases their chances of stimulating further emissions of photons. The result of this avalanche effect is the release of an intense burst of **laser light**.

Properties of laser light
- Photons produced by stimulated emission have precisely the same energy as the photons which stimulated the emission, so the associated light waves have the same frequency and wavelength. In other words, laser light is truly **monochromatic**.
- Laser light waves are *in step* (or *in phase*) with each other (see Fig. 15.12). When atoms are stimulated to emit light, the waves representing the stimulated emission *add* to the waves which stimulated the emission, thereby increasing or *amplifying* their amplitude. (The word *laser* is an acronym for light amplification by stimulated emission of radiation.)
- A beam of laser light is said to be **coherent**, meaning that *all* the waves contributing to such a beam are in phase. Spontaneously emitted radiation waves lack any such phase relationship because they are emitted randomly.
- A laser beam is *parallel* rather than divergent. Its intensity is therefore maintained over long distances and is not subject to reduction by the inverse square law (Section 14.3.5).

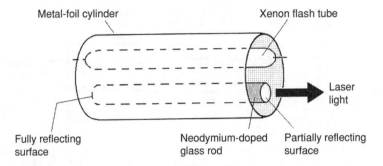

Fig. 15.13 A neodymium–glass solid-state laser pumped by light from a xenon flash tube. In this close-coupled design, the metal-foil-lined cylinder focuses light from the xenon flash tube onto a glass rod doped with the rare earth element neodymium. This creates population inversion in the glass rod and stimulated emission of photons occurs. The photons are reflected back and forth from one end of the rod to the other, triggering more stimulated emissions. Coherent laser light is emitted in a narrow near-parallel beam through the partially reflecting surface at one end of the glass rod.

Types of lasers
Lasers are described as solid-state, semiconductor, gas, or liquid according to the nature of the laser medium used. The following are three common examples:

- **Solid-state lasers** use a neodymium-doped glass rod, which may be up to 1 m long. The parallel ends of the rod are coated with a reflecting film (Fig. 15.13). Population inversion in the rod is created by pumping with light from xenon flash tubes (like the light source in an electronic flash unit on a camera). A solid-state laser can be designed to produce 3-ms pulses of infrared, visible or ultraviolet light with energies of up to 5 kJ.

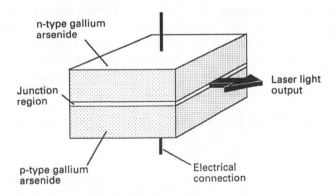

Fig. 15.14 A gallium arsenide semiconductor laser pumped by the flow of electric current. The laser consists of a specially designed p–n junction diode. A forward-biased electrical supply drives current through the junction, creating a population inversion around the junction. Internal reflections confine the laser emission to the 2-μm-thick junction region. Laser light is emitted from one edge of the junction as shown. The side length of such a laser is less than 0.5 mm.

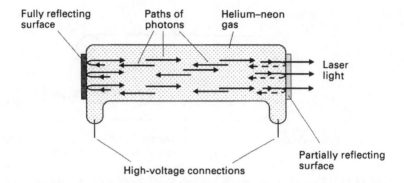

Fully reflecting surface

Paths of photons

Helium–neon gas

Laser light

High-voltage connections

Partially reflecting surface

Fig. 15.15   A helium–neon gas laser. Population inversion is created by particle collisions as high-voltage electrical discharge takes place. Photons produced by stimulated emission are reflected back and forth through the gas, triggering more stimulated emissions. Laser light emerges through the partially reflecting surface at one end of the discharge tube.

- **Semiconductor lasers** consist of a forward-biased p–n junction between layers of a semiconducting material such as gallium arsenide (Fig. 15.14). Population inversion is created in the region of the junction by the passage of an electric current (less than 500 mA) through the junction. Semiconducting lasers have a long working life and are more compact than other types. They can generate a continuous output of up to 40 mJ s^{-1} (40 mW) at wavelengths up to 900 nm (infrared). They are used widely in laser imagers, laser printers and the disk drives, which read data from (and write data to) the optical discs, compact discs (CDs) and digital versatile discs (DVDs) used for data storage.
- **Gas lasers** consist typically of a sealed tube containing a 10:1 mixture of helium and neon gas (Fig. 15.15). Population inversion is created by electrical discharge in the tube, with the presence of helium helping to excite the neon gas. The laser transitions take place in the neon and generate a continuous output of up to 10 mW. Being simple to operate, helium–neon (**He–Ne**) lasers are very common and are used in some laser imagers.

Table 15.2 summarises the characteristics of the principle types of lasers.

Table 15.2   Characteristics of the types of lasers described in the text

Type	Medium	Wavelength(s) (nm)	Output
Solid-state	Neodymium–glass	1060	100 mJ–100 J (pulsed)
Semiconductor	Gallium arsenide	750–905	1–40 mW (continuous)
Gas	Helium–neon	633	0.1–50 mW (continuous)

Source: Watson (1988).

Are lasers safe?
The dangers associated with laser devices arise from two sources, electrical and radiation.

- **Electrical hazards.** Some types of lasers (e.g. gas discharge type) involve high-voltage electricity, which carries its own potential risks. If it is operated sensibly, the design of laser equipment eliminates any electrical risk.
- **Radiation hazards.** The light from a laser is intense and may focus large amounts of energy onto a very small area, which may be capable of causing tissue damage or blindness. Laser devices are therefore classified according to the nature and power of their laser output (see Table 15.3). Every laser device should carry an appropriate warning label indicating its classification. For example, domestic CD players are marked to indicate that they contain a Class 1 laser.

Table 15.3   Classification of lasers for safety purposes

Classification	Description
Class 1	No risk to eyes or skin Very low power output Inherently safe
Class 1M	Low risk to eyes; no risk to skin Safe in normal operations, including direct viewing of the laser beam, unless the user employs optics that could concentrate the laser output into the eye
Class 2	Low risk to eyes; no risk to skin Emits visible light for which the natural aversion response to bright light (including the blink reflex) prevents retinal injury, including direct viewing of the laser beam with optics that could concentrate the laser output into the eye. These lasers do, however, present a dazzle hazard
Class 3R	Low risk to eyes; low risk to skin Lasers whose output is up to a factor of five over the maximum allowed for Class 1 or Class 2. Because of safety factors built into the limits for these classes, the risk of injury for direct viewing of a Class 3R laser beam remains low
Class 3B	Medium risk to eyes; low risk to skin Direct exposure of the eye is hazardous, even taking aversion responses into account, but scattered laser light is usually safe. The higher power Class 3B lasers are also a skin hazard, but the natural aversion response to localised heating generally prevents a skin burn
Class 4	High risk to eyes and skin Direct exposure of the eye and skin is hazardous and scattered laser light may be hazardous to the eyes. Such lasers are also a fire hazard

Source: IEC (2001).

15.3.2.6   Photon-stimulated luminescence

The process of **photon-stimulated luminescence (photostimulable emission)** is similar in many respects to thermoluminescence (Section 15.3.2.3). When a phosphor such as europium-activated barium fluorohalide is exposed to ionising radiation, it stores the energy absorbed from the radiation. If the phosphor is later stimulated by exposure to an appropriate light source, e.g. light from a red-emitting (633-nm) helium–neon laser, the energy stored in the phosphor is released as visible (blue) light. The brightness of the light emission is proportional to the magnitude of the original ionising radiation exposure. Further exposure to the stimulating light releases *all* the stored energy from the phosphor, which can then be reused. Photon-stimulated luminescence is the principle of operation of the image receptors used in some types of **computed radiography** (Ball & Price, 1995).

From the work we have studied so far in this chapter, we know that light has at least two important effects:

(1)   The human eye responds to it; i.e. we can *see* light.
(2)   Photographic film responds to it; i.e. light causes chemical changes to occur in photographic emulsion, which can be used to record images.

There are other effects such as **photosynthesis** in green plants and the synthesis of vitamin D in human skin. While these are not appropriate for studying here, a phenomenon known as the photoelectric effect *is* relevant.

15.4   Photoelectric effect

The term **photoelectric effect** refers to the process of release of electrically charged particles (usually electrons) as a result of irradiation of matter by light or other electromagnetic radiation. The term includes several types of related interactions:

- External photoelectric effect
- Photoconduction
- Photovoltaic effect
- Photoionisation

15.4.1   *External photoelectric effect*

In this process, electrons are released from the surface of a metal by the absorption of energy from light shining on the surface of the metal. The effect is rather like the thermionic emission of electrons described in Chapter 11, but in photoelectric emission the electrons absorb energy from light rather than from internal energy. As we saw in Section 14.5.4, photoelectric emission can occur only if individual incident light photons have sufficient energy to liberate an electron. The photoelectric effect is demonstrated in a vacuum tube device known as a

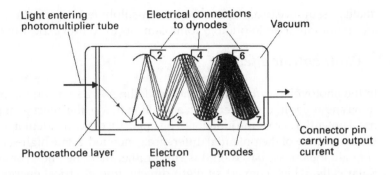

Light entering photomultiplier tube

Electrical connections to dynodes

Vacuum

Connector pin carrying output current

Photocathode layer

Electron paths

Dynodes

Fig. 15.16   A photomultiplier tube (PMT). The evacuated tube contains a photocathode and a series of specially shaped anodes known as **dynodes**, which are charged to progressively more positive potentials. (Dynode 2 is more positive than dynode 1, dynode 3 is more positive than dynode 2, and so on.) The photocathode and the dynodes are coated with a photoemissive layer. A photon of light entering from the left triggers the release, by photoelectric emission, of one or more electrons from the surface of the photocathode. On release, the electron is attracted to the first dynode, where, by the same process, it releases more electrons (two in the diagram). They, in turn, are attracted to the second dynode, where they trigger the release of more electrons (four in the diagram). By the time the seventh dynode is reached, 64 electrons will have arrived, giving a multiplication factor of 64. In an actual PMT, *more* than seven dynodes may be used, and each dynode may emit six times more electrons than it receives. A total multiplication effect approaching 100 million can be achieved, enabling the PM tube to detect the arrival of very small numbers of light photons.

photoelectric cell, in which electrons are released by photoelectric emission from an externally illuminated, negatively charged photocathode. The electrons are then drawn across the vacuum to a positively charged anode under the influence of an electric field. The electron current created depends directly on the intensity of the incident light and the device can therefore be used to monitor the brightness of light. When the light is of very low intensity, a particularly sensitive form of photocell known as a **photomultiplier (PM) tube** is required (Fig. 15.16). PM tubes are used to detect scintillation events in a gamma camera (Section 20.6.2.1) and to monitor the image brightness of an X-ray image intensifier (Ball & Price, 1995). Photoelectric emission of electrons also takes place from the photocathode of an image intensifier (Carter, 1994).

15.4.2   *Photoconduction*

In this process, valence electrons in a semiconductor absorb energy from incident light photons, and are raised into the conduction band, thereby increasing its ability to conduct an electric current. Assuming the photons of light have sufficient energy to achieve this effect, the electrical resistance of the semiconductor varies with the intensity of the incident light: an increase in light intensity results in a fall in resistance. Such solid-state devices, known as **photoresistors**, have many applications. For example, photoresistors are found in some types of optical **densitometers** used to measure film blackening as part of a film-processor quality-assurance programme. Cadmium-sulphide-photoresistive **light meters** are commonly used in photographic cameras to control exposure factors.

15.4.3   *Photovoltaic effect*

In the photovoltaic effect, light photons falling on a semiconductor create electrons and holes in the material. In a junction diode, the effect generates an electrical potential across the junction. The intensity of the incident light determines the magnitude of the potential difference generated. Some high-sensitivity camera light meters are based on this effect rather than the photoconductive effect. **Solar cells**, which convert sunlight directly into electrical energy, employ the photovoltaic effect in silicon or gallium arsenide diodes; they are used, for example, as a power source in some electronic calculators and in space probes and satellites.

15.4.4   *Photoionisation*

Photoionisation is the *ionisation* of a material by exposure to light or other electromagnetic radiation. In this effect, the incident photons must possess enough energy to release completely one or more electrons from an atom. The electrons so liberated are known as **photoelectrons**. The photoelectric effect and the ionisation resulting from exposure to X- and gamma radiation are discussed further in Section 17.2.2.

   With one notable exception, we have now covered most aspects of the properties of light which impinge on diagnostic imaging. The major omission is **optics**, the study of the way light is reflected and refracted by lenses and mirrors and the way it is diffracted when passing through narrow apertures. We refer the reader to sources such as Muncaster (1993) for a general treatment of geometrical optics, to Jenkins & White (2001) for a mathematical approach and to Ball & Price (1995) for a largely non-mathematical treatment of areas of optics particularly relevant to radiographers. In the next chapter we begin our study of the high-energy radiation produced by X-ray tubes on which much of the work of a radiographer relies.

Chapter 16
X-Rays

We are now in a position to be able to study X-rays: how they are produced and the properties they possess.

16.1   Production of X-rays

There are two types of events which can lead to X-ray production:

(1)   An electron travelling at high speed may experience a sudden change in its direction of motion.
(2)   An electron in an atom may undergo a transition from a high-energy state to a lower energy state.

Most of the output of an X-ray tube is the result of the first type of event taking place, but in some circumstances (e.g. in mammography equipment) the second type of event may contribute significantly to the total X-ray output.

The X-ray tube is a device which is designed to produce fast-moving electrons and cause them to deviate violently. In Chapter 12 we studied the construction of the X-ray tube in detail. Let us now remind ourselves of the basic features illustrated in Fig. 16.1. The tube contains:

- A heated filament, which releases negative electrons by thermionic emission
- A positive anode, which attracts them
- A high-tension supply, which accelerates the electrons to very high speeds
- A target (part of the anode), whose job is to force the fast-moving electrons to deviate very rapidly, thus causing X-rays to be emitted

16.1.1   Interactions at the target

What actually happens at the target? Electrons reaching the target from the filament of a diagnostic X-ray tube may possess up to 150 keV of kinetic energy, depending on the kilovoltage applied across the X-ray tube. These high-energy electrons interact with the atoms of target material in a number of ways, most

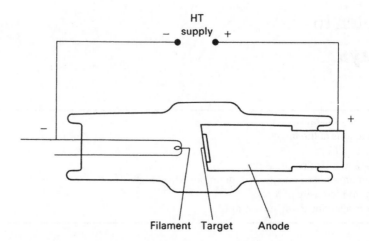

Fig. 16.1 The key features of a simple X-ray tube insert. The heated filament provides a supply of electrons which are accelerated by the high-voltage (HT) towards the anode. The high-energy electrons bombard the target of the anode, thereby producing X-radiation.

of which merely serve to increase the temperature of the target. However, there are *two* types of interactions which result in the emission of X-rays. Unfortunately, the heat-producing interactions are far more likely to occur than X-ray-producing interactions, and less than 1% of the energy deposited on the target of an X-ray tube is converted into X-radiation (Hay, 1982).

The X-rays produced at the target of an X-ray tube are described as **Bremsstrahlung** radiation, or **characteristic** radiation, according to the nature of the interactions involved.

16.1.1.1   Bremsstrahlung ('braking') radiation

Consider one high-energy electron arriving from the filament and entering the target (Fig. 16.2). Its path takes it deep inside a target atom such that it passes close enough to the nucleus for it to be influenced by the electric field around the nucleus. The negatively charged electron experiences an electric force of attraction to the positively charged nucleus, making it deviate towards the nucleus. The sudden change in motion of the electron constitutes a violent acceleration which disturbs the electromagnetic field and a photon of X-radiation is emitted (Section 14.1). The electron now continues on its new course. The principle of conservation of energy (Section 1.1.1.1) tells us that in producing an X-ray photon, the electron has lost some of its kinetic energy:

Final KE of electron = initial KE of electron − energy of photon

Consequently, the electron must now be travelling more slowly than before the interaction. Note that the slowing down of the electron is the *consequence* rather than the *cause* of the emission of an X-ray photon.

This slowing down of the electron, which accompanies the emission of an X-ray photon, provides the origin of the term **braking radiation**, sometimes

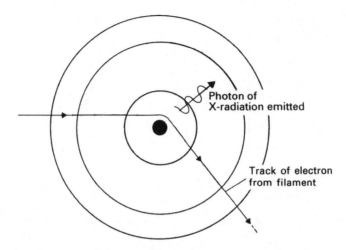

Fig. 16.2   The production of Bremsstrahlung radiation. The diagram shows a high-energy electron from the filament passing close to the nucleus of an atom in the target. The sudden deviation in the track of the electron prompts it to emit an X-ray photon. The electron continues, but at reduced speed.

given to X-radiation arising from this type of interaction. More commonly, the German word **Bremsstrahlung**, meaning slowing down, is applied to X-radiation produced in this way.

The interaction of an incident electron with an atomic nucleus in the target varies in its severity according to how powerful an electric field the nucleus produces and how close to the nucleus the electron passes. At one extreme, the electron may not be influenced at all, because it does not penetrate deep enough into the atom. At the other extreme, the electron may be so severely affected that *all* its kinetic energy is consumed in producing the X-ray photon and the electron is brought to rest! The energy of photons of Bremsstrahlung radiation may therefore be of *any* value between zero and a maximum equal to the initial kinetic energy of the incident electron. When we make an X-ray exposure, millions of electrons undergo Bremsstrahlung interactions, so photons of *all* energies in this range are created. The result is an X-ray beam having a **continuous spectrum** (Fig. 16.3).

16.1.1.2   Characteristic radiation

Consider another high-energy electron from the filament of the X-ray tube arriving at the tube target. This time, its path causes it to interact with an *inner-shell* (e.g. K-shell) electron in one of the atoms of the target material, transferring enough of its kinetic energy to the target electron to eject it from the atom (Fig. 16.4). In other words, the atom has been **ionised** and an electron vacancy has been created in its K shell. Clearly, for this process to take place, the kinetic energy of the incident electron must be at least equal to the ionisation energy of the target electron (Section 4.3.5.6). For a tungsten target, the K-shell ionisation energy is 69.5 keV, so an incident electron must have at least this amount of energy to free an electron from the K shell of a tungsten atom.

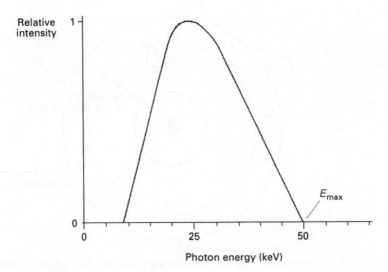

Fig. 16.3   The continuous spectrum of Bremsstrahlung X-radiation. In this case, the maximum energy of the radiation (E_{max}) is 50 keV, indicating that none of the electrons arriving at the target had more than 50 keV of kinetic energy.

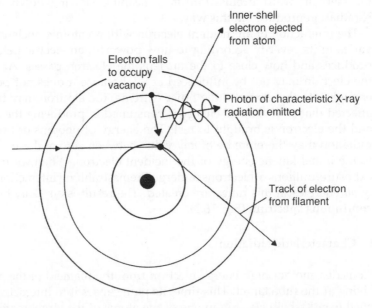

Fig. 16.4   The production of characteristic X-radiation. The diagram shows a high-energy electron from the filament ionising an atom of target material by interacting with one of its K-shell electrons. As the electron is ejected, a vacancy is created in the K shell. The vacancy is immediately filled by the downward transition of an electron from a higher energy level (in this case, the L shell). The excess energy of the electron from the L shell is released as a photon of characteristic X-radiation.

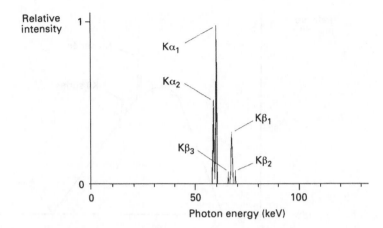

Fig. 16.5   The characteristic X-ray spectrum for the element tungsten, which is commonly used as an X-ray tube target material. The two prominent emission lines (labelled $K\alpha_1$ and $K\alpha_2$) at about 58 and 59 keV are due to electron transitions from the L shell to the K shell. The emission lines (labelled $K\beta_1$, $K\beta_2$ and $K\beta_3$) around 67 keV are the result of M- to K-shell transitions.

Once a target atom has been ionised in this way, its electrons immediately adjust their energy levels. One can imagine the electrons behaving rather like patients in an X-ray waiting room changing seats when someone gets up to leave. In terms of the Bohr model of the atom (Section 4.3.4), these adjustments can be visualised as the movement of an upper-shell electron into the vacancy created in the inner shell. This downward transition of an electron involves the *release* of energy because the inner shell represents a lower energy state than the upper shell. The energy is released *either* by transferring the energy to another orbital electron which is ejected (then known as an **Auger electron**) *or* by the emission of a photon of electromagnetic radiation.

If a photon of radiation *is* emitted, its energy is equal to the difference between the energy levels of the two shells involved in the electron transition. Furthermore, in the case of an X-ray tube target material, the magnitude of the energy difference ensures that the radiation emitted is in the X-ray part of the electromagnetic spectrum. The *precise* energy of the X-ray photon depends not only on which particular electron energy levels were involved in the transition, but on the **proton number** of the atom concerned. For example, in a tungsten target, electron transitions from the L shell to the K shell produce X-ray photons having 57.98 and 59.32 keV of energy (Kaye & Laby, 1995). The spectrum of radiation produced by this type of interaction is therefore a **line spectrum**, which is characteristic of the target material employed (Fig. 16.5).

16.1.2   *X-ray spectrum*

As we have discovered, both line and continuous spectra can be produced. However, unlike light, the X-ray line spectrum can never be produced alone in an X-ray tube. If present, it is always superimposed on a continuous spectrum (Figs. 16.6 and 16.7).

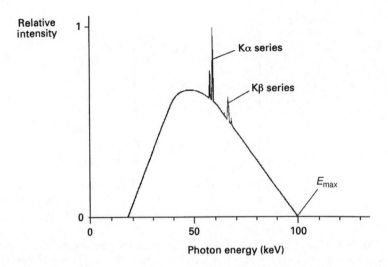

Fig. 16.6   An X-ray photon energy spectrum showing tungsten characteristic line spectra superimposed on a continuous spectrum. As in Fig. 16.5, the most prominent tungsten emission lines are the Kα series at 58 and 59 keV, resulting from L- to K-shell transitions (see Section 16.1.2.1). The spectrum represents an X-ray beam generated by an X-ray tube operating at 100 kV. The beam has a maximum photon energy of 100 keV because electrons from the filament, accelerated through a potential difference of 100 kV, will have acquired 100 keV of kinetic energy by the time they reach the target. They are therefore incapable of producing any X-ray photons with more than 100 keV of energy (see Section 16.1.2.3).

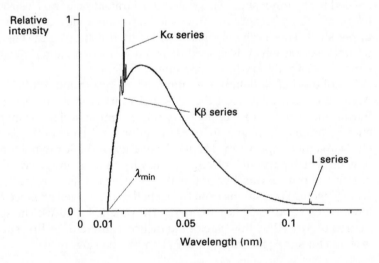

Fig. 16.7   An X-ray wavelength spectrum showing tungsten characteristic line spectra superimposed on a continuous spectrum. This wavelength spectrum is an alternative way of depicting the beam shown in Fig. 16.6. The Kα emissions occur at wavelengths around 0.021 nm and the smaller Kβ emissions around 0.018 nm. L-series emissions (resulting from transitions into the L shell) have also been included, but their contribution to the total X-ray output of the tube is negligible. The Duane–Hunt relationship (Section 16.1.2.3) tells us that this X-ray beam, generated at a tube voltage of 100 kV, has a minimum wavelength (λ_{min}) of 0.0124 nm.

Table 16.1   Probabilities, line spectra and photon energies for the most common electron transitions involved in K-series emissions from a tungsten X-ray tube target

Transition[a]	Probability[b]	Emission line[c]	Photon energy[d] (keV)
L–K	0.5	$K\alpha_1$	59.32
L–K	0.25	$K\alpha_2$	57.98
M–K	0.15	$K\beta_1$	67.24
M–K	0.05	$K\beta_2$	69.10
M–K	0.05	$K\beta_3$	66.95

[a] The most common electron transitions involved in the production of K-series emissions from a tungsten X-ray tube target.

[b] Probability of a particular transition occurring (e.g. 0.5 means one in two transitions are of this type).

[c] Line spectra produced. Because each electron shell includes more than one energy level (Section 4.3.5.1), transitions between the same two shells may produce more than one emission line. The different emission lines are named according to the normal convention employed in spectroscopy: $K\alpha$ indicates an L-to-K transition, $K\beta$ indicates an M-to-K transition, etc.; the subscript (1, 2, 3, etc.) indicates different energy changes within a particular shell transition.

[d] Photon energy of the radiation emitted.

Source: Kaye & Laby (1995).

16.1.2.1   K-series emissions

The most prominent line spectra arising from a tungsten target are caused by electrons filling vacancies in the K shell. Such vacancies are most likely to be filled by L- or M-shell electrons, and the group of line spectra so created are known as **K-series emissions**. Table 16.1 indicates the probability of each of the possible L-to-K and M-to-K transitions in a tungsten target and the energy of the photons emitted in each case. We can see from the table that by far the greatest contribution to X-ray output arises from the two L-to-K transitions because they are the most likely to occur. By contrast, M-to-K transitions are less likely and make a relatively minor contribution. Electron transitions into the K shell from even higher shells are possible (e.g. N-to-K transitions), but their probabilities are so low that they do not contribute significantly to the output of an X-ray tube and we can safely ignore them.

16.1.2.2   L-series and M-series emissions

Characteristic radiation resulting from electron transitions into the L shell creates the **L-series emissions**, while that from transitions into the M shell produces the **M-series emissions**. For a tungsten target, the L-series photons have energies in the range 11–8 keV and the M-series photons have energies less than 2 keV. X-ray photons with such low energies contribute neither to image formation nor to patient radiation dose. This is because in a normal diagnostic X-ray tube the attenuating effect of **inherent filtration** prevents low-energy photons from escaping through the output port (Section 17.3.2).

16.1.2.3   Maximum photon energy and minimum wavelength

Another feature of the X-ray spectrum is the presence of an upper photon energy limit (or minimum wavelength). For any particular tube voltage there will be a corresponding upper photon energy limit or minimum wavelength. This is because the tube voltage determines the amount of kinetic energy possessed by electrons arriving at the target from the filament and therefore the maximum energy of the X-ray photons produced by the Bremsstrahlung process (Section 16.1.1.1). An electron accelerated by a tube voltage of (say) 50 kV will acquire 50 keV of kinetic energy. If *all* this energy is transformed into an X-ray photon in a single Bremsstrahlung interaction, the photon will have 50 keV of energy. Where the X-ray tube is supplied by a pulsating rather than constant voltage, the maximum energy acquired by the electrons is determined by the *peak* value of tube voltage. Consequently, the maximum energy (E_{MAX}) of the resulting X-ray photons is set by the peak tube kilovoltage (kVp). For example, at a peak tube voltage of 86 kV, the maximum photon energy will be 86 keV.

By using the relationship $E = hc/\lambda$ derived from Planck's law (Section 14.5.3), we can calculate the value of the minimum wavelength (λ_{min}) if we know the peak value of the tube voltage. When simplified, the relationship can be stated as:

$$\lambda_{min} = 1.24/kVp \text{ nm}$$

This relationship is sometimes known as the **Duane–Hunt law**. As the tube voltage is increased, maximum photon energy is increased and minimum wavelength is decreased.

N.B. The apparent similarities between the units we are using to express X-ray tube voltages and X-ray photon energies can lead to confusion. In the examples quoted in the preceding paragraphs, the tube voltage (in kV or kVp) is *numerically equal* to the maximum photon energy (in keV). This situation is often the case. Unfortunately, it is only too easy for this to deceive the unwary into believing that kilovolts (kV) and kiloelectronvolts (keV) are interchangeable units. In fact, these units are quite different. The kilovolt (kV) and the peak kilovolt (kVp) are measures of **electrical potential difference**, whereas the electronvolt (eV) and kiloelectronvolt (keV) are measures of **energy**. Readers must therefore always be alert to the possibility of confusion or error when discussing the influence of tube voltage on radiation energy.

16.2   Quality and intensity of X-rays

16.2.1   *Quality*

The term 'quality' describes the penetrating power of an X-ray beam. It is not the same as the *quantity* or amount of radiation involved, just as the colour of light is not the same as its brightness. It is helpful to keep this comparison in mind when discussing X-ray beams and to think of quality as being the 'colour' of the X-ray beam.

If radiation is **monoenergetic** (**monochromatic** or **homogeneous**), by which we mean it contains only a single value of photon energy, its quality can be indicated simply by quoting the photon energy or the wavelength of the radiation. X-ray beams, however, are invariably **heterogeneous** (i.e. having a range of different photon energies) and to describe completely the quality of such a beam, it would be necessary to give the spectrum of the radiation. In practice, in radiography it is more usual to quote one or more of the following characteristics:

- The generating voltage
- The half-value thickness
- The beam filtration
- The effective photon energy

We shall be discussing these aspects in detail in Chapter 19.

16.2.2 *Intensity*

This is a measure of the quantity (amount) of radiation energy flowing in unit time (Section 14.3.3). It can be usefully compared with the brightness of light; the 'brightness' of an X-ray beam is related to its intensity. Intensity is defined as the quantity of energy flowing in unit time through a unit area when measured at right angles to the direction of the beam. Its units are watts per square metre ($W\ m^{-2}$). Figure 16.8 illustrates the situation referred to in the definition.

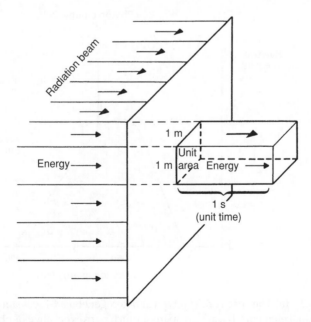

Fig. 16.8 A diagram illustrating the concept of X-ray beam intensity. The intensity of an X-ray beam is the amount of energy flowing per unit time per unit area measured at right angles to the direction of the beam. In SI units, intensity is measured in watts per square metre ($W\ m^{-2}$).

The total intensity of an X-ray beam is represented by the sum of the intensities of the separate components of the beam. A complex heterogeneous beam such as an X-ray beam, consisting of a wide range of different photon energies, can be thought of as a combination of a large number of separate monochromatic (homogeneous) components, each possessing its own individual intensity. The *total* intensity of the heterogeneous beam is then seen as the sum of the intensities of its individual components. In terms of the spectral emission curve of the beam from an X-ray tube, the total intensity of the beam is proportional to the area enclosed by the curve (Fig. 16.9).

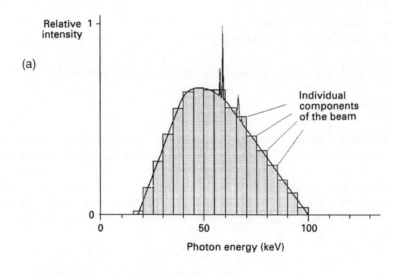

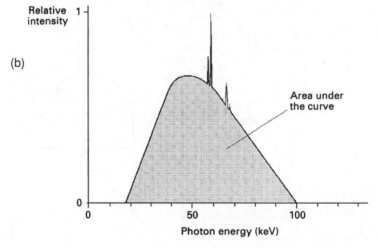

Fig. 16.9   (a) The spectrum of a typical heterogeneous X-ray beam analysed into 17 individual elements. Because it spans a much narrower range of photon energy, each element approximates to a monochromatic component of the beam. The total intensity of the beam is proportional to the sum of the areas (shaded) of each component. (b) If the beam was analysed into a much larger number of components, the total intensity would be proportional to the area (shaded) under the curve of the spectrum.

Unfortunately, there are practical difficulties in directly measuring the intensity of an X-ray beam. For this reason, in radiography we usually prefer to measure the quantity of radiation in terms of one of its effects rather than in terms of intensity; e.g. the ionising effect on air, which we call **exposure**, is measured in coulombs per kilogram (C kg^{-1}), not in the basic units of intensity (Section 19.2.1.1).

16.2.3   Factors affecting X-ray output

Five factors are involved here:

- Tube kilovoltage (kV)
- Tube current (mA)
- Filtration
- Tube target material
- Distance from source

16.2.3.1   X-ray tube kilovoltage

Tube voltage affects both quality and intensity. It affects quality because the maximum photon energy is determined by the peak tube voltage. The higher the tube kilovoltage, the more penetrating the beam becomes.

Tube voltage affects the presence or absence of line spectra because if the tube voltage is below a critical value, none of the electrons hitting the target will possess enough energy to cause K-series emissions. The electrons must possess energy at least equal to the **K-shell ionisation energy** of the target material in order to remove K-shell electrons and thereby promote transitions into the K shell (Section 4.3.5.6). For a tungsten target, the critical energy required is just under 70 keV (69.5 keV) and the tube voltage must therefore reach a peak of at least 70 kV for K-series emissions to occur. For a molybdenum target, K-series emissions are generated only if the peak tube voltage is over 20 kV.

It is easy to spot the presence or absence of K lines on diagrams of X-ray spectra such as Figs. 16.3 and 16.6. Does, however, the presence of K-series emissions make a *significant* difference to the output intensity of an X-ray tube? It has been claimed that for an X-ray tube with a tungsten target operating at voltages between 80 and 150 kV, K-series emissions contribute no more than 10% of the total tube output (Epp & Weiss, 1966). At tube voltages *below* 70 kV, they make no contribution whatsoever because as we have seen, no tungsten K-series emissions can occur at these voltages. However, the situation is very different in **mammography** (soft-tissue radiography of the breast), where much lower voltages (between 20 and 30 kV) are employed. An X-ray tube with a molybdenum target is used and the molybdenum K-series emissions (at energies between 17.5 and 19.6 keV) make a very worthwhile contribution to the tube output.

Intensity is also affected because higher voltages give the electrons more energy and the X-ray process becomes more efficient; thus, the beam carries more energy. Figure 16.10 shows the effect on the X-ray spectrum of altering the tube voltage. The type of high-voltage rectification, which determines the

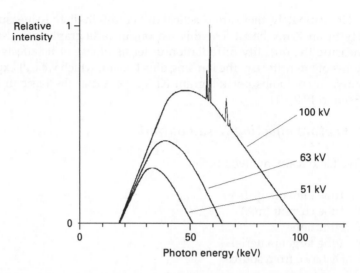

Fig. 16.10 The effect on the X-ray spectrum of changing the tube kilovoltage. The diagram illustrates the spectra obtained from an X-ray tube with a tungsten target when operated at 51, 63, and 100 kV. The tungsten Kα and Kβ emission lines are present on the spectrum of the beam generated at 100 kV. When a pulsating voltage is applied to the X-ray tube, the spectrum of the beam changes from moment to moment during the X-ray exposure. Note the four changes in the spectra due to the change in kilovolts: (1) the maximum photon energy of the beam increases as the tube voltage increases; (2) the average photon energy of the beam increases as the tube voltage increases; (3) the overall intensity of the beam increases as the tube voltage increases; (4) there are no K-series emission spectra when the tube voltage is at 63 and 51 kV.

voltage waveform, also affects both quality and intensity. If the tube voltage is not constant, the spectrum is continually changing and the average spectrum is always of lower quality than that produced by the peak voltage. The intensity of an X-ray beam is approximately proportional to the square of tube voltage.

16.2.3.2   X-ray tube current

The value of tube current (mA) affects only the intensity of the beam; it does *not* affect its quality. Because current is the rate of flow of electric charge (Section 3.3.3), X-ray tube current is a measure of the rate of flow of charge carriers (i.e. electrons) from the filament to the anode. For example, a tube current of 1000 mA (1 A) means that charge is arriving at the anode at the rate of 1 C s^{-1}. Each individual electron carries 1.6×10^{-19} C of charge; consequently, when a tube current of 1000 mA is flowing, electrons hit the target of the anode at the rate of about 6×10^{18} (i.e. 6 million million million) per second! If the current is halved (to 500 mA), only 3×10^{18} electrons will be arriving per second and only half the number of X-ray-producing interactions can take place. The X-ray output is therefore halved (Fig. 16.11).

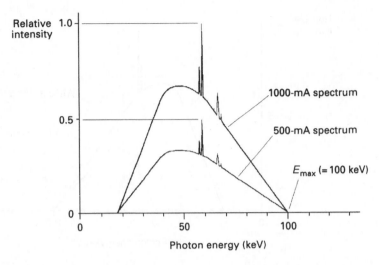

Fig. 16.11   The effect on a 100-kV X-ray beam of changing the tube current from 500 to 1000 mA. It is assumed that no other exposure factors have been altered. The result is a doubling of intensity across all photon energies in the spectrum. This has the effect of doubling the area enclosed by the curve and therefore confirms that the total output has doubled (see Section 16.2.2). Note that although the tungsten K-series emissions have doubled in intensity, they still appear at precisely the same photon energy. There is no change in the quality of the beam.

In general, the intensity (I) of an X-ray beam is *directly proportional* to tube current (mA):

$$I \propto \text{mA}$$

In cases where the current is pulsating, the *average* intensity of the beam is directly proportional to the *average* value of the current.

Altering tube current has no effect on the energy gained by individual electrons, as they accelerate from filament to anode. (Their energy is determined by the tube *voltage*.) The *quality* of an X-ray beam is therefore not influenced in any way by a change in tube current. Figure 16.11 confirms that reducing the tube current from 1000 to 500 mA has produced no changes in the maximum photon energy (E_{max}), nor in the distribution of photon energies, nor in the nature of the characteristic emission. Both X-ray beams have exactly the same quality.

16.2.3.3   Beam filtration

Until now, we have discussed X-ray beams in their virgin state, unaffected by any interactions they may suffer as they pass through matter. In practice, all X-ray beams are modified to a greater or lesser extent by such interactions even before they emerge from the output port of the X-ray tube (Section 17.3.2). Moreover, diagnostic X-ray beams suffer further modifications because they must negotiate their way through one or more metal **filters** before they reach the patient.

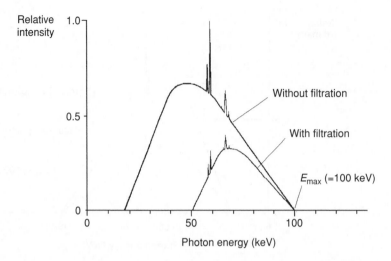

Fig. 16.12 The effect of filtration on a 100-kV X-ray beam. The low-energy part of the beam has been preferentially filtered out, leaving a beam which, although reduced in intensity, has a higher average photon energy and is therefore of higher quality. Because the spread of photon energies has been reduced, the beam has become less heterogeneous. Adding extra filtration would further reduce the energy spread and the beam would approximate more closely to a monochromatic (homogeneous) state, although its intensity would be seriously compromised. Note that the value of E_{max} is unchanged. Note, too, that the tungsten K-series emissions appear at the same photon energy levels, but their intensity has been reduced by the effect of filtration.

Filters are materials deliberately inserted into the X-ray beam to improve the *quality* of the beam. Unfortunately, they also reduce the beam's intensity. A filter consists of a thin sheet of metal, such as aluminium, copper, molybdenum or palladium, which has the effect of absorbing most of the low-energy (long-wavelength) radiation and yet transmitting most of the high-energy (short-wavelength) radiation. The purpose of such filters is to reduce unwanted radiation doses to the patient's skin. Figure 16.12 illustrates the effect on the X-ray spectrum of adding beam filtration (see also Chapter 17).

16.2.3.4 Distance from source

A diverging beam, such as that produced by an X-ray tube, is subject to a reduction of intensity with distance as described in Section 14.3.5. During its passage through the air between the X-ray tube and the patient, the intensity (I) of an X-ray beam adheres approximately to an **inverse-square-law** relationship with distance (d) from the source of X-rays:

$$I \propto \frac{1}{d^2}$$

The intensity of the beam therefore falls off rapidly with increasing distance. Note that this reduction in intensity is due to the *divergence* of the beam rather than to any interactions between the beam and atoms of atmospheric gases. Because air is such a tenuous medium, over the distances encountered in radiography diagnostic X-ray beams suffer relatively few such interactions. Consequently, for practical purposes we can assume that the passage of an X-ray beam through air affects neither its intensity nor its quality.

16.2.3.5 Target material

The proton number of the target material affects the intensity of the beam produced. Atoms with high proton numbers have a greater effect on the electrons from the filament because their nuclei have a greater positive electric charge. Also, using a different target material modifies the photon energy of the characteristic radiation and therefore affects the quality of the beam. The target material does not alter the *quality* of the Bremsstrahlung radiation, only its intensity. The effect on the X-ray spectrum of a change in target material is shown in Fig. 16.13.

Although we have been discussing the effect on X-ray output of using different target materials, it is of course not possible to change the target once an X-ray tube has been assembled. Target material is one of many features of tube design which affect its performance. The manufacturers select a target material to suit the conditions under which the tube will be operated in order to maximise its output. As we saw in Sections 12.4.1.3 and 12.5.2.1, the target focal track of most X-ray tubes is made from a tungsten–rhenium alloy. Only in mammography X-ray tubes, designed to operate at low kilovoltages, are alternative target

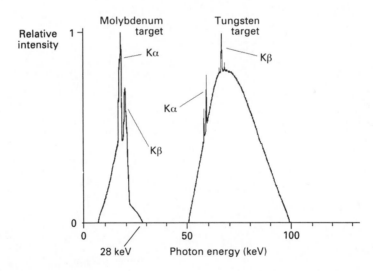

Fig. 16.13 The photon energy spectra of X-ray beams generated by two different target materials. In each case, the X-ray beam has been modified by filtration appropriate to the operating conditions of the tube. Left: the tube with a molybdenum target was operating at 28 kV (giving an E_{max} of 28 keV); its spectrum shows the molybdenum Kα and Kβ emissions (at 17.5 and 19.6 keV, respectively), which make a valuable contribution to the total output. Right: the tube with a tungsten target was operating at 100 kV (giving an E_{max} of 100 keV); its spectrum shows the tungsten Kα and Kβ emissions (at 59 and 67 keV): their contribution to total output is minimal.

Table 16.2   Summary of factors affecting X-ray tube output

Changing factor	Quality	Intensity
Raising tube voltage	Increased	Increased
Reducing tube voltage ripple	Increased	Increased
Raising tube current	No effect	Increased
Increasing beam filtration	Increased	Reduced
Increasing distance from source	No effect	Reduced
Using target with higher proton number	Changes line emissions only	Increased

materials (molybdenum or rhodium) employed. The various factors which influence the quality and intensity of an X-ray beam are summarised in Table 16.2.

Having described the processes by which X-rays are generated, in the next chapter we explore the ways in which ionising radiations such as X- and gamma rays interact with matter.

Chapter 17

Interaction of X-Rays and Gamma Rays with Matter

In this chapter we investigate what happens when a beam of X- or gamma rays is directed at matter. We shall then be in a position to explain how these radiations behave when they interact with living tissues.

A beam of radiation may be transmitted through a medium; e.g. light passes through glass and X-rays pass through wood. However, in each case the intensity of the beam is reduced after it has passed through the medium and we say the beam has been **attenuated** (made weaker). The loss in intensity may be very small or very great, but there is always *some* loss of energy from the beam.

Why is this so? What has happened to the radiation energy which is missing? There are two possibilities:

(1)   As the beam passes through matter, some of its energy is **absorbed**; i.e. the energy is transferred to matter, as shown in Fig. 17.1. In living tissues this can be a reason for the harmful effects of some radiations.

(2)   As the beam passes through the matter, some of its photons are **scattered**; i.e. they collide with atomic particles and are forced to change course. They may then emerge but travelling in directions different from the original beam, as shown in Fig. 17.2.

Both these interactions take place when an X- or gamma-ray beam penetrates into matter.

17.1   Transmission of X- or gamma rays through a medium

We saw in Chapter 16 that beams of radiation may be homogeneous (consisting of photons all of the same energy) or heterogeneous (consisting of photons of a

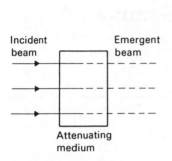

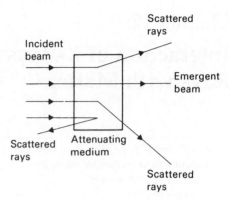

Fig. 17.1 Energy of a beam being absorbed in an attenuating medium.

Fig. 17.2 Energy of a beam being scattered out of the beam.

whole range of energies). X-ray beams are always heterogeneous but gamma-ray beams can be homogeneous.

We shall consider firstly what happens when a homogeneous beam passes through a medium and then later expand the explanation to cover the behaviour of heterogeneous beams.

17.1.1 Experiment to investigate attenuation

As we have seen, when a beam of X-rays passes into matter it is attenuated by being absorbed and scattered. How can we investigate the amount of attenuation that takes place? Let us consider an experimental set-up (Fig. 17.3) that we could use. It consists of an X-ray source, a radiation-measuring device and a selection of different thicknesses of a suitable medium, such as aluminium, to insert in the beam. The radiation-measuring device (a dosimeter) will tell us the quantity of radiation transmitted when the beam is attenuated by a known thickness of aluminium. Suitable exposure factors are first determined, ensuring that even with the maximum thickness of attenuator in place, a measurable reading is obtained

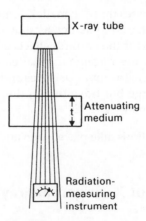

Fig. 17.3 Experimental set-up for measuring attenuation of an X-ray beam.

on the dosimeter. We then proceed by making a series of *identical* exposures on the X-ray tube, taking a dosimeter reading after each exposure. The first dosimeter reading (Q_0) is taken with *no* attenuator in the path of the beam. Before each subsequent exposure we zero the dosimeter and insert a different thickness (x) of attenuator in the beam, e.g. 0.5 mm, 1.0 mm, 1.5 mm, etc., until we have exhausted the supply of attenuators. The increasing thicknesses are built up by using multiple layers of attenuator; e.g. a 1.5-mm thickness is achieved by using three 0.5-mm thicknesses. As each exposure is made, we record the reading (Q) on the dosimeter and the total thickness (x) of attenuator. Table 17.1 shows the sort of data we might collect from such an experiment. The data are then plotted on a graph (Fig. 17.4). As common sense suggests, as thicker attenuating material is inserted, the dosimeter reading reduces. The graph is the familiar shape that we encountered in Chapter 7, relating to the charging and discharging of capacitors; it is an **exponential decay curve**. Plotting the *logarithmic* values of the dosimeter readings produces a straight-line graph (Fig. 17.5), confirming that there is an exponential relationship between Q and x. We can express this in the form:

$$Q \propto e^{-\mu x}$$

where μ is a constant. If we assume that the dosimeter reading is proportional to the intensity (I) of the X-ray beam, the expression can be written:

$$I \propto e^{-\mu x}$$

and

$$I = \text{constant} \times e^{-\mu x}$$

Table 17.1 Data[a] collected during an experiment to investigate the attenuation of an X-ray beam

Attenuator thickness, x (mm)	Dosimeter reading, Q[b]	Relative dose[c] (%)	Log_e relative dose[c]
0.0	24.0	100.0	4.6
0.5	19.6	81.7	4.4
1.0	16.0	66.7	4.2
1.5	13.2	55.0	4.0
2.0	10.8	45.0	3.8
2.5	8.8	36.7	3.6
3.0	7.2	30.0	3.4
3.5	6.0	25.0	3.2
4.0	4.8	20.0	3.0
4.5	3.8	15.8	2.8
5.0	3.2	13.3	2.6

[a] All figures are quoted to an accuracy of one decimal place.
[b] In arbitrary dose units.
[c] Value expressed as a percentage of the unattenuated dose.
[d] Natural logarithms of relative doses (obtained from the 'ln' function on an electronic calculator).

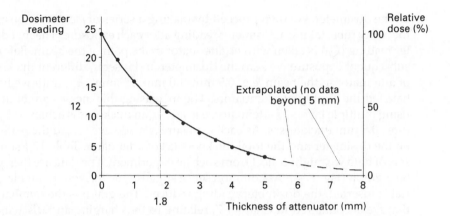

Fig. 17.4 A graph of dosimeter readings plotted against attenuator thickness, using data from Table 17.1. The vertical scale on the right-hand side represents dose readings expressed as a percentage of the maximum reading. The percentages are therefore relative values and have no units. The dashed line is a tentative extrapolation (prediction) of the dose values beyond the maximum attenuator thickness included in the experiment. It is difficult to extend such a curved line accurately. From the graph, the attenuator thickness which would have halved the original dose reading has been obtained. Its value is about 1.8 mm (see worked example in Section 17.1.2.1).

When $x = 0$, i.e. when there was *no* attenuator present, the expression $e^{-\mu x}$ is equal to e^0 and has the value 1 because *any* number raised to the power zero is 1. The equation then becomes:

$$I = \text{constant}$$

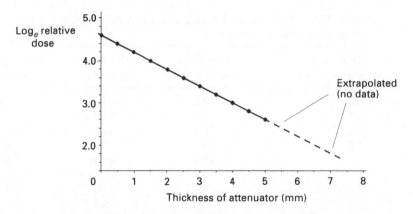

Fig. 17.5 A graph of the natural logarithm value of relative dose plotted against attenuator thickness (data from Table 17.1). The fact that this graph is a straight line tells us that an exponential relationship exists between dose (Q) and attenuator thickness (x). The relationship takes the form $Q \propto e^{-\mu x}$ (see text for details). The dashed line is an extrapolation beyond the maximum attenuator thickness used in the experiment. Extending a straight line accurately is far easier than attempting (as in Fig. 17.4) to extend a curved line. We can therefore rely with more confidence on a prediction made from a straight-line graph.

However, with no attenuator present, the intensity was at its maximum and could be determined from the initial dosimeter reading (Q_0) that we obtained. We shall call this unattenuated intensity I_0. It then follows that I_0 is the constant of proportionality. We can therefore write the general equation as:

$$I = I_0\, e^{-\mu x}$$

where I is the intensity of radiation detected when an attenuator of thickness x is inserted in the beam, I_0 is the intensity of radiation that is detected when *no* attenuator is present, e is the symbol for the exponential constant (its value is approximately 2.72), μ (the Greek letter 'mu') is a quantity which is related to the attenuating properties of the medium through which the beam has passed (it has a different value for different attenuating media and is known as the **total linear attenuation coefficient**) and x is the thickness of the attenuating material in the beam.

As a true exponential decay curve never reaches the horizontal axis, in theory no matter how thick the attenuating medium the radiation intensity never reduces to zero.

17.1.2 Attenuation coefficients

Attenuation coefficients tell us about the effectiveness of different materials as attenuators of radiation. There are several forms of attenuation coefficients employed.

17.1.2.1 Total linear attenuation coefficient

The total linear attenuation coefficient (μ) takes into account the total attenuation caused by all the various absorption and scattering processes involved. It is called a *linear* coefficient because it is linked with a linear dimension, i.e. the thickness (x) of the attenuating medium.

It is possible to rearrange the exponential relationship derived in Section 17.1.1 to separate out the term μ in order to understand what exactly it represents:

$$\mu = -\frac{1}{x}\log_e\frac{I}{I_0}$$

In this equation, the expression I/I_0 represents the factor or fraction by which the intensity of the beam has been reduced as a result of passing through an attenuator of thickness x. The term $1/x$ means *per unit thickness* of attenuator. (The negative sign, which is a consequence of the way we have chosen to express the ratio of intensities, is 'corrected' when we obtain the log value of the ratio.) We can now see the origin of the definition of the total linear attenuation coefficient of a medium:

The total linear attenuation coefficient (μ) is the fraction of X-rays removed from the beam per unit thickness of a medium (Graham et al., 2007).

However, note that μ depends on the *logarithmic* value of the fractional reduction in beam intensity ($\log_e I / I_0$) rather than on the fraction itself.

Table 17.2 Examples of attenuation coefficients for a 50-keV beam

Attenuating medium	Density (kg m^{-3})	Total linear attenuation coefficient (cm^{-1})	Total mass attenuation coefficient (m^2 kg^{-1})
Air[a]	1	0.0002	0.02
Water	1000	0.2	0.02
Aluminium	2700	1.0	0.04
Calcium	1500	1.5	0.1
Lead	11 300	90.0	0.8

[a] Density of air quoted is approximate value at a typical atmospheric pressure of 100 kPa (1000 millibars) and a temperature of 20°C.
Data adapted from Ridgway & Thumm (1973) and Kaye & Laby (1995).

The SI unit of linear attenuation coefficient is *per metre* (m^{-1}), although it is common to see the coefficient quoted in per centimetre (cm^{-1}) (see Table 17.2).

Worked example
As an example, let us refer to the experimental data displayed in Table 17.1 and Figs 17.4 and 17.5. Here, the beam intensity would have been reduced to one-half of its former value as a result of passing through about 1.8 mm of aluminium. Thus, the term $I/I_0 = 0.5$ and the thickness $x = 1.8$ mm. The 'ln' function on an electronic calculator tells us that the natural log value of 0.5 (i.e. $\log_e 0.5$) is -0.693. We can now substitute these values in the expression for μ:

$$\mu = -\frac{1}{x} \log_e \frac{I}{I_0}$$

which then becomes

$$\mu = -\frac{1}{1.8} \times (-0.693)$$

$$= 0.38 \text{ mm}^{-1} \quad (3.8 \text{ cm}^{-1} \text{ or } 380 \text{ m}^{-1})$$

We conclude that for the beam energy employed in the experiment, the total linear attenuation coefficient of aluminium is about 380 m^{-1}. We have included the phrase *for the beam energy employed in the experiment* because the value of the linear attenuation coefficient of an attenuator is different at different beam energies (see Section 17.1.2.3).

The value of the total linear attenuation coefficient depends on the probability of interactions or 'encounters' taking place between the X-ray photons in the beam and the atoms of the attenuating medium. The number of encounters per unit distance travelled through the medium depends on two fundamental properties of the attenuating medium:

(1) *The 'target area' presented to the incoming X-ray photons by each of the atoms in the medium.* Photons are more likely to interact with large atoms (which present them with a bigger target area) than with small atoms. Consequently, the photons are more likely to suffer encounters in a medium with a high proton number (whose atoms possess lots of orbital electrons) than in a medium with a low proton number.

(2)   *The spacing between the atoms in the medium.* Encounters are more likely to occur in a medium in which the atoms are densely packed than in one in which the atoms are more widely spaced. A dense medium therefore provides a higher probability of encounters than a less dense medium even if it has the same proton number.

The linear attenuation coefficient of a medium therefore varies with density *even for the same medium*. This makes it extremely difficult to provide tables of linear attenuation coefficients, because not only must different values be provided to correspond with different beam energies, but the possibility of changes in the density (ρ) of the medium must also be considered. (ρ is the Greek letter 'rho'.)

17.1.2.2   Total mass attenuation coefficient

In order to eliminate the complicating effect of density on linear attenuation coefficient it is usual to divide it by density. The result (μ/ρ) is known as the **mass attenuation coefficient** and its value for a given medium is quite independent of density. The SI unit of mass attenuation coefficient is the *square metre per kilogram* ($m^2\ kg^{-1}$), although it is still sometimes quoted in $cm^2\ g^{-1}$, where ($1\ cm^2\ g^{-1} = 0.1\ m^2\ kg^{-1}$).

   N.B. The authors have found it a helpful teaching strategy to use the acronym **MAC** as an abbreviation for mass attenuation coefficient and **TMAC** for total mass attenuation coefficient. While this practice has proved effective and popular with students, please be warned that the use of these abbreviations is not widely accepted and they should not be quoted in written assignments and research papers!

17.1.2.3   Dependence of attenuation coefficients on beam energy

Table 17.2 shows examples of the values of attenuating coefficients for four different materials when measured using an X-ray beam with a photon energy of 50 keV. It is important to realise that as the photon energy of the beam increases, a greater fraction of the beam will be transmitted through an attenuating medium. The values of μ and TMAC (μ/ρ) will therefore change if the photon energy of the beam is altered. For example, the value of TMAC (μ/ρ) for aluminium, which is $0.3\ m^2\ kg^{-1}$ at a beam energy of 20 keV, falls to less than $0.015\ m^2\ kg^{-1}$ at 150 keV (Kaye & Laby, 1995).

   So far, we have assumed that the photon energy of the beam of radiation does not change during its passage through an attenuator. We have assumed, for example, that if a 50-keV beam enters an attenuator, its photon energy is still 50 keV when it emerges, although its intensity is (of course) reduced. In fact, only a *homogeneous* (monochromatic) beam would behave in this way.

   As we have seen, an X-ray beam is essentially **heterogeneous** (Section 16.2.1). The low-energy component of an X-ray beam is attenuated more severely than the high-energy component, and the effective photon energy of the beam increases as it penetrates further through an attenuator. Consequently, the relationship between the transmitted intensity of such a beam and attenuator thickness does not follow precisely the exponential pattern we have described.

Fortunately, the beam which emerges from a diagnostic X-ray tube has usually been heavily filtered (Section 16.2.3.3) and it approximates quite closely to a monochromatic beam. We therefore find that the intensity of a diagnostic X-ray beam may not, after all, depart *too* drastically from that predicted by the exponential relationship (Hay, 1982).

Worked example
Estimate the percentage reduction in intensity suffered by a near-homogeneous 60-keV X-ray beam when it passes through a sheet of lead 0.25 mm thick. Assume that the TMAC of lead is 0.5 m^2 kg^{-1} for a 60-keV beam. The density of lead is 11.3×10^3 kg m^{-3}.

Because TMAC $(\mu/\rho) = 0.5$

$$\mu = 0.5 \times \rho$$
$$= 0.5 \times 11.3 \times 10^3$$
$$= 5.65 \times 10^3 \text{ m}^{-1}$$

The thickness of attenuator, $x = 0.25$ mm $= 0.25 \times 10^{-3}$. Then from:

$$I = I_0 \, e^{-\mu x}$$

the fractional reduction in intensity, I/I_0, is given by:

$$I/I_0 = e^{-\mu x}$$
$$= e^{-1.41} \text{ (because } \mu x = 5.65 \times 10^3 \times 0.25 \times 10^{-3} = 1.41)$$
$$= 0.24 \text{ (using the } e^x \text{ function on an electronic calculator)}$$

Because the *fractional* reduction in intensity is 0.24, the *percentage* reduction must be 24%. The 0.25-mm sheet of lead therefore reduces the radiation intensity to 24% of its former value.

17.1.2.4 Hounsfield units

Attenuation coefficient measurements are fundamental to the technique of **computerised tomography** (CT). A CT scan involves surveying a series of transverse sections of the patient to compute the total linear attenuation coefficient of each tiny volume element (**voxel**) of tissue comprising the section. These values of attenuation coefficient are used to determine the shade of grey with which the corresponding picture element (**pixel**) is displayed in the CT image.

During the development of CT technology, begun by Godfrey Hounsfield's team in the late 1960s, it was common to express linear attenuation coefficients not in the traditional units we have described, such as cm^{-1} or m^{-1}, but in *arbitrary* measures, which were later to become known as **Hounsfield or CT numbers**. This system of measurement is based on a comparison between the linear attenuation coefficient of a medium (μ_{medium}) and that of water (μ_{water}). The CT number (H) of a medium (usually a type of tissue) is given by:

$$H = 1000 \, (\mu_{medium}/\mu_{water} - 1)$$

On this scale, water has a CT value of *zero* Hounsfield units (0 HU). Substances which attenuate X-rays *more* than water have *positive* values (e.g. the CT number

Table 17.3 Approximate CT numbers for different tissues

Tissue	CT number[a] (HU)
Air	−1000
Fat	−65
Water	0
Kidney	+30
Muscle	+45
Blood (normal)	+55
(coagulated)	+80
Bone (cancellous)	+130
(compact)	>+250

[a] Apart from water, CT numbers may change if X-ray beam energy is altered. The CT numbers quoted represent the centre of the range of values commonly encountered.
Source: Wegener (1992).

for bone is approximately +1000 HU). Substances which attenuate X-rays *less* than water have *negative* values (e.g. the CT number for air is −1000 HU). All the remaining types of body tissues have CT values lying within this range. The tissues examined during a CT scan may therefore span a range of about 2000 HU.

CT numbers are beam energy dependent. Consequently, they may differ for the same tissue on different CT scanners according to the quality of the X-ray beam employed, although, by definition, the CT number of water is always zero. Table 17.3 shows typical CT values for a range of different tissue types. CT numbers and Hounsfield units have been firmly established in CT for many years, but they are not employed outside this field.

Attenuation coefficients help us to predict how much attenuation will occur in a particular set of circumstances. However, they do not help us to explain how or why attenuation occurs. To answer these questions we need to explain the processes which contribute to attenuation.

17.2 Processes of attenuation

Attenuation is caused by absorption and scatter. Four processes need to be described to explain how absorption and scatter occur:

- Unmodified scatter (also known as classical or elastic scatter)
- Photoelectric absorption
- Compton scatter (also known as modified scatter)
- Pair production

We shall now consider each of these processes in detail.

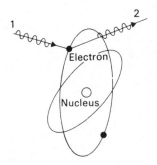

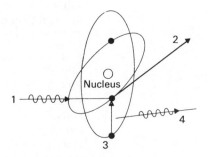

Fig. 17.6 Unmodified scattering of low-energy photon: (1) path of incoming low-energy photon; (2) photon deflected by collision with electron (without loss of energy).

Fig. 17.7 Stages in the process of photoelectric absorption (photoionisation): (1) X-ray photon collides with orbital electron; (2) electron ejected from shell; (3) electron from outer shell fills vacancy; (4) photon of characteristic radiation emitted.

17.2.1   *Unmodified scatter*

This process occurs when the energy of photons in the beam is small compared with the ionisation energy of the atoms of the attenuating medium; i.e. it occurs with *low-energy* radiation. Figure 17.6 shows a photon of radiation interacting with an electron in an atom and 'rebounding' away in a different direction. The photon does not have enough energy to release the electron from its shell, so *none* of its energy is transferred to the electron. The photon does not lose energy, the only change being one of direction, hence the term *unmodified* scatter. This process is not a significant cause of attenuation at the X-ray energies normally used in radiography.

17.2.2   *Photoelectric absorption*

This process of **photoionisation** (Section 15.4.4) occurs when the energy of photons in the beam is equal to or not much greater than the ionisation energy of the atoms of the attenuating medium. The photon transfers *all* its energy to an electron. The electron is then ejected from the atom (Fig. 17.7). The electron ejected is known as a **photoelectron**. Because the photon has given up all its energy, it no longer exists; i.e. true absorption has taken place.

The photoelectric absorption process leaves the ionised atom with an electron vacancy. This is filled by electron transition from a higher energy level, accompanied by the emission of a photon of characteristic radiation. The photon of radiation emitted has an energy which depends on the difference in energy between the two energy states involved in the transition; e.g. an M- to K-shell transition would produce a photon of higher energy than an L- to K-shell transition. The energy also depends on the proton number of the atom in the attenuating medium because it is that which determines the energy levels of the electron shells (Section 4.3.6).

The photon energy of this **characteristic radiation** is generally very low because the materials (e.g. body tissues) with which an X-ray beam interacts usually contain elements (e.g. carbon, oxygen and hydrogen) with low proton numbers and low ionisation energies. This low-energy characteristic radiation itself is quickly absorbed, slightly increasing the internal energy of the medium and producing a very small rise in temperature. The **photoelectron**, which is a by-product of photoionisation, continues onwards through the medium, suffering successive encounters with other atoms, at each stage adding further to the internal energy of the medium. Eventually, when all its kinetic energy is exhausted, the photoelectron is captured by a nearby atom. As a result of these events, *all of* the energy originally carried by the incident X-ray photon is absorbed in the medium.

When photoelectric absorption occurs in materials with *high* proton numbers, electrons are occasionally ejected from the *inner* shells of atoms. The characteristic radiation emitted may then be in the X-ray part of the electromagnetic spectrum. This process is very similar to the production of **characteristic X-rays** in an X-ray tube previously described in Section 16.1.1.2, except that the ionising agents were then high-energy *electrons* from the tube filament rather than X-ray *photons*.

17.2.2.1   Effect of photon energy on photoelectric absorption

The probability of photoelectric absorption occurring is greatest when the energy of the incoming photon just equals the ionisation energy of the atom with which it interacts. If the photon energy is less than the ionisation energy, the process cannot occur. If the photon energy is much above the ionisation energy, the chances of the process occurring are reduced. A golfing analogy may be helpful here.

A golfing analogy
A golfer trying to hole a putt must ensure that the ball is struck at the correct speed as well as in the right direction. If the ball is hit too weakly, it will not reach the hole and therefore cannot drop in. If the ball is hit too strongly, it may pass straight over the hole without dropping in. However, if the ball is struck correctly, with just the right force, its chances of falling into the hole are very much greater, assuming, of course, that its direction is correct. However, we should remind ourselves that this *is* an analogy and that it is the *energy*, rather than the speed of photons, which must be within certain limits for photoelectric absorption to occur. *All* photons, whatever their energy, travel at the same speed, i.e. 3×10^8 m s^{-1}.

Let us return to our golfing analogy. Suppose the golfer decides to visit his golf club's practice putting green. The greenkeeper has produced a remarkably level putting surface, but for reasons best known to himself, he has positioned the three practice holes in a rather unusual manner such that although the holes are placed at different distances from the tee, they are all in exactly the same direction (Fig. 17.8). To reach the more distant holes, the golfer must therefore strike the ball hard enough for it to pass directly over the nearer holes. Our intrepid golfer has no problem striking the ball in the right direction, but he has

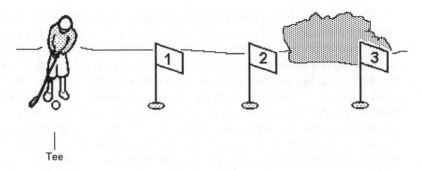

Fig. 17.8 The practice green described in the golfing analogy. All three holes are in line with the teeing off point. Consequently, to reach hole 2, the ball must pass over hole 1 and to reach hole 3, the ball must pass over holes 1 and 2. A ball travelling too quickly to drop into hole 1 may nevertheless be travelling too slowly to reach hole 2.

an unfortunate tendency to overhit or underhit the ball. He therefore decides to concentrate on this aspect of his game. His caddie provides him with a large collection of golf balls and suggests that he try hitting the balls towards the holes with gradually increasing force.

The golfer strikes the first few balls so weakly that they do not even *reach* the first hole! Then things start to improve. He is now striking the balls sufficiently hard to reach the first hole and begins to hole his putts. Success at last!

Still following the caddie's advice, the golfer continues by striking the balls even harder, but now his success rate falls: an increasing number of balls pass right over the first hole instead of falling in. Yet, they do not have sufficient momentum to take them on to the second hole. The golfer becomes despondent. The harder he strikes the balls, the lower his success rate becomes until, suddenly, he begins to strike the balls hard enough to reach and drop into the second hole. At long last his success rate recovers.

When the golfer continues to persevere and strikes the balls with ever-increasing force, his success rate again falls away until he strikes the balls hard enough to reach the third hole and the pattern is repeated. Figure 17.9 shows graphically how the golfer's success rate at holing his putts varies with the force he uses to strike the ball. But what has this to do with photoelectric absorption?

The experiences of the golf balls are analogous to those of X-ray photons interacting with matter. To an incident photon of X-radiation (the golf ball), an atom presents a number of potential targets (the holes) that the photon can interact with (drop into) to produce photoionisation. Interactions which require *low* energy generally involve the *outer-shell* electrons of atoms (represented by the nearer holes on the putting green), whose ionisation energies are low. Interactions requiring *greater* energy involve *inner-shell* electrons (represented by the more distant holes on the putting green), whose ionisation energies are much higher.

Very low energy photons may not have enough energy even to remove electrons from the outer shells of atoms. This is the case with **non-ionising radiation**, such as visible light. However, as the energy of the incoming photons increases, a point is reached where such ionisation suddenly begins to occur. (The success

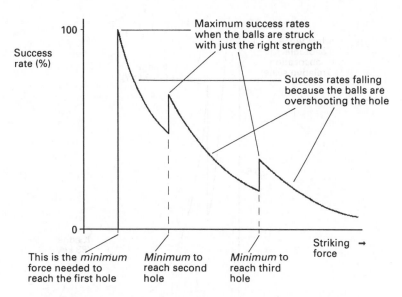

Fig. 17.9   The golfer's record of success at holing his putts on the practice green. He must hit the ball with a certain minimum force even to reach the first hole. Below that minimum level his success rate will be zero because none of his attempts will reach the hole. Hitting the ball slightly too hard results in some attempts passing over hole 1 (but stopping before hole 2). His success rate therefore reduces as his striking force increases. Hitting with a force equal to the hole 2 minimum suddenly raises the success rate because balls can now reach and drop into hole 2. A similar pattern of changes in success rate occurs when the striking force is increased further.

rate suddenly rises.) Further increases in photon energy result in a reduction in the likelihood of ionisation (the balls passing over the hole) until the *next* energy threshold is reached and electrons can be ejected from that level (the balls now reaching the second hole).

   This pattern of change – a gradual fall leading to a sudden increase – in the likelihood of photoelectric absorption occurring is repeated again and again as photon energy increases, until the highest ionisation energy of the atom is reached (the final hole). Further increases in photon energy then result in a final gradual decrease in incidence of photoelectric absorption (Fig. 17.10).

   If the incidence of photoelectric absorption is high, more attenuation will take place, so the MAC will be correspondingly higher. The TMAC is the sum of several coefficients, each related to a different attenuation process. Thus, part of TMAC is due to the attenuation from photoelectric absorption; we shall use the abbreviation PEMAC to represent photoelectric mass attenuation coefficient. The component of the total *linear* attenuation coefficient (μ) due to photoelectric absorption is normally represented by the symbol τ (the Greek letter 'tau'). However, as we saw in Section 17.1.2.2, MAC is the result of dividing the linear attenuation coefficient by density (ρ). Consequently, the value of the PEMAC is τ/ρ. Figure 17.11 shows how PEMAC (τ/ρ) changes with photon energy. Clearly, this is very similar to Fig. 17.10. The discontinuities, where attenuation is suddenly increased, are called **'absorption edges'**. The photon energies at

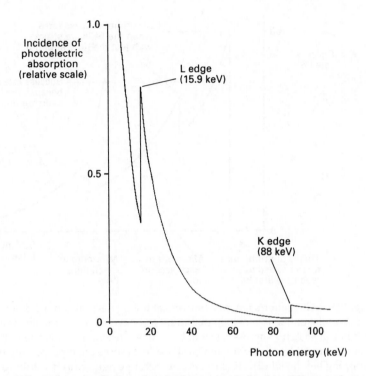

Fig. 17.10   The incidence of photoelectric absorption in lead at different photon energies. The graph shows that (1) the probability of a photoelectric interaction occurring decreases markedly as photon energy increases; (2) there are sudden changes in probability (known as **absorption edges**) at specific photon energies, characteristic of the absorbing material (e.g. 15.9 and 88.0 keV for lead). The overall pattern of change has similarities to that shown in Fig. 17.9.

which they occur depend on the ionisation energies of the medium concerned. Apart from these anomalies, the value of PEMAC is inversely proportional to the cube of the photon energy (E); i.e.

$$\tau/\rho \propto \frac{1}{E^3}$$

Quite small increases in photon energy can therefore produce significant reductions in the amount of photoelectric absorption taking place; e.g. if E is doubled, τ/ρ will be reduced to one-eighth of its former value.

17.2.2.2   Effect of attenuating medium on photoelectric absorption

If the photon energy is kept constant, and a range of different attenuating media are considered, photoelectric absorption occurs to a much greater degree in materials having a high proton number. It has been found that the value of PEMAC is directly proportional to the cube of the proton number (Z) of the attenuator:

$$\tau/\rho \propto Z^3$$

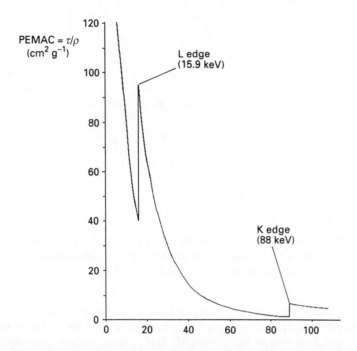

Fig. 17.11 The variation in the photoelectric mass attenuation coefficient (PEMAC) for lead at different photon energies. The value of PEMAC (τ/ρ) for lead falls from around 120 cm^2 g^{-1} at 5 keV to 5 cm^2 g^{-1} at 110 keV. Sudden increases in the value of τ/ρ occur at absorption edges when a further shell of electrons becomes susceptible to photoelectric interactions. For lead ($Z = 82$), at beam energies above 15.9 keV, all the orbital electrons except those in the K shell are potential targets for photoelectric interactions. Above 88 keV, all 82 orbital electrons are potential targets. Note that only two absorption edges are illustrated in the diagram: lead has further L and M edges (e.g. at 13.0, 3.0 and 2.5 keV), but these are grouped too closely together to show clearly on the photon energy scale employed above.

The significance of this is that for this form of attenuation, a slight change in the proton number of the medium produces a large change in the intensity of the transmitted beam of radiation (e.g. if Z is doubled, PEMAC will increase by a factor of eight). This sensitivity of photoelectric absorption to the proton number of the attenuator is of great significance in diagnostic radiography, as we shall see in Chapter 18.

Let us now consider the third of the four attenuation processes.

17.2.3 Compton (modified) scatter

If an X-ray photon has an energy *very much greater* than the ionisation energy of the electron with which it interacts, Compton scattering can take place. Figure 17.12 shows such a photon colliding with an electron. As the photon energy is so great, the electron recoils from the collision and is ejected at speed from its atom. It is sometimes referred to as a *Compton recoil electron* and like the photoelectron described in Section 17.2.2, it may continue to interact with other atoms in the

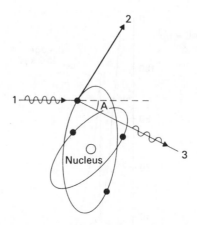

Fig. 17.12 Stages in the process of Compton scattering: (1) X-ray photon collides with orbital electron; (2) electron ejected from atom; (3) photon scattered through angle *A* continues with reduced energy and longer wavelength.

attenuator before finally coming to rest. The photon has transferred some of its energy to the electron in the form of the electron's kinetic energy, so some *absorption* of energy has occurred. The photon suffers a change of direction as a result of the collision, so *scattering* of the photon has also taken place. The photon's energy is reduced, giving the electromagnetic wave with which it is associated a lower frequency and a longer wavelength.

17.2.3.1   Effect of photon energy and attenuating medium on Compton scatter

The loss of energy of the photon depends on the angle (*A*) through which it is scattered (Fig. 17.12). It is greatest when $A = 180°$, i.e. when the photon is scattered back along its original path. The associated wavelength increase does not depend on the photon's original wavelength, nor on the attenuating medium, but the scattering angle *A* tends to be smaller for photons with high energies (short wavelengths) as they are less likely to be deflected off course by collisions with electrons. The incidence of Compton scatter decreases as the photon energy of the beam increases. This affects the mass attenuation coefficient due to the Compton effect (CEMAC), which also decreases as the photon energy is raised. The value of linear attenuation due to Compton effect is usually represented by σ (the Greek letter 'sigma'), so the value of CEMAC is σ/ρ, and

$$\frac{\sigma}{\rho} \propto \frac{1}{E}$$

In contrast to PEMAC, at a fixed photon energy the value of CEMAC depends on the density of the attenuator rather than its proton number.

17.2.4   Pair production

This absorption process can occur only when the photon energy exceeds 1.02 mega electronvolts (MeV). As the photon passes close to the nucleus of an atom in the attenuator, it experiences the strong electric forces around the nucleus caused

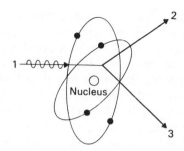

Fig. 17.13 Transformation of a photon into two particles of matter by pair production: (1) X-ray photon passes close to nucleus; (2) negative electron (negatron); (3) positive electron (positron).

by the positive charges on the nuclear protons. As a result, the photon undergoes a dramatic change of state: its energy is transformed into two minute particles of matter, as shown in Fig. 17.13; hence, the process is called **pair production**. The two particles created are electrons. One of the particles is a normal electron, carrying a negative electric charge: it is sometimes referred to as a **negatron**. The other particle is an **anti-electron** or **positron**, which is the anti-matter equivalent of an electron (see Section 4.5.2). A positron has the same mass as that of a negatron, but it carries a *positive* electric charge. The original photon of radiation carried no electric charge. Because the charges on a negatron and positron are equal and opposite in magnitude ($+$ and -1.60×10^{-19} C), the *total* electric charge both before and after the pair-production process is zero; i.e. there has been no *net* gain or loss of electric charge.

Why must the incident photon possess at least 1.02 MeV to trigger pair production? The answer lies in Einstein's equation $E = mc^2$, which enables us to work out the energy equivalent of matter (Section 1.1.3). The pair-production process creates two particles whose total mass (m) is twice the mass of an electron. We know that the mass of an electron is 9.11×10^{-31} kg (Section 4.3). Therefore:

$$m = 2 \times 9.11 \times 10^{-31}$$
$$= 18.22 \times 10^{-31} \text{ kg}$$

Consequently, the energy equivalent (E) of the two particles created during pair production is given by:

$$E = mc^2$$

where the speed of light is $c = 3 \times 10^8$ m s^{-1}.

$$E = 18.22 \times 10^{-31} \times (3 \times 10^8)^2$$
$$= 1.64 \times 10^{-13} \text{ J}$$

However, $1 \text{ eV} = 1.60 \times 10^{-19}$ J. Therefore:

$$E = \frac{1.64 \times 10^{-13}}{1.60 \times 10^{-19}}$$
$$= 1.02 \times 10^6 \text{ eV}$$
$$= 1.02 \text{ MeV}$$

Hence, the combined mass of the negatron and positron created during pair production has a total energy equivalent of 1.02 MeV. Consequently, *at least* 1.02 MeV of energy is required to produce these two particles. The photon of radiation must therefore carry at least 1.02 MeV to trigger pair production.

If the incident photon possesses *more* than 1.02 MeV of energy, the excess is shared equally between the negatron and the positron as kinetic energy. Because all the original energy of the photon has been transferred, the photon no longer exists. The negatron and positron proceed to impart their kinetic energy to other atoms in a series of collisions, which slightly raise the internal energy of the attenuating medium.

17.2.4.1   Annihilation radiation

When the negative electron eventually comes to rest, it is captured by a nearby atom. However, when the positron comes to rest, a much more dramatic fate awaits it! It combines with a normal electron and the two particles annihilate each other in a burst of radiation (Section 4.5.2). The combined mass of the two particles is converted into energy in the form of two photons of **annihilation radiation** (Fig. 17.14). Because a mass equal to twice the mass of an electron has been converted, the total energy released is 1.02 MeV. This energy is equally shared between the two photons of annihilation radiation; i.e. they each possess 0.51 MeV of energy.

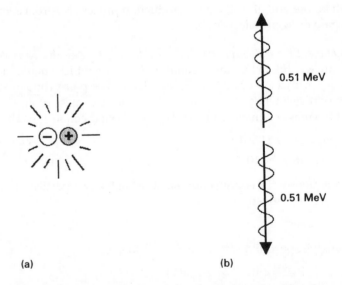

(a)   (b)

Fig. 17.14   (a) A negatron (negative electron) and a positron (positive electron) about to undergo mutual annihilation. Having virtually no kinetic energy, the only energy possessed by the two anti-particles is that stored in their combined mass $(18.2 \times 10^{-31}$ kg), which, according to Einstein's equation $E = mc^2$, is equivalent to 1.02 MeV. (b) Following annihilation, two photons of electromagnetic annihilation radiation are emitted in opposite directions, each carrying precisely half of the 1.02 MeV of available energy.

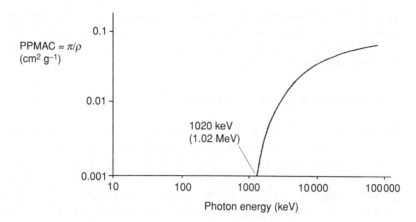

Fig. 17.15 Variation in the pair-production mass attenuation coefficient (PPMAC $= \pi/\rho$) for lead at different photon energies. Note that on this occasion we have used logarithmic scales on both axes. The value of π/ρ is zero at energies below 1.02 MeV because pair production cannot take place unless at least 1.02 MeV of energy is available (see Section 17.2.4). Note that unlike the other processes of attenuation, pair production *increases* as photon energy increases.

Pair production is a process of true absorption because all the energy of the original photon is transformed.

17.2.4.2 Effect of photon energy and attenuating medium on pair production

The mass attenuation coefficient due to pair production (PPMAC) is zero at photon energies below 1.02 MeV and increases as energy increases above that value (Fig. 17.15). The value of linear attenuation coefficient due to pair production is usually represented by π (the Greek letter 'pi'), so the value of PPMAC is π/ρ. For a fixed photon energy, PPMAC is directly proportional to the proton number (Z) of the attenuating material; i.e.

$$\pi/\rho \propto Z$$

It is important to stress that pair production *never* occurs with the X- or gamma-ray energies used in diagnostic radiography.

17.2.5 *Relative importance of the attenuation processes*

We have described four processes of interaction between a beam of ionising radiation and matter: (1) elastic (unmodified) scatter, (2) photoelectric absorption (photoionisation), (3) Compton (modified) scatter and (4) pair production. Which has the greatest effect on the X- and gamma-ray beams used in clinical radiography?

For the radiation energies employed in diagnostic imaging, we can immediately exclude two of the above processes. **Unmodified scatter** can be excluded because its contribution is so small as to be negligible (Graham et al., 2007). **Pair production** can be excluded because it does not take place at all in the diagnostic energy range. We are therefore left with **photoelectric absorption** and **Compton scatter** as the crucial processes of attenuation: which of these is the more important? There is no single, all-embracing answer for this, and depends on the conditions ruling at the time.

17.2.5.1   Consequences of energy dependence

We have seen that both photoelectric and Compton processes are *photon energy dependent* and both processes become less likely as photon energy increases. However, the *manner* in which their influence decreases with photon energy (E) is not the same. Photoelectric absorption decreases steeply with increasing photon energy ($\tau/\rho \propto E^{-3}$), while Compton scatter decreases less dramatically ($\sigma/\rho \propto E^{-1}$). Furthermore, at critical energies which depend on the nature of the attenuating medium, **absorption edges** make the fall in photoelectric absorption quite erratic (Section 17.2.2.1). Figure 17.16 shows an example of how the MACs for photoelectric and Compton effects change with increasing photon energy over the diagnostic range of energies. At the low-energy end of the range, representing the low-kilovolt X-rays used for **mammography**, up to 75% of the beam attenuation in the soft tissues of the body can be attributed to the effect of photoelectric absorption, with the Compton effect playing a relatively minor role.

Conversely, at the high-energy end of the range, representing the high-kilovolt X-rays sometimes used for chest radiography and the gamma-ray energies used in **radionuclide imaging**, only 15–20% of beam attenuation in soft tissues is attributable to photoelectric absorption. The Compton effect plays a dominant role at these energies.

At a beam energy between 30 and 40 keV, representing X-rays generated at around 55 kV, photoelectric and Compton effects make a roughly equal contribution to attenuation in soft tissues (Hay, 1982).

In radiotherapy, where beam energies extending well beyond 1 MeV are employed, the Compton effect and pair production are the dominant attenuation processes.

17.2.5.2   Consequences of attenuator dependence

We have seen that as well as being photon energy dependent, the photoelectric and Compton mass attenuation coefficients (τ/ρ and σ/ρ) are affected by the nature of the attenuating medium in which the interactions take place. Photoelectric attenuation increases rapidly with the effective proton number (A) of the attenuator:

$$\tau/\rho \propto A^3$$

while Compton attenuation increases with its density (ρ):

$$\sigma/\rho \propto \rho$$

The result is that the relative importance of photoelectric and Compton attenuation changes for different materials even at the same photon energy (Fig. 17.16).

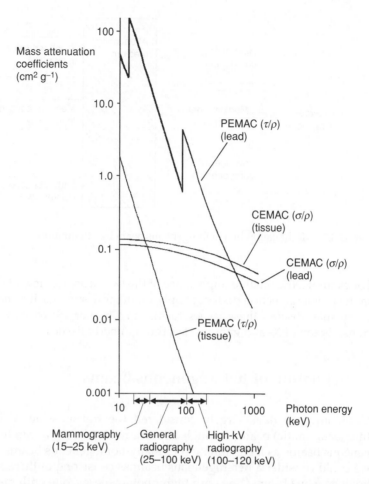

Fig. 17.16 The variations in Compton and photoelectric mass attenuation coefficients (CEMAC and PEMAC) at different photon energies. Curves for two different materials (lead and body tissue) have been included. Because Compton scatter depends on density rather than proton number, its linear attenuation coefficient (σ) is only density dependent. The values of the mass attenuation coefficient (σ/ρ) for the two materials are therefore very similar. Note the steady reduction in CEMAC as photon energy increases. In contrast, at a given photon energy, PEMAC depends greatly on proton number ($\tau/\rho \propto Z^3$). The values of τ/ρ for tissue ($Z \approx 7$) are therefore very much less than the values for lead ($Z \approx 82$). Note the steep reduction in PEMAC as photon energy increases. Note also the absence of absorption edges on the tissue curve. This is because the ionisation energies of the elements from which tissue is formed are extremely low (measured in electronvolts rather than kiloelectronvolts). They therefore do not appear in the energy range depicted. The dominant roles of photoelectric attenuation in mammography, and Compton attenuation in high-kilovolt radiography, are also demonstrated (see Section 17.2.5.1).

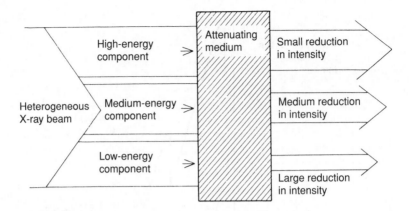

Fig. 17.17   Modification of a heterogeneous beam by attenuation.

For example, the relative importance of the two processes in soft tissues quoted in the previous section does *not* apply for other tissues, such as bone.

We shall discuss these issues further in Chapter 18, when we explore the transmission of X- and gamma rays through body tissues.

17.3   Attenuation of heterogeneous beams

Until now, we have largely considered the transmission of homogeneous (monochromatic) beams through a medium. However, we can think of heterogeneous beams as a combination of many homogeneous beams. For example, we could consider a heterogeneous beam as consisting of three superimposed homogeneous beams: one with high photon energy, one with medium photon energy and one with low photon energy.

Figure 17.17 shows such a beam being transmitted through an attenuating medium. We can see that the high-energy component of the beam is attenuated to a lesser degree than the low-energy component. The transmitted (emergent) beam, although reduced in intensity, contains a greater proportion of high-energy photons than did the original beam before attenuation. Most of the low-energy photons are absorbed or scattered from the beam. With sufficient attenuation we can transform a beam which contains a wide range of photon energies into a beam which is almost homogeneous, mainly containing high-energy photons.

A similar effect can be seen if a beam of white light is passed through a coloured sheet of glass. The white light is heterogeneous because it contains many different photon energies, but after passing through the glass only a narrow range of photon energies remain and the emergent light beam is essentially homogeneous (monochromatic).

The effect of attenuation we have been describing is termed **filtration**, and the attenuators used for the purpose of modifying the beam in this way are known as filters. An analogy from the world of athletics may help with our understanding of the idea of filtration. In athletic competitions, preliminary rounds known as 'heats' are used to 'filter out' the weaker competitors, so that by the time the final round is reached the quality of those taking part is high. We can think of filters of radiation as having the same sort of effect on X-ray photons as athletic heats do on the competitors.

17.3.1 Do photons suffer exhaustion?

Those successful contenders who reach the final round in our imaginary athletic competition may experience some exhaustion from the effort of having to qualify through the early rounds. It is interesting to realise that photons of electromagnetic radiation have no corresponding experience. Photons in the emergent beam shown in Fig. 17.17 have successfully negotiated the attenuator because they managed to pass through it completely unscathed, without suffering *any* interactions at all. The photons which emerge from the attenuator are in exactly the same state (and carry the same energy) as when they entered, but of course they are reduced in number. When an X-ray intensifying screen is exposed in its cassette, the primary-beam X-ray photons causing it to fluoresce have travelled from the target of the X-ray tube through the tube filters and through the patient, without suffering a single interaction with matter. Perhaps even more surprising is the thought that the photons of starlight that we see in the night sky may have travelled billions upon billions of miles for millions upon millions of years before reaching us. In all that time, and over all that distance, they have suffered not a single interaction with matter until they encounter the retina at the back of our eye. These observations perhaps confirm that matter is a relatively rare occurrence in the universe and that matter itself mainly consists of the empty space between its particles!

17.3.2 Filtration

Any medium through which a heterogeneous beam of radiation passes modifies the spectrum of the beam. Figure 17.18 illustrates the spectrum of a beam of X-rays before and after passing through a filter. It shows that although the

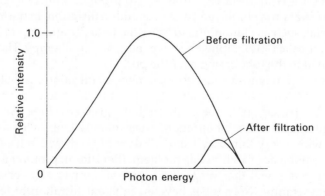

Fig. 17.18   The effect of filtration on the spectrum of a heterogeneous X-ray beam.

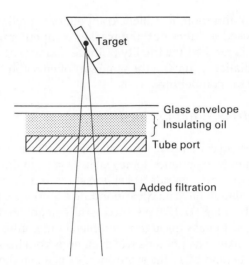

Fig. 17.19   Attenuation of an X-ray beam as it leaves the X-ray tube.

intensity of the beam is reduced, its quality is improved because the low-energy component is virtually removed from the beam. Very low energy photons are not needed in the beam because in radiotherapy they do not penetrate to the deeper tissues of the body, which are often being treated, and in diagnostic work they do not reach the X-ray film and therefore do not contribute to the formation of the radiographic image. In both branches of radiography, low-energy photons are positively harmful, as they produce undesirable doses of radiation to the patient's skin.

For biological safety reasons, therefore, beam filtration is an important feature of equipment design. Some degree of filtration is inevitable because an X-ray beam has to pass through parts of the X-ray tube itself before emerging from the tube port, e.g. (a) the target, (b) the glass envelope, (c) the insulating oil and (d) the tube port. Figure 17.19 shows the passage of a beam from the tube target.

In general-purpose diagnostic X-ray tubes, this *inherent* filtration is equivalent to the filtration due to a layer of aluminium at least 1 mm thick; i.e. the inherent filtration is equivalent to '1-mm Al'. To produce sufficient effect on the beam, extra filtration is employed, known as **added filtration**, in the form of thin sheets of metal, such as aluminium, to bring the total filtration up to 2.0- or 2.5-mm Al in diagnostic radiography and even more in radiotherapy. The added filters are attached to the tube casing over the port.

For some diagnostic purposes, an inherent filtration equivalent to 1-mm Al is far too high and the X-ray tube design is modified to minimise inherent filtration. The passage of the beam through the glass envelope makes a considerable contribution to inherent filtration. Consequently, employing a **metal tube envelope** with a very thin **beryllium window** through which the beam can emerge is a common approach to this problem. (Beryllium, proton number 4, is a more radiolucent metal than aluminium, proton number 13.) For example, modern mammography X-ray tubes have an inherent filtration of less than 1 mm of beryllium.

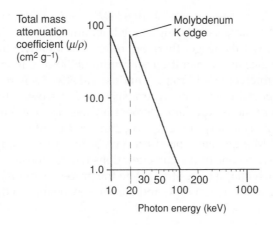

Fig. 17.20 Variation in the total mass attenuation coefficient (TMAC $= \mu/\rho$) for molybdenum at different photon energies. Logarithmic scales have been employed. The molybdenum K absorption edge occurs at 20.002 keV. At energies just below this value, μ/ρ is low and attenuation is minimal even though the radiation is of low penetration. This relatively transparent 'window' allows the characteristic radiation, emitted by a molybdenum X-ray tube target, to be transmitted with minimal attenuation (see Section 17.3.2.1).

Filter materials have to be chosen with care to ensure that the beam is modified in the way desired and to ensure that the added filtration is not so thin as to be impractical to manufacture accurately. Aluminium is the most common filter used in diagnostic radiography, while copper, tin and lead may be used in radiotherapy.

17.3.2.1 Effect of absorption edges in a filter

A filter may exhibit rather unusual behaviour at beam energies close to the energies of its **absorption edges** (Section 17.2.2.1). Let us take the element molybdenum as an example. Figure 17.20 shows the way the attenuation coefficient of molybdenum changes at different photon energies. Consider, particularly, the molybdenum K absorption edge, which occurs at an energy of 20.002 keV. At photon energies *just below* this level, the attenuation coefficient is at a minimum and transmission through molybdenum is at a maximum. In other words, molybdenum is almost transparent to radiation whose photon energy is just under 20.002 keV. Molybdenum is a much better attenuator (and a much worse transmitter) of radiation, whose energy is above 20.002 keV or significantly below 20.002 keV. For the energy range from (say) 17 to 20 keV, molybdenum therefore presents a transparent *window* of transmission, while for energies outside this range molybdenum is relatively opaque.

The molybdenum transmission window finds a particular application in mammography. X-ray tubes designed to operate at the low kilovoltages employed in mammography commonly use molybdenum as their target material because its K-series characteristic X-ray emissions make a valuable contribution to X-ray output (Section 16.2.3.1). The photon energies of the most prominent of these emissions lie in the range 17.4–19.6 keV, *energies to which a molybdenum filter is preferentially transparent*. Using a molybdenum filter in conjunction with a molybdenum X-ray tube target therefore offers special advantages. The most useful X-ray energies are transmitted with minimal loss of intensity, while the lower energies which only add to patient dose are effectively removed. Molybdenum is not a special case in being transparent to its own characteristic radiation. K-series emissions from *any* element always occur at energies just below the energy of its K absorption edge; the same is true of the L series and L edge, M series and M edge, etc. The effect on a beam of the K edge of a filter material must always be one of the considerations when choosing beam filtration.

In the next chapter, we shall relate the processes of interaction we have been describing to the action of X- and gamma-ray beams on living tissues.

Chapter 18

X-Ray and Gamma-Ray Interaction with Tissues

Transmission of X- and gamma-ray beams through body tissues
  Tissue differentiation in the radiographic image
Effects of scattered radiation on patient dose, staff dose and image quality
  Practical points about scatter

Having explained the processes of attenuation which occur when a radiation beam interacts with matter, we can investigate the particular case of a beam passing through living body tissues. We shall then be better able to understand how the beam which is transmitted through the patient may be used to produce an image.

18.1 Transmission of X- and gamma-ray beams through body tissues

We have seen that when a beam of diagnostic X- or gamma rays interacts with matter, two attenuation processes occur:

(1) Photoelectric absorption
(2) Compton (modified) scatter

Because living tissue is a form of matter, consisting of the same kinds of atoms and fundamental particles, it is reasonable to suppose that these two same processes occur when body tissues are exposed to radiation. We saw in Chapter 17 that different materials produce different degrees of attenuation, according to the values of their total attenuation coefficients. Different types of body tissues have different total attenuation coefficients too and therefore attenuate X- or gamma-ray beams differently. We know that the value of the total attenuation coefficient of a substance depends largely on its proton number (Z). Let us therefore examine the proton numbers of some types of body tissues. Tissues are composed of many different chemical elements, each with its own specific value of proton number, but we can make an estimate of the average or effective proton number of a particular tissue, taking into account the individual elements present and their relative abundance in the tissue. For example:

(1) Bone has an effective proton number of about 14 because bone contains calcium ($Z = 20$) and phosphorus ($Z = 15$) as well as lighter elements.

(2) Soft tissues (muscle, fat, etc.) have an effective proton number of about 7 because the heavier elements are less abundant.

If we assume, then, that for bone, $Z = 14$ and for soft tissue, $Z = 7$, we can see how X- or gamma-ray beams would be affected by interaction with each of these tissues.

The photoelectric absorption process is very dependent on the proton number of the absorbing medium. We saw in Section 17.2.2.2 that for its attenuation coefficient PEMAC, τ/ρ is proportional to Z^3. We may infer, therefore, that at a particular beam energy, PEMAC for bone is eight times (2^3) higher than PEMAC for soft tissue because the proton number of bone is twice that of soft tissue. Hence, bone causes a lot more photoelectric absorption than does soft tissue.

The Compton scattering process is relatively independent of the proton number of the scattering medium. Consequently, we may infer that bone and soft tissue cause roughly the same amount of Compton scattering of an X- or gamma-ray beam.

Let us now see what this means in practice.

18.1.1 Tissue differentiation in the radiographic image

In diagnostic radiography, X-ray beams are generated over a wide range of tube voltages, extending from as low as 20 kV (e.g. for mammography) to as much as 150 kV (e.g. for high-kilovoltage chest radiography). Depending on the type of high-tension generator used, this range of tube kilovoltage may represent a range of effective photon energies, which extends from about 15 to 100 keV (Hay, 1982). As we saw in Section 17.2.5.1, the relative importance of the two main attenuation processes changes considerably over this range. We shall, therefore, separately consider the upper and lower parts of this kilovoltage and photon energy range.

18.1.1.1 Lower range of beam energies

If we use a beam energy for which photoelectric absorption is the main process of attenuation (i.e. the lower range energies used in diagnostic radiography), soft tissues will transmit a much greater part of the beam than will bone. In Fig. 18.1, the parts of the X-ray film receiving radiation which has passed through soft tissue will be exposed to a far greater extent than the parts which receive the radiation transmitted through bone. When processed, the film will show dark areas where the beam passed through soft tissues and light areas where the beam passed through bone. Because of this contrast of tones a recognisable image of the bone will be produced.

Of course, the thickness of the tissue through which the beam passes also affects the amount of transmission. A thick layer of soft tissue may produce the same attenuation of the beam as a thin layer of bone. However, as long as we use beam energies for which photoelectric absorption is the main cause of attenuation, on our radiographs we can expect to be able to differentiate

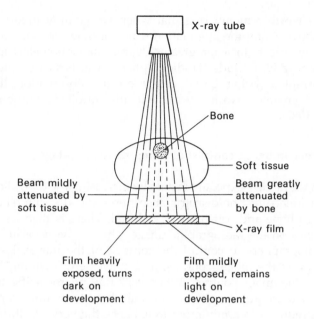

Fig. 18.1   Formation of diagnostic image on X-ray film due to differential absorption in tissues.

well between different types and different thicknesses of tissues. This is why tube voltages of 20–65 kV (giving effective beam energies of 15–40 keV) provide such excellent bone and soft-tissue differentiation in the radiographic image.

18.1.1.2   Upper range of beam energies

If we use higher beam energies, for which the Compton effect is the dominant attenuation process, the differentiation between bone and soft tissue is considerably reduced, sometimes to the point where bone seems almost invisible against a soft-tissue background. This is because the marked difference in effective proton number between bone (or other calcified tissue) and soft tissue is no longer relevant: Compton attenuation depends on *density* rather than on proton number (Section 17.2.3.1). However, tissue differentiation is still present and in some instances, may even be enhanced at high kilovoltages. For example, the differences between low-density air-filled structures (e.g. the airways of the respiratory tract) and their higher density surroundings are well differentiated, and peripheral pulmonary blood vessels are well demonstrated against air-filled lung tissue in a high-kilovoltage chest radiograph (Jackson, 1964). This ability of the Compton effect to differentiate air-filled structures may be the rationale behind the use of high-kilovoltage techniques in plain radiography of the larynx and trachea. It is also one of the justifications for high-kilovoltage chest radiography (Evans, 1991).

It is worth remembering that when we employ tube voltages of 100 kV and above, Compton attenuation is responsible for tissue differentiation (and image contrast) to a far greater degree than photoelectric attenuation. The rather negative attitude of radiographers towards the Compton effect is perhaps unwarranted, being based solely on the observation that the Compton effect generates scatter which, if uncontrolled, reduces image contrast (Hay, 1982).

18.1.1.3 Effect on image contrast of changing tube voltage

When we modify exposure factors by increasing the tube kilovoltage, we lower the incidence of photoelectric absorption and the difference in transmission through bone and soft tissue is reduced. There is then less contrast between the tones on the radiographic image. This is a very useful method available to radiographers to control the contrast of the image. Raising the kilovoltage lowers the image contrast, and conversely, lowering the kilovoltage increases the image contrast. When very tiny **microcalcifications** are being examined, as in radiography of the female breast (mammography), tube kilovoltage is reduced to a minimum to enhance the very small differences in attenuation so that they may be recorded on the X-ray film. Modification of milliampere seconds *without* changing the kilovoltage does *not* cause alterations in image contrast, because in this case the photon energy of the beam is not affected, and there is therefore no change in the incidence of photoelectric absorption.

18.2 Effects of scattered radiation

As a beam of X- or gamma radiation passes through tissues, some of the photons are scattered due to the Compton process. This scattered radiation makes an important contribution to the energy or **dose** absorbed by the tissue. The total dose received by the tissues is the sum of the dose caused by absorption of the primary beam and the dose caused by absorption of the scattered radiation.

Any radiation doses to living tissues can be damaging, whether from scattered radiation or the primary beam (Section 21.2.2). Therefore, in diagnostic radiography, every effort must be made to ensure that the tissues receive only the very minimum dose consistent with the production of a useful radiograph. To control scatter effectively we need to know what determines how much scatter will be generated.

Because scattered radiation arises from the Compton effect, the amount of scatter generated depends on how much Compton scattering takes place. The volume of tissue irradiated by the primary beam also has an important influence on the quantity of scatter produced. Clearly, more scattered radiation would be generated if a large volume of tissue were irradiated than if a small volume of tissue were irradiated. In practice, therefore, the radiation beam field size (i.e.

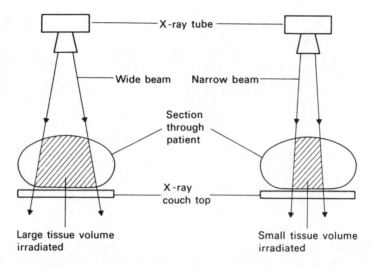

Fig. 18.2 The effect of beam collimation reducing the volume of tissue irradiated.

the diaphragm, cone or collimator setting) can be used to limit the quantity of scattered radiation produced.

In radiographic imaging, scatter has three important effects:

(1) It contributes to the radiation dose received by the patient.
(2) It contributes to the radiation dose received by the staff.
(3) It degrades the quality of the radiographic image by reducing contrast.

18.2.1   *Effect of scatter on patient dose*

The amount of scatter generated inside the patient may be minimised by beam collimation ('coning down') because this reduces the volume of tissue irradiated by the primary beam (Fig. 18.2). When the energy of the primary beam is low, i.e. at low kilovoltages, the scattered radiation is also of low energy and is likely to be absorbed in the patient in regions close to the area under examination. If the primary beam energy is raised, by increasing the tube kilovoltage, the scatter becomes more penetrating. More scatter will then escape from the patient and more will produce radiation doses in parts of the patient remote from the original exposure. Figure 18.3 illustrates how the dose received by the gonads during chest radiography may be affected by beam energy.

18.2.2   *Effect of scatter on staff dose*

With low-kilovoltage exposures little scattered radiation leaves the deep tissues of the patient. (It is mostly absorbed inside the patient.). With high-kilovoltage exposure more of the scatter escapes from the patient and becomes a hazard

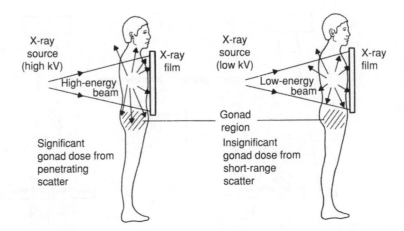

Fig. 18.3   The effect of X-ray tube kilovoltage (and therefore beam energy) on gonad dose. Owing to the more penetrating nature of high-kilovoltage scatter, the gonad region may receive a higher radiation dose than from low-kilovoltage scatter. However, the situation is far more complicated than the diagrams suggest. Backscatter from the film support, forward scatter from the beam collimator and the use of a lead-rubber waist apron may further modify the gonad dose.

to the members of staff in the vicinity. Beam collimation is again an effective method of reducing the danger, but ray-proof barriers and protective clothing offer extra protection.

18.2.3   Effect of scatter on image quality

Scattered radiation reaching the X-ray film or other image receptor causes overall fogging of the image, reducing the information it records. The radiographer can overcome this by reducing the amount of scatter being produced, e.g. by beam collimation and, in some cases, by applying 'compression' techniques to displace overlying tissues, thus reducing the volume of tissue irradiated, as shown in Fig. 18.4 (Ball & Price, 1995). The radiographer can also protect the film from scattered radiation by the use of secondary radiation grids (Fig. 18.5) and backscatter protection underneath the film (Fig. 18.6) (Ball & Price, 1995).

18.2.4   Practical points about scatter

Before we leave the topic of scattered radiation it is worth pointing out three of the practical consequences of the properties of scattered radiation:

(1)   The photon energy of scattered radiation is less than the photon energy of the primary beam from which it is derived. If we are exposed to scattered radiation, we are likely to absorb it because it is of low energy and it therefore constitutes a serious hazard to health.

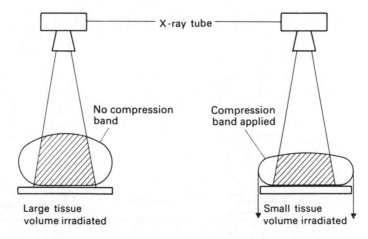

Fig. 18.4 The effect of a compression band in reducing the volume of tissue irradiated. Note that the effect is one of *displacement* of tissue rather than true compression.

(2) As beam energy increases, the angle at which scatter is emitted tends to reduce (Section 17.2.3.1). Consequently, at high tube voltages more of the scattered radiation is emitted in the general direction of the primary beam than at lower voltages; i.e. there is more **forward scatter** generated in high-kilovoltage radiography than in low-kilovoltage radiography. Because the film is in the direct path of forward scatter, image fogging may cause serious problems in high-kilovoltage radiography. In these circumstances, great care must be taken to protect the film from forward scatter, either by using

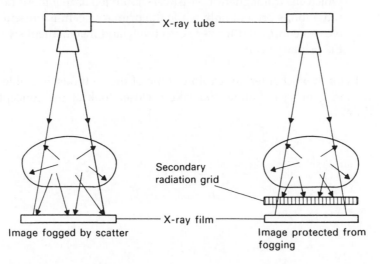

Fig. 18.5 The action of a secondary radiation grid in protecting the radiographic image from fogging by scatter from patient.

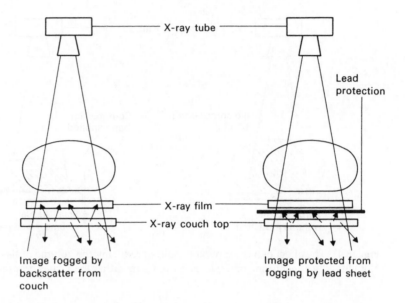

Fig. 18.6   The action of lead backing layer in protecting the image from fogging by backscatter from the couch top.

an efficient secondary radiation grid or by using an **air-gap technique** (Ball & Price, 1995).

(3)   It is not unknown for visitors to the imaging department, with limited knowledge of radiation science, to imagine that scattered radiation wanders around the X-ray room, or is released from the body of a patient, for some time after the X-ray exposure has ended. Consideration of the speed at which electromagnetic rays travel should tell us that this is not so. Scattered radiation is present only while the primary beam is present. In that sense we can control scatter very effectively and instantaneously by turning off the primary beam.

   In our next chapter, we explore some of the methods available for *measuring* X- and gamma radiation and take a closer look at the concept of radiation dose.

Chapter 19

X-Ray and Gamma-Ray
Measurements (Dosimetry)

19.1   Absorbed dose

When matter is irradiated with ionising radiation it is important to know how much energy is transferred from the radiation to the material exposed. This is particularly so where the material is living tissue because the effect of radiation on tissue is closely related to the amount of energy it absorbs. The quantity of energy transferred from radiation is known as the **absorbed dose** and is defined as the energy absorbed per unit mass of the medium.

19.1.1   Units of absorbed dose

The SI unit of absorbed dose is the **gray** (Gy), which represents 1 joule of energy absorbed per kilogram of material. An older unit of absorbed dose called the rad may still be encountered:

$$1 \text{ rad} = 10^{-2} \text{ Gy}$$

In diagnostic imaging, the levels of absorbed dose are likely to be expressed in milligray (mGy) or microgray (μGy).

The value of absorbed dose depends on both the photon energy of the beam and the type of absorbing medium. A high-energy beam produces *less* absorbed dose than does a low-energy beam of the same intensity because more of its photons are transmitted without absorption. A material having a high effective proton number receives a higher absorbed dose than does a material of low proton number exposed to the same beam because more absorption interactions take place.

Dose can be expressed either in terms of a cumulative value, totalled over a period of time quoted in grays, or in terms of dose rate, which is the dose absorbed per unit time, quoted in grays per second (Gy s^{-1}). Cumulative dose and dose rate are related: if dose rate is constant, then:

Cumulative dose = dose rate × time

where time represents the length of time over which the dose is measured.

Worked examples

(1) A dose rate of l0 mGy h^{-1} continuing for 30 min would give:

$$\text{Cumulative dose} = 10 \times \frac{30}{60}$$

$$= 5\,\text{mGy}$$

(2) If a total dose of 45 μGy is received in a time of 15 min, the dose rate is given by:

$$\text{Dose rate} = \frac{\text{total dose}}{\text{time}}$$

$$= \frac{45}{15}$$

$$= 3\,\mu\text{Gy min}^{-1}$$

There is another method of expressing radiation dose, which more closely reflects the effects of radiation on living tissues. This measurement, known as **dose equivalent**, is discussed in Chapter 21 when we explore the principles of radiation protection.

19.2 Measurement of dose

To measure directly the quantity of energy a medium absorbs due to exposure to radiation is technically a very difficult task, which is not feasible to undertake in the clinical situation. In practice, therefore, the value of absorbed dose is determined indirectly by using one of the effects of radiation which can be more easily measured. Suitable effects include the following:

(1) Ionisation of air
(2) Fogging of photographic emulsion
(3) Thermoluminescence

(4) Scintillation
(5) Ionisation of a semiconductor

Measuring instruments which employ any of these effects as a means of arriving at an estimation of absorbed dose are known as dosemeters or dosimeters. We shall now look further at the first three effects noted above and examine how they are used as the basis of working dosimeters. Scintillation has a special application in the detection of gamma-ray photons in radionuclide imaging. We shall explore this application in Chapter 20.

19.2.1   Ionisation of air

Air in its normal state is a good electrical insulator because it contains no conduction electrons. If, however, air is exposed to X- or gamma rays, some of the photons of radiation release electrons from the atoms in the air, ionising it and enabling it to conduct electricity. The more radiation to which the air is exposed, the better able it is to conduct electric current. By measuring the electrical conductivity of the air the quantity of radiation causing the ionisation may be estimated.

19.2.1.1   Exposure

The measure of the strength of an X- or gamma-ray beam by the quantity of charge (Q) on the ions produced per unit mass (m) of air is called **exposure** (E). Consequently:

$$E = \frac{Q}{m}$$

Note that this use of the term 'exposure' is rather different from its more general usage in radiography as a shortened form of 'exposure factors'.

Exposure unit
The SI unit of radiation exposure is the coulomb per kilogram ($C\ kg^{-1}$), which is defined as the X- or gamma-ray exposure which produces a total positive or negative ion charge of 1 coulomb per kilogram of dry air. An older unit of exposure, the roentgen (R) is still quite popular:

$$1\ R = 2.58 \times 10^{-4}\ C\ kg^{-1}$$

It is possible to convert an exposure measurement into the value of absorbed dose, which it represents by the use of a conversion factor; e.g.

Absorbed dose = exposure × conversion factor

However, this is not quite as straightforward as it seems, because the conversion factor is not constant. Its value is not only different for different materials, but it may also vary for the *same* material at different beam energies.

The dosimeters which employ the air ionisation effect of radiation use an **ionisation chamber** as the detection device. We shall look at two types of ionisation-chamber dosimeters, the 'free-air' ionisation chamber and the 'thimble' chamber. The first is a laboratory instrument, while the second is used as a clinical dosimeter.

19.2.1.2 Free-air ionisation chamber

Although this instrument is not used in hospitals, it demonstrates more clearly than other dosimeters the principles of how ionisation-chamber measurements are made. The free-air chamber is used to measure radiation exposure. It essentially consists of a box of air. A known mass of air is exposed to a beam of X- or gamma rays and the ions produced in the air are collected on two electrically charged metal plates. The total charge collected is measured with an instrument called an electrometer. The amount of charge (Q) is therefore known and the mass of air (m) from which it was collected is also known. Calculating the value of Q/m gives a direct measure of exposure.

Worked example
A free-air ionisation chamber was irradiated with X-rays. The total resulting electric charge, collected on the plates of the ionisation chamber, was 5 μC. The charge originated from the ionisation created a 1-litre volume of dry air. The density of air was 1.18 kg m^{-3} under the prevailing conditions of atmospheric pressure and temperature. Calculate the radiation exposure involved.

To calculate exposure (E), we need to know the mass (m) of the irradiated air from which charge was collected and the total electric charge (Q) created by the ions released in that mass of air. From the data we are given, the value of charge collected was:

$$Q = 5 \; \mu C$$
$$= 5 \times 10^{-6} \; C$$

We can derive the mass of air from the figures provided for its density (ρ) and volume (V):

$$m = \rho \times V$$

where $\rho = 1.18$ kg m^{-3} and $V = 1 \, L = 1000 \, cm^3 = 10^{-3} \, m^3$.

$$m = 1.18 \times 10^{-3} \; kg$$

We can now calculate the exposure (E):

$$E = \frac{Q}{m}$$
$$= \frac{5 \times 10^{-6}}{1.18 \times 10^{-3}}$$
$$= 4.2 \times 10^{-3} \; C \, kg^{-1}$$

The exposure concerned was therefore 4.2 mC kg^{-1} (equivalent to about 16 R). Note that the value for air density changes with temperature and pressure. The value quoted is for dry air at a temperature of 20°C and an atmospheric pressure of 100 kPa or 1000 millibars (Kaye & Laby, 1995). Temperature and

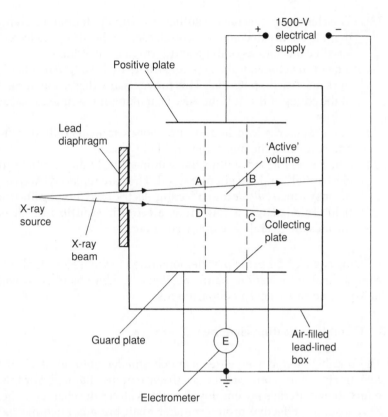

Fig. 19.1   The free-air ionisation chamber. Charges resulting from ionisation of the air in the volume ABCD are largely confined within the collecting electric field (bounded by dashed lines). Those charges which stray beyond the collecting field, and are therefore 'lost', are replaced by an equal number of charges straying *into* the collecting field from outside its boundaries. The sensitive electrometer is thus able to monitor correctly the total charge originating from ionisation of the air in ABCD.

pressure therefore need to be monitored and, if necessary, the value of air density modified accordingly.

Design features of the free-air chamber
Figure 19.1 shows the basic design of the free-air chamber. Some of the features on the diagram require further explanation.

(1)   The lead diaphragm restricts the size and shape of the radiation beam passing through the chamber. The dimensions of the beam must be known so that the volume ABCD and therefore the mass of air from which ions are collected can be calculated.
(2)   The electrically charged plates are sufficiently far apart to allow ions released by the ionising effect of the radiation to dissipate their kinetic energy by undergoing collisions with other atoms. This increases to a maximum the total charge produced.

(3) The charged plates have a sufficiently high potential difference applied to them to ensure that *all* the ions released in the air are collected before they have a chance to recombine and form neutral atoms.

(4) One of the charged plates is constructed with a 'guard plate' around it at the same (earth) potential. This prevents any distortion of the electric field at the edges of the volume ABCD, making it possible to calculate its exact volume.

(5) The chamber is lead lined to prevent extraneous radiation from entering and distorting the measurements being made.

(6) Some ions formed within the volume ABCD move out of the collecting electric field and are not measured. They are replaced by an equal number of ions formed *outside* the collecting electric field moving into the measuring field. This balance is known as **electronic equilibrium**. It is this which dictates the overall size of the chamber.

Using some of the principles demonstrated in the free-air ionisation chamber, a much smaller ionisation chamber called a thimble chamber is available for use in X-ray and radiotherapy departments.

19.2.1.3 Thimble ionisation chamber

The thimble chamber encloses a much smaller volume of air than does the free-air chamber in order to reduce the size of the chamber. For this reason, **air-equivalent** materials are employed in the walls of the chamber. These materials have a similar effective proton number to air but are much more dense. Thus, they allow the chamber to behave as if it contained a much greater volume of air than is actually present. When exposed to radiation, ions are liberated from the walls of the chamber as well as from the air inside the chamber, so maintaining electronic equilibrium. Because of the use of air-equivalent chamber walls, the size of the chamber can be dramatically reduced from a cumbersome laboratory instrument to a small chamber which may be the size of a thimble. A larger chamber can be employed if greater sensitivity is required.

Figure 19.2 shows the construction of a typical thimble chamber. The wall or *cap* is made of bakelite or plastic coated on the inside with a layer of graphite.

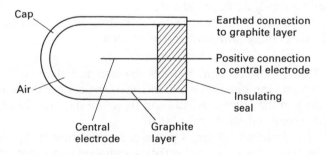

Fig. 19.2   Construction of a thimble chamber.

Both of these combinations are air equivalent. Graphite is included to act as an electrical conductor forming part of the electric circuit needed to collect the ions liberated by the exposure to radiation.

The central electrode is a thin rod of aluminium. It forms the other part of the ion collecting circuit. The central electrode is made positive with respect to the earthed graphite, so electrons released from the cap and from the air inside the chamber are collected on the central rod. The rod is held in position by an insulating seal which closes off the chamber.

On some models, the chamber is connected by a cable to the electrical measuring instrument and power supply. Alternatively, the ionisation chamber (no longer thimble shaped) may be built into the same housing as the battery-powered miniaturised electronic circuitry. Such an **integrated design** offers a compact, robust and easy-to-use instrument, which is ideally suited for the regular monitoring of X-ray tube output forming part of a departmental **quality-assurance** (QA) programme. Probably, the most appropriate application of these instruments is in the monitoring of *changes* in exposure (or 'absorbed dose') over a period of time rather than in providing absolute measurements of these quantities.

Readings from ionisation-chamber dosimeters are susceptible to errors due to changing temperature, atmospheric pressure and humidity. **Correction factors** may need to be applied if conditions vary significantly from those under which the instruments were calibrated.

Modes of operation
Ionisation-chamber instruments may be used in either of two modes of operation:

(1) As a dosimeter, it measures the total exposure over a specific time period. Used in this way, the charge collected on the central electrode is stored on a capacitor. The amount of charge collected is measured and the total exposure read off from a digital liquid crystal display (LCD). This mode is suitable for monitoring radiographic exposures.

(2) As a dose-rate meter, it measures the exposure produced per unit time. The charge collected per second by the central electrode is found by measuring the electric current flowing in the circuit (remembering that charge/time = current). The exposure rate is displayed on the LCD. This mode could be used to check exposure rate during fluoroscopy (screening), where the X-ray exposure is continuous.

Despite the introduction of SI units, it is still common to see radiation exposure expressed in roentgens (R) rather than in coulombs per kilogram ($C\ kg^{-1}$), particularly on instruments manufactured in North America. However, some instruments express their readings in units such as micrograys (μGy), which suggests they are measuring absorbed dose rather than exposure. In fact, they are probably displaying a radiation measurement known as **kerma**.

19.2.1.4   Kerma measurements

Exposure is a measurement which is strictly only obtainable from a free-air ionisation chamber in which true **electronic equilibrium** is achieved. Only in these circumstances can we be sure that we have accounted for and recorded *all* the energy deposited in the attenuating medium (in this case air) and can therefore convert exposure into an absorbed dose measurement. In practical dosimeters, having much smaller dimensions, we are unable to record all the energy deposited because some of this energy will escape outside the volume of attenuator we are monitoring. For example, the photoelectrons and Compton recoil electrons resulting from X-ray interactions with matter may travel some distance before coming to rest and therefore be out of range of our charge-collecting system. In such cases, the amount of energy we are able to record is *less* than the total energy removed from the beam.

The quantity which we actually measure, with our relatively small volume of attenuator, is known as the **kerma** (kinetic energy released per unit mass). Like absorbed dose, it is measured in joules per kilogram (i.e. in gray) but it represents the energy deposited in a *small* volume of attenuator. For diagnostic radiation the values of kerma and absorbed dose are practically identical, but when the radiation is of high energy (i.e. megaelectronvolts) they may differ considerably. The concept of kerma can be applied to *any* attenuating medium, but if kerma measurements are derived from the deposition of energy in air (e.g. in an ionisation chamber), they are known as **air kerma**.

Dosimeters are normally calibrated to indicate either *exposure, absorbed dose in air* or *air kerma*. They can therefore give an accurate indication of the energy deposited in a medium only if it has the same mass attenuation coefficient as air.

19.2.1.5   Dose-area product meters

Ionisation-chamber dosimetry has found a specialised application in monitoring the intensity and field size of the beam emerging from the collimators of an X-ray tube. A flat radiolucent ionisation chamber (sometimes known as a *Diamentor*) positioned over the output window of the light-beam diaphragm is used to monitor not only the **air kerma** (often referred to as 'dose') of the X-ray beam, but also the **area** over which it is spread. The two factors are combined into an **air kerma area product**, or **dose-area product** reading, where

Dose-area product = dose × area

The *air kerma* or 'dose' component of the product depends on the X-ray tube exposure factors: kV, mAs, high-tension (HT) waveform and beam filtration. The *area* component depends on the amount of **beam collimation** the radiographer or radiologist has employed. The combined reading, usually expressed in centigray centimetre squared ($cGy\ cm^2$) or decigray centimetre squared ($dGy\ cm^2$), gives an indication of (but is not equal to) the radiation dose received by the patient. Dose-area product monitoring is used during radiographic *and* fluoroscopic (screening) investigations and provides graphic evidence of the effect of beam collimation on patient dose. For example, for the same selected radiographic exposure factors, collimating the beam to cover an 18 cm × 24 cm film rather than a 24 cm × 30 cm film results in a reduction of the dose-area product to 60% of its former value. This is because the area of an 18 cm × 24 cm film is only three-fifths (60%) of the area of a 24 cm × 30 cm film.

19.2.1.6   Automatic exposure control (*iontomats*)

Another application of ionisation-chamber dosimetry is in equipment used to provide automatic control of diagnostic X-ray exposures. An ionisation chamber forms a key element in most of the control systems known as **automatic exposure devices** (AEDs) or, more commonly, *iontomats*. A set of radiolucent ionisation chambers is incorporated into the X-ray table or bucky stand. During a radiographic exposure, one (or more) of the chambers is used to monitor the levels of radiation arriving at the X-ray cassette. When sufficient radiation has been received to produce a correctly exposed image, the control circuitry automatically terminates the X-ray exposure. Used sensibly, *iontomats* can reduce the incidence of wrongly exposed radiographs, minimise the number of repeat exposures required and therefore benefit the patient, the radiographer and the radiology manager (Carter, 1994). The *Iontomat* or AED is not a *true* dosimeter, since it provides no indication of the amount of radiation to which it has been exposed.

   N.B. The term *Iontomat* is a trade name first used by *Siemens PLC* for its own system of automatic exposure control. For many years, radiographers have used the term to describe the AED of *any* manufacturer, rather in the way that all domestic vacuum cleaners are called *Hoovers*.

19.2.1.7   Geiger–Müller counters

Some ionisation-chamber instruments are designed to detect the arrival of *individual* photons of ionising radiation or *individual* high-energy particles. The **Geiger–Müller** counter, often known as a **Geiger counter** or **GM tube**, is one of the most versatile and widely used instruments of this type. Figure 19.3 shows the main design features of a GM tube. The ionisation chamber is filled with a gas, such as air or argon, at low pressure. The cylindrical metal wall of the tube and a metal rod or wire extending lengthways along the axis of the tube form the electrodes between which a strong electric field is established by the application of a high voltage (e.g. 400 V). When an ionising photon or high-energy particle enters the tube through its mica window, it ionises an atom of the low-pressure gas. The pairs of ions created are rapidly accelerated by the electric field. If the electric field is sufficiently strong, their kinetic energy is increased to such an extent that when, inevitably, they collide with other gas atoms, *more* ions are produced. These ions, in turn, are also accelerated and undergo more ionising collisions with gas atoms. The result is an **avalanche** or **gas-multiplication effect**, in which the arrival of a single photon or high-energy particle triggers the release of a sizeable pulse of ionisation current. The electrical pulse, caused by the detection of each single photon, is amplified electronically and then actuates an electronic counting circuit. The rate of production of pulses is presented as

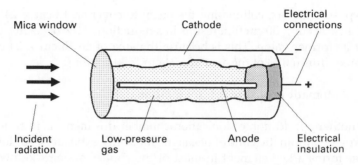

Fig. 19.3 The main features of a Geiger–Müller tube. Radiation photons or high-energy particles enter the tube through its radiolucent mica window. Ions created in the low-pressure gas are accelerated by an electric field set up between anode and cathode. An avalanche effect occurs, creating a significant pulse of ionisation current even from a single encounter with an ionising particle or photon (see text for details of operation).

the **count rate** on an analogue scale or digital display. The counter output is often applied to a loudspeaker circuit, providing a series of audible *clicks*, each one triggered by the arrival of a single photon of radiation.

Dead time
For a short period after the detection of a photon or high-energy particle, while the ionisation current is being **quenched** (extinguished) and the gas ions in the GM tube recombine, the tube cannot detect the arrival of further photons. This recovery period is known as the **dead time** of the GM tube and is typically around 100 µs. The dead time effectively prevents this type of instrument from measuring count rates above $10\,000\ \text{s}^{-1}$.

Applications of GM tubes
A GM tube generates the same size of electrical pulse whatever the energy of the photon or particle it has detected. GM tubes are therefore *detectors* of ionising radiation, rather than true dosimeters. They are particularly useful for detecting the presence of **radioactive contamination** and are a familiar sight in departments of radionuclide imaging, where unsealed sources of radioactivity are available (Section 20.6).

We shall now consider the photographic effect, which is also used as a means of measuring radiation doses.

19.2.2 *Photographic effect*

The sensitive emulsion on photographic film contains microscopic particles of silver bromide. When this emulsion is irradiated with X- or gamma rays, invisible changes occur in the structure of the silver bromide molecules. When the film is chemically developed, the particles of silver bromide which were affected by the radiation are converted into particles of metallic silver. When the film is fixed, any remaining silver bromide is dissolved out of the emulsion. The resulting film therefore contains particles of silver in the parts which have been exposed to radiation, and no silver in unexposed regions. High exposure produces more silver than does low exposure (see Ball & Price, 1995).

If the film is held against a light source such as an X-ray illuminator ('viewing box'), light is transmitted by the unexposed parts of the film and absorbed by the exposed parts; i.e. exposed parts appear grey or black. It has been found that the degree of blackening (optical density) of the film is related to the radiation exposure it has received. By measuring the optical density of the emulsion it is possible to arrive at an estimate of exposure and dose.

The personnel radiation-monitoring film badge is an example of the use of the photographic effect in dosimetry. Unfortunately, the blackening of film due to radiation depends very greatly on the quality of the radiation as well as on its intensity. Much greater blackening is caused by the beam energies used in diagnostic radiography than by high-energy radiotherapy beams. A particular degree of blackening, for example, may be caused either by a small exposure to diagnostic X-rays or by a larger exposure to a radiotherapy beam. When using photographic methods of dosimetry, it is therefore necessary to devise some way of estimating the quality of the radiation for which a dose reading is required. In the film badge which houses the radiation-monitoring film, plastic and metal filters are incorporated to enable a check to be made on radiation quality. We shall be investigating the film badge dosimeter in more detail when discussing radiation protection in Chapter 21.

19.2.3 *Thermoluminescent effect*

In Section 15.3.2.3, we outlined the phenomenon of **thermoluminescence** exhibited by certain phosphors, and it may be helpful if the reader reviews the *whole* of Section 15.3.2 on luminescence before proceeding further.

When exposed to ionising radiation, valence electrons in a thermoluminescent phosphor are raised to the conduction band and become trapped in the forbidden gap while attempting to return to the valence band. Only if the phosphor is subsequently heated is its internal energy increased sufficiently for the trapped electrons to escape to the conduction band. From there they can descend (via luminescence centres) and produce light. Part of the energy absorbed by the phosphor when it was first stimulated is therefore stored until the phosphor is heated, at which point the energy is released as light. The way in which the intensity of light emission changes with increasing temperature is illustrated by means of a graph known as a **glow curve** (Fig. 19.4). It has been found that the *peak* light intensity is proportional to the radiation dose received by the thermoluminescent phosphor. Measurement of the peak light intensity therefore enables an estimate to be made of the radiation dose. This process forms the basis for thermoluminescent dosimetry.

19.2.3.1 Thermoluminescent dosimetry

A number of thermoluminescent phosphors are available, each with its own particular characteristics and advantages. However, we shall confine this

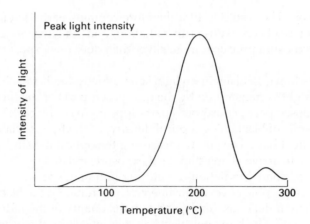

Fig. 19.4   The glow curve produced by heating a lithium fluoride TLD.

discussion to one commonly used thermoluminescent phosphor, **lithium fluoride** (LiF). Lithium fluoride is available as a fine powder, but for dosimetry it is more convenient to use rods, discs or *chips* made of teflon (PTFE) impregnated with lithium fluoride. In these forms the thermoluminescent dosimeter (TLD) may be used in a variety of ways, e.g. worn on the person, stuck on the wall or on equipment, or even inserted into a body cavity. To determine the radiation dose it has received, the TLD is inserted into a device called a 'TLD reader'. Here the lithium fluoride is heated in an electric oven and the peak intensity of light it emits is measured with a sensitive **photomultiplier (PM)** tube (Section 15.4.1). The measurement from the TLD reader is then checked against a calibration chart from which an estimate of absorbed dose, or dose equivalent (Section 21.3.1.2), can be obtained.

Before they are used again for dose-monitoring purposes, lithium fluoride TLDs are subjected to a simple **annealing process** to release any residual energy stored from the previous exposure. A typical annealing regime consists of a heating cycle in which the TLDs are raised to a temperature of 400°C for 1 h followed by 300°C for 3 h.

Advantages of thermoluminescent dosimetry
- As long as TLDs are annealed before each application, they can be used over and over again, possibly up to 300 times.
- Lithium fluoride TLDs are particularly suitable for monitoring of tissue dose because the effective proton number of LiF (8.1) is close to that of human tissue (7.4).
- Lithium fluoride TLDs suffer negligible fading of stored dose information, even after several weeks, because of the relatively high temperature (210°C) at which peak light emission from LiF occurs.
- A wide range of doses varying from about 10 μGy to 1 kGy can be monitored.
- Once loaded into a TLD reader, LiF chips can be read automatically.

19.2.4   Scintillation

In Section 15.3.2.4, we described the phenomenon of scintillation. In this process, the interaction of a single photon of ionising radiation with a **scintillation crystal** causes the simultaneous emission of hundreds of photons of visible light, perceived as a tiny flash of light. Detecting and amplifying such scintillations with a **PM tube** enables an electronic counting circuit to be activated, which provides either a record of the total count over a given period of time or a measure of the count rate. Scintillation counters incorporate a device known as a **pulse height analyser** (PHA). The function of the PHA is to apply some discrimination to the pulses of electrical output from the PM tube. Only those pulses whose height (i.e. magnitude) lies within a specified range are counted. This enables, for example, scintillations due to scattered radiation to be distinguished from those due to primary radiation (Ott et al., 1988).

Like **Geiger–Müller counters** (Section 19.2.1.7), scintillation counters are used to monitor levels of radioactivity rather than to measure exposure or absorbed dose. They do not suffer the GM counter's limitation on count rate and are therefore able to register much higher count rates.

A large thallium-activated sodium-iodide scintillation crystal with a multiple array of PM tubes is a key design feature of the **gamma cameras** used in radionuclide imaging (Section 20.6.2.1).

19.2.5   Ionisation of semiconductor materials

Electrical conduction in a semiconductor is limited by the availability of charge carriers. The introduction of a doping agent increases the number of electrons (in an *n-type* material) and holes (in a *p-type* material), thereby improving conductivity (Section 6.1.1.2). When a semiconducting material is exposed to ionising radiation, ions created in the semiconductor cause a further increase in its electrical conductivity. If a potential difference is applied across the semiconductor, exposure to radiation will generate a pulse of **ionisation current**, whose magnitude depends on the absorbed dose of radiation in the semiconductor. Semiconductor dosimeters often use silicon, whose proton number ($Z = 14$) is closer to that of tissue than the alternative material, germanium ($Z = 32$). The response of silicon is therefore less radiation energy dependent than that of germanium.

A semiconductor detector functions very much like a *solid-state* ionisation chamber. Because its ionisation energy is much smaller than that of air (e.g. 3 eV instead of 33 eV), more ion pairs are created for each radiation photon absorbed. Consequently, semiconductor detectors produce higher ionisation currents than air-ionisation chambers, thus providing more precise readings, which are less susceptible to statistical fluctuations.

Semiconductor detectors may be used in diagnostic radiography for monitoring the output of an X-ray tube for QA or fault-diagnosis purposes. The detector is placed in the X-ray beam and its output cable is connected to an oscilloscope. The oscilloscope displays the variation of X-ray beam intensity with time and allows the X-ray generator waveform to be examined (Siel, undated).

Until now, we have considered methods of measuring the exposure and absorbed dose produced by ionising radiations. It is sometimes necessary to consider the quality as well as the quantity of radiation.

19.3   Evaluation of beam quality

The quality of a heterogeneous beam of radiation is most completely described by reference to its spectrum (see Section 16.1.2). What is needed in practice is a quicker and simpler method of indicating the main characteristics of a beam on which its quality depends. Three features may be chosen.

19.3.1   *Maximum photon energy*

We may specify the maximum energy of photons in the beam (or the minimum wavelength of the radiation). This is easily accomplished with an X-ray beam because the maximum energy photons are produced when electrons reaching the target convert all their energy into X-rays in one Bremsstrahlung interaction. They have a maximum energy (E_{MAX}) which is related to the *peak kilovoltage* (kVp) applied to the X-ray tube; E_{MAX} (in kiloelectronvolts) is numerically equal to the peak tube voltage (in kilovolts). The minimum wavelength (λ_{min}) is given by the Duane–Hunt law:

$$\lambda_{min} = \frac{1.24}{kVp} \text{ nm}$$

We must not forget that the tube voltage waveform and beam filtration can also influence beam quality. However, since most modern diagnostic X-ray units employ constant or near-constant voltage HT generators, their tube voltage waveforms are very similar. Nor does the beam filtration of different general-purpose units vary greatly. Consequently, by quoting the peak kilovoltage applied to the X-ray tube we give a good indication of the quality of the beam. This is therefore the most common method used to express beam quality in diagnostic radiography. Quoting the tube kilovoltage is a particularly convenient and straightforward method because kilovoltage is one of the exposure factors considered routinely by radiographers in their everyday work and is a quantity which is readily displayed on the control console of an X-ray set.

19.3.2   *Effective photon energy*

We may specify the **effective photon energy** of the beam. This represents the photon energy of a *monochromatic* or *monoenergic* beam which has the same penetrating effect as the heterogeneous beam being considered. For example, if a heterogeneous X-ray beam generated at 100 kV has the same ability to penetrate matter as that of a monochromatic (single energy) beam with a photon energy of 60 keV, the effective photon energy of the 100 kV beam is 60 keV. This method of expressing beam quality is not one which radiographers are likely to encounter frequently in staff-room or viewing-room discussion! This is because unlike tube kilovoltage, the value of effective photon energy is not immediately available to

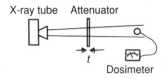

X-ray tube   Attenuator

Dosimeter

Fig. 19.5   An experimental set-up to determine the half-value thickness of an X-ray beam (see Section 17.1.1 for a more detailed description).

the radiographer. Furthermore, there is no constant relationship between it and the maximum photon energy of an X-ray beam because both voltage waveform and beam filtration are complicating factors. However, as a rough guide the effective photon energy of a diagnostic X-ray beam is between 60 and 70% of its maximum photon energy in the tube voltage range 40–150 kV (Hay, 1982).

19.3.3   Half-value thickness

We may specify the thickness of attenuator required to halve the intensity of the beam. This will give us an indication of its ability to penetrate. For example, if one beam needs a copper sheet 2 mm thick to halve its intensity, while a second beam needs 6 mm of copper to reduce its intensity by the same fraction, we would conclude that the second beam is more penetrating than the first. The thickness of attenuator described above is known as the half-value thickness (HVT) or half-value layer (HVL) of the beam.

We define HVT as the thickness of attenuator which, when inserted into a radiation beam, will reduce its intensity by 50%. We can devise a simple practical test to determine the HVT of an X-ray beam. Figure 19.5 shows the basic requirements for the test.

19.3.3.1   Measurement of half-value thickness

The experimental procedure is the same as that described earlier to investigate the attenuation of an X-ray beam and we recommend the reader refer back to Section 17.1.1 before proceeding further.

A series of identical X-ray exposures is made onto the ionisation chamber of a dosimeter. The X-ray beam is made to penetrate through progressively thicker layers of a suitable attenuator (e.g. aluminium). The attenuator thickness and dosimeter reading are recorded for each exposure and a graph is plotted of dosimeter reading against attenuator thickness. The result is the familiar **exponential decay** curve (Fig. 19.6). To obtain the HVT of the beam, a horizontal line is drawn on the graph from a point on the dose axis representing exactly half the dose reading obtained when no attenuator was present. The thickness of attenuator which produced this 50% reduction in dose can then be read off (HVT = 1.8 mm Al in the example shown in Fig. 19.6). It is recommended that **relative dose** values are plotted rather than the readings taken directly from the dosimeter. A graph of relative dose demonstrates more clearly the fractional (or percentage) reduction in dose produced by different thicknesses of attenuator, and the HVT may be read off at the 50% level of relative dose. Relative dose

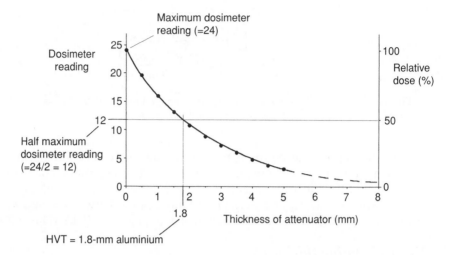

Fig. 19.6 A graph of dosimeter readings plotted against attenuator thickness, using data obtained from an experiment to measure the half-value thickness (HVT) of an X-ray beam. The vertical scale on the right-hand side represents relative dose expressed as a percentage of the maximum reading. From the graph, the thickness of aluminium which would halve the original dose reading is about 1.8 mm. The HVT of the beam is therefore said to be 1.8-mm Al.

values are obtained by dividing each dose reading by the *maximum* dose reading. Relative dose can be expressed either as a decimal (e.g. 0.5) or as a percentage (e.g. 50%).

Using logarithmic scales

As we noted in Section 17.1.1, because of possible difficulties in drawing an exponential curve accurately, it is often better experimental practice to plot the dose values on a *logarithmic* rather than a *linear* scale. A true exponential relationship plotted in this way produces a straight-line graph, which is much easier to draw. The logarithmic graph can be achieved in several ways, e.g.

(1) By plotting the dose values (preferably as *relative* values) on the log scale of **log-linear graph paper**. The HVT can be directly read off the graph at the 50% relative dose level (Fig. 19.7).
(2) By converting each dose reading (or preferably *relative* dose reading) to its log value and then plotting the log values on **linear graph paper**. The log value for 50% relative dose must then be obtained (from a calculator) and the HVT can then be read off (Fig. 19.8).

The first of these methods requires less use of the calculator, but care is needed when plotting values on, and reading values from, logarithmic graph paper, particularly if such a technique is used infrequently. It may prove helpful at this stage if we work through a simple example involving the use of HVT.

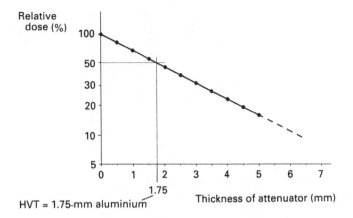

Fig. 19.7   A graph of the relative dose plotted against attenuator thickness on a log-linear paper. The vertical (relative dose) scale is logarithmic, while the horizontal (attenuator thickness) scale is linear. Note the non-linear spacing of the vertical scale. The straight-line nature of the graph tells us that an exponential relationship exists between dose and attenuator thickness. The half-value thickness (HVT) appears to be about 1.75-mm Al. We can often obtain a more reliable reading from a straight-line graph than that from a curved graph, such as shown in Fig. 19.6.

Worked example
The HVT of a homogeneous beam of radiation is quoted as 3 mm of tin. What percentage of the beam will be transmitted through a tin sheet 9 mm thick?

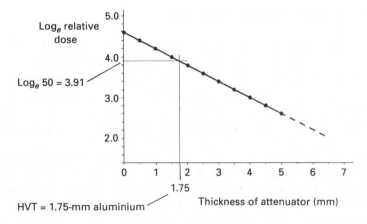

Fig. 19.8   An alternative way of producing a straight-line graph is to plot the logarithmic values of relative dose (obtained by using the 'ln' function on an electronic calculator). $\log_e 100$ is about 4.6, so the maximum dose (=100%) is plotted at 4.6 on the vertical scale. Each of the other relative dose values is converted in a similar fashion and a straight line drawn through the plotted points. $\log_e 50$ is 3.91, so 50% relative dose is represented by 3.91 on the vertical scale. It is this level which enables us to determine the half-value thickness (HVT = 1.75-mm Al).

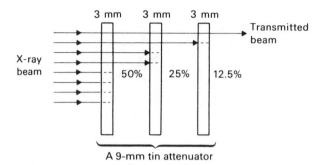

Fig. 19.9   A 9-mm attenuator containing three half-value thicknesses, transmitting 12.5% of the incident X-ray beam.

Remember that if the HVT is inserted, the beam intensity is reduced by 50%. We can consider 9 mm as being three separate layers each of thickness 3 mm. The first 3 mm will reduce the beam to 50%. The second 3 mm will reduce the beam by 50% again, i.e. to 25%. The third 3 mm will reduce the beam by 50% again, i.e. to 12.5%.

We can conclude, therefore, that a 9-mm tin sheet will cut the intensity of the beam to 12.5% of its original value. Figure 19.9 illustrates the method we have used to solve this problem. We have provided the answer in the form of **percentage transmission**.

It is also possible to quote the answer as a **fractional transmission** value rather than a percentage. In this case we would say the fractional transmission is 1/8, since 12.5% represents the fraction one-eighth.

19.3.3.2   Changes in half-value thickness

As we have seen, HVT is a measure of *the penetrating power* of a beam of radiation: it is an indicator of *beam quality*. When a monochromatic (homogeneous) beam penetrates through matter, its intensity reduces but its quality, and therefore its HVT, remains the same. However, with a *heterogeneous* beam the situation is more complicated. The further through matter a heterogeneous beam penetrates, the higher its quality and its HVT become. This was the principle underlying the use of beam filtration described in Section 17.3.2.

Let us consider again the worked example we have just studied (Fig 19.9). We were careful to state initially that the beam involved was homogeneous, but suppose it had been a *heterogeneous* beam. After passing through the first HVT (3 mm of tin), the beam would emerge at half its former intensity, but with higher quality than previously. In other words, its HVT would have increase to *more* than 3 mm (say, 3.3 mm). Consequently, when the beam encounters the next 3-mm thickness of tin, *more than 50%* would be transmitted, i.e. more than 25% of its *original* intensity. By the time the beam emerges from the final 3-mm layer, its HVT would be still greater (say, 3.4 mm), resulting in the transmission of significantly more than 12.5% of its original intensity.

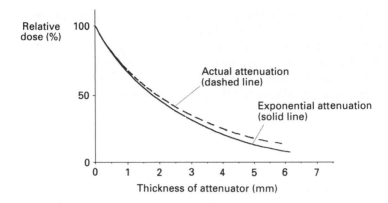

Fig. 19.10 Attenuation of a heterogeneous X-ray beam. The lower line (solid) shows the amount of attenuation predicted by the exponential law of attenuation. The upper line (dashed) shows the actual attenuation of a heterogeneous X-ray beam. The graph shows that the amount of attenuation is slightly less than predicted. This is because although reducing in intensity, the beam gets progressively more penetrating as it passes through matter (see also Section 17.3.2).

This complication is an unfortunate drawback to using the HVT method for specifying the quality of a heterogeneous beam. The HVT of 3-mm tin, quoted in the worked example, is an example of what is known as the **first HVT** of the beam. Subsequent higher values of HVT which apply as the beam is attenuated more and more are known as the **second HVT**, the **third HVT**, and so on.

The anomalous behaviour we have described indicates that the relationship between the transmitted intensity of a heterogeneous X-ray beam and the thickness of attenuator has departed from the precise **exponential law** described in Section 17.1.1. The fall in intensity is not quite as great as the exponential law predicts (Fig. 19.10), and a logarithmic graph of relative dose plotted against attenuator thickness will not *quite* produce a straight line. In practice, the X-ray beams encountered in diagnostic radiography are normally so heavily filtered that these departures from the exponential law of attenuation are relatively insignificant.

19.4 Conclusions

We have described three possible methods of indicating the quality of a radiation beam, but which of the methods is used in practice? As we shall see in the next chapter, gamma rays emitted from a radioactive sample consist of a few specific photon energies of which one energy is often dominant. Such radiation is essentially homogeneous and its quality can be expressed by quoting the dominant photon energy (usually in kiloelectronvolts or megaelectronvolts). Because X-ray beams are more or less *heterogeneous*, the expression of quality is less straightforward than that with gamma rays. As we pointed out, the peak

X-ray tube kilovoltage is generally quoted in diagnostic radiography. In radio-therapy it is usual with X-ray beams having energies up to 2 MeV to specify both the generating voltage (or effective photon energy) and the HVT. Above 2 MeV only the effective photon energy need be specified.

In our next chapter we shall examine the phenomenon of radioactivity, the radiations it produces and its applications in diagnostic imaging.

Chapter 20

Radioactivity and Radionuclide Imaging

Causes of radioactivity
Radioactive transformation processes
   Alpha-particle emission
   Negative- and positive beta-particle emissions
   Gamma-ray emission
   Internal conversion
   Electron capture
   Branching transformations
Radioactive decay rates
   Activity
   Decay of activity
   Decay constant
   Radioactive half-life
   Specific activity
Production of radionuclides
   Nuclear-fission products
   Neutron activation
   Bombardment in particle accelerators
   Radionuclide generator
Medical applications of radionuclides
   Therapeutic applications
   Diagnostic applications
Radionuclide imaging
   Radiopharmaceuticals
   Biological and effective half-life
   Gamma camera

Chapter 4 should be reviewed before studying this section of work on radioactivity.

In Section 4.3.3, we said that the nuclei of some atoms are unstable and they tend to disintegrate, emitting radiation and fast-moving particles. We called these unstable nuclides **radionuclides** and described them as being **radioactive**.

Radionuclides have been used as radiotherapy sources since the early days of such treatment, but in recent years they have become important in the diagnosis of disease, particularly in that branch of nuclear medicine known as **radionuclide imaging**. We shall outline the principles of this technique for producing diagnostic images in Section 20.6.

20.1 Radioactivity

Radioactivity, or radioactive decay, is defined as a process whereby some nuclides undergo spontaneous changes in the structure of their nuclei, accompanied by the emission of particles and radiation.

Radioactivity is a nuclear process; i.e. it involves the nuclei of atoms rather than the electrons in orbit around the nuclei. Thus, radioactivity is not influenced by chemical changes that may be occurring, nor by changes in the physical environment, such as variations in temperature or pressure. It is therefore not possible to control the rate of radioactive breakdown of a nuclide.

20.1.1   Causes of radioactivity

Why do some nuclides disintegrate, while others are stable? The nuclei of atoms contain two kinds of fundamental particles: positively charged protons and uncharged neutrons (Section 4.3). Because the protons carry similar charges, electric forces are set up between them, which cause them to repel each other. If unrestrained, the protons would separate, causing the nucleus to break up. However, the presence of neutrons in the nucleus is associated with strong nuclear forces of attraction, which counteract this tendency, and as a result the nucleus may survive intact.

In order for the repulsion forces to be overcome in a particular nucleus, there must be a specific number of neutrons present. The 'neutron:proton ratio' must be correct. If too many or too few neutrons are present, sooner or later nuclear disintegration will take place.

Some nuclides, particularly ones having high proton numbers, are unstable no matter how many neutrons are present; e.g. uranium, whose proton number is 92, has no stable isotopes.

After the disintegration of a radionuclide, a new nuclide is formed, which may or may not be stable. The nuclides which result from radioactive transformations are known as *daughter products*. In some instances, a whole series of transformations may be involved before a stable daughter nuclide is achieved.

20.1.1.1   Natural and artificial radioisotopes

Many unstable isotopes occur naturally in the earth, in living organisms and in the atmosphere, e.g. $^{238}_{92}U$ (uranium), $^{226}_{88}Ra$ (radium), $^{40}_{19}K$ (potassium) and $^{14}_{6}C$ (carbon). Other radioisotopes have been produced by man in nuclear reactors, nuclear bombs and high-energy machines called particle accelerators, e.g. $^{131}_{53}I$ (iodine), $^{90}_{38}Sr$ (strontium), $^{60}_{27}Co$ (cobalt) and $^{99}_{43}Tc$ (technetium).

20.2   Transformation processes

When radionuclides break down, several different types of emissions may be produced, depending on which particular process of decay has occurred. Let us now examine some of these transformation processes.

20.2.1   Alpha-particle (α) emission

The emission of an alpha particle is associated with the breakdown of heavy elements such as uranium and radium. The alpha particle is a combination of four fundamental particles, two protons and two neutrons; i.e. an alpha particle is identical in structure to the nucleus of a helium atom ($^4_2$He). The decay of radium is an example of alpha-particle emission:

$$^{226}_{88}\text{Ra (radium)} \rightarrow\ ^{226}_{88}\text{Rn (radon)} + ^4_2\alpha \text{ (alpha particle)}$$

The alpha particle is ejected at high speed from the nucleus. Notice that the proton numbers and the nucleon numbers balance on both sides of the equation ($86 + 2 = 88$ and $222 + 4 = 226$). Notice also that in this process the nucleon number of the nuclide has reduced by *four* and its proton number has reduced by *two*.

The daughter product radon (a chemically inert gas) is also radioactive and undergoes a further alpha-particle emission. After a sequence of nine successive transformations, a stable nuclide is formed, one of the isotopes of lead.

20.2.1.1   Decay schemes

The decay of radium, and of any other radionuclide, is often depicted graphically as a form of energy diagram known as a **decay scheme**. The decay scheme for radium is shown in Fig. 20.1. The height of the horizontal lines in the decay scheme represents different nuclear-energy states: radioactive transformations involve a downward transition from a high-energy state to a low-energy state. Changes in proton number are represented by horizontal displacement on the decay scheme; e.g. the decrease in proton number associated with alpha-particle emission is shown as a displacement to the left.

20.2.1.2   Properties of alpha particles

Alpha particles carry a positive electric charge and cause intense ionisation in matter through which they pass. They are the heaviest of the particle emissions. Because they are electrically charged, their course is influenced by both electric and magnetic fields; e.g. they would be attracted towards a negatively charged electrode.

Alpha particles have a very short range. Even in air their energy will become attenuated after travelling only a few centimetres. A sheet of paper would stop them completely. The effect of alpha particles on living tissues is intense, but very localised.

20.2.2   *Negative beta-particle (β^-) emission*

The emission of a negatively charged beta particle is associated with the breakdown of nuclides which have too many neutrons; i.e. nuclides whose neutron:proton ratio is too high. The negative beta particle is identical to an electron having the same mass and carrying the same charge.

For a particular nuclide decaying by β^- emission, the *total* energy released from the nucleus is always the same. The β^- particle may carry *all* of this energy, or it may carry only a *part* of the energy released. In the latter case, the 'missing' energy is carried by another particle, known as an **antineutrino**, which is ejected from the nucleus at the same time as the β^- particle. The antineutrino is

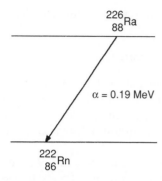

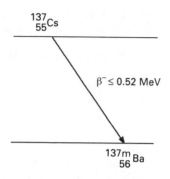

Fig. 20.1   The decay scheme for radium-226. The horizontal lines represent energy states in the nucleus. The diagram shows that the radium nucleus emits an alpha particle carrying 0.19 MeV of energy. The arrow pointing to the left indicates that the proton number of the daughter nuclide (radon-222) is less than that of the parent nuclide. Radon-222 undergoes a complex series of transformations, eventually producing a stable nuclide of lead.

Fig. 20.2   The decay scheme for caesium-137. The caesium nucleus releases about 0.52 MeV of energy by emitting a negative beta particle and an antineutrino. The division of energy between these two particles is variable, but as the total energy is always 0.52 MeV, the energy of the beta particle can never be greater than 0.52 MeV. The arrow pointing to the right shows that the proton number of the daughter nuclide (barium-137m) is greater than that of the parent. Barium-137m is a metastable radionuclide (see Section 20.2.4).

represented by the symbol $\bar{v}$. (v is the Greek letter 'nu' and the bar over the letter signifies that it is an antiparticle; the combined symbol is pronounced 'new bar'.) The β^- particle results from the transformation of a neutron (n) in the nucleus into a proton (p); i.e.

$$^1_0\text{n} \rightarrow {}^1_{+1}\text{p} + {}^0_{-1}\beta + \bar{v}$$

As a result of the transformation, the number of neutrons in the nucleus is reduced by 1, while the number of protons is increased by 1, thus decreasing the neutron:proton ratio. The breakdown of radioactive caesium ($^{137}_{55}\text{Cs}$) is an example of β^- emission:

$$^{137}_{55}\text{Cs (caesium)} \rightarrow {}^{137}_{56}\text{Ba (barium)} + {}^0_{-1}\beta + {}^0_0\bar{v}$$

Notice that in this process the nucleon number remains the same, while the proton number increases by 1. The decay scheme for caesium-137 is shown in Fig. 20.2.

20.2.2.1   Properties of β^- particles

Negative beta particles cause ionisation in any medium they traverse. They can be deflected by electric and magnetic fields, but in the opposite sense to alpha particles; e.g. they would be repelled away from a negatively charged electrode.

Beta particles have a greater range than alpha particles and would not be much attenuated by a sheet of paper, but would be stopped by a layer of aluminium a few millimetres thick. Beta particles also have a localised damaging effect on body tissues.

20.2.2.2 Properties of antineutrinos

The **antineutrino** ($\bar{\nu}$) is a rather mysterious particle, whose existence was first suggested (by Wolfgang Pauli in 1931) to resolve the apparent energy imbalance during transformations involving β^- particle emission. The antineutrino is the antimatter equivalent of the **neutrino** (see Sections 4.5.2 and 20.2.3). The particle carries no electric charge and when it is at rest it has no mass either! However, it possesses energy when in motion, a property normally associated with mass (kinetic energy $= \frac{1}{2}mv^2$). Antineutrinos are highly unlikely to interact with matter. Consequently, they are extremely penetrating, have no significant ionising effect and are so elusive that 25 years elapsed before they were detected experimentally (Hey & Walters, 2003).

We have described the emission of negatively charged beta particles (β^-), but positive beta particles (β^+) can also be emitted through a rather different process, which we shall now describe.

20.2.3 Positive beta-particle (β^+) emission

The emission of *positive* beta particle is associated with the breakdown of nuclides which have too many protons, i.e. nuclides whose neutron:proton ratio is too low. The β^+ particle is identical to a positively charged electron, i.e. a **positron** (Section 17.2.4). It has the same mass as that of an electron, but is of opposite electric charge. The β^+ emission results from the transformation of a proton in the nucleus into a neutron and is accompanied by the emission of a **neutrino** (ν); i.e.

$$_{+1}^{1}p \rightarrow {}_{0}^{1}n + {}_{+1}^{0}\beta + {}_{0}^{0}\nu$$

As a result of the transformation, the number of neutrons in the nucleus is increased by 1, while the number of protons is reduced by 1, thus *increasing* the neutron:proton ratio. The breakdown of radioactive oxygen ($_{8}^{15}O$) is an example of β^+ emission:

$$_{8}^{15}O \text{ (oxygen)} \rightarrow {}_{7}^{15}N \text{ (nitrogen)} + {}_{+1}^{0}\beta + {}_{0}^{0}\nu$$

Notice that in this process the nucleon number remains the same, while the proton number reduces by 1. The decay scheme for oxygen-15 is shown in Fig. 20.3.

20.2.3.1 Properties of β^+ particles

Positive beta particles interact with matter in a similar way to the negative beta particles, as described in Section 20.2.2.1. However, they are deflected by electric and magnetic fields in the opposite direction to β^- particles. Like the positrons described in Section 17.2.4.1, β^+ particles eventually combine with negative electrons and disappear in a burst of **annihilation radiation**.

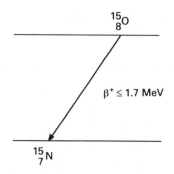

Fig. 20.3 The decay scheme for oxygen-15. The oxygen nucleus sheds 1.7 MeV of energy shared between a positive beta particle and a neutrino. The energy of the beta particle can therefore never be greater than 1.7 MeV. The daughter nuclide is nitrogen-15.

20.2.3.2 Properties of neutrinos

Neutrinos (ν) are just as elusive as antineutrinos, their antimatter equivalent. They carry no electric charge and have zero rest mass. They possess energy only when in motion. The difference between neutrinos and antineutrinos is visualised as a difference in the direction of their intrinsic spinning motion. Neutrinos rarely interact with matter, have no significant ionising effect and are extremely penetrating.

20.2.4 Gamma-ray (γ) emission

Beta decay processes often leave the daughter nucleus in an excited state, still having too much energy. The nucleus sheds its surplus energy by emitting one or more photons of high-energy electromagnetic radiation called gamma (γ) radiation. In cases of *prompt* gamma decay, there is no measurable delay between the emission of the beta particle and the emission of a gamma-ray photon. In other cases, the excited state may remain for some time before, eventually, gamma-ray emission occurs and the nuclide becomes stable. The temporary excited condition of the radionuclide is known as a **metastable state** and the subsequent transformation from metastable to stable state is called an **isomeric transition**. The isotope of barium ($^{137}_{56}$Ba), which was produced as a daughter product in our example of β^- emission, behaves in this way:

$$^{137m}_{56}\text{Ba} \rightarrow\ ^{137}_{56}\text{Ba} + \gamma$$

The *m* is used to indicate that a nuclide is in a metastable state. The decay scheme for barium-137m is shown in Fig. 20.4. Notice that unlike alpha and beta decay, gamma-ray emission involves no alteration in the proton number or nucleon number.

The energy of gamma-ray emission is always the same for a particular nuclide; i.e. it is characteristic of a specific transformation and produces a line spectrum rather than continuous spectrum (Section 14.7.5).

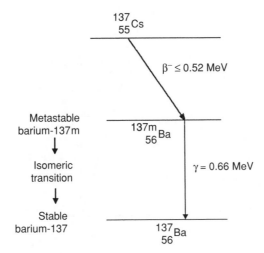

Fig. 20.4   The decay scheme previously shown in Fig. 20.2 is now extended to include the isomeric transition of the metastable nuclide barium-137m into stable barium-137. The transition is accompanied by the emission of a 0.66-MeV gamma-ray photon. Nuclides, such as barium-137m and barium-137, which have the same proton numbers and the same nucleon numbers but different energy states, are known as **isomers,** hence the term **isomeric transition**.

20.2.4.1   Properties of gamma rays

Gamma-ray photons have no mass and carry no electric charge, being electromagnetic radiation rather than matter. They are not influenced by electric or magnetic fields, but they do have an ionising effect on matter, interacting with it in the same way as X-rays (see Chapters 17 and 18).

Depending on their energy, gamma rays can be far more penetrating than alpha or beta particles, requiring the equivalent of several millimetres of lead to produce significant attenuation. Gamma rays are able to penetrate into body tissues and are therefore used in the radiotherapy of deep-lying lesions. Radioactive cobalt ($^{60}_{27}$Co) has been used as a source of gamma rays for this purpose. Gamma-ray emitters are also used extensively for diagnostic purposes in the field of **nuclear medicine**. We explore the imaging aspects of nuclear medicine later in this chapter (Section 20.6).

20.2.5   *Internal conversion*

This is another means by which an excited nucleus can release energy. In this case, the excess energy is transferred to one of the electrons (usually from the K shell) orbiting around the nucleus. This electron is then ejected from the atom and its place is filled by downward transitions of electrons similar to those associated with **photoionisation (photoelectric effect)** described in Section 17.2.2. The characteristic radiation (sometimes known as **fluorescent radiation**) emitted may interact with outer electrons of the atom, releasing them as **Auger electrons**.

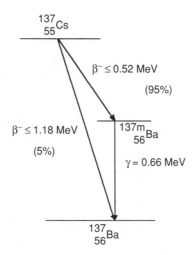

Fig. 20.5   A more complete decay scheme for caesium-137, showing the branching transformations by which it decays to stable barium-137. In a sample of caesium-137, 95% of the nuclei decay via a two-stage route, emitting a β^- particle and a 0.66-MeV gamma-ray photon. The remaining 5% of the caesium-137 nuclei decay via a single β^- transformation.

20.2.6   Electron capture

Like β^+ decay (Section 20.2.3.1), this process occurs in nuclides which have too many protons. Here, the nucleus captures one of the K-shell electrons and combines it with a proton to form a neutron:

$$_{+1}^{1}\mathrm{p} + {}_{-1}^{0}\mathrm{e} \rightarrow {}_{0}^{1}\mathrm{n}$$

20.2.7   Branching transformations

Many radionuclides decay by more than one transformation process. For example, caesium-137 decays to barium-137 in two ways (Fig. 20.5):

(1) By a β^- decay in which 1.18 MeV of energy is released from the nucleus by the emission of a single negative beta particle and antineutrino.
(2) By a β^- decay in which 0.52 MeV is released as a negative beta particle and antineutrino. The nuclide is then in a temporary, **metastable state**. This is followed by an **isomeric transition**, in which the emission of a gamma-ray photon sheds the remaining 0.66 MeV of energy ($0.52 + 0.66 = 1.18$ MeV).

In such branching transformations, the different transformations always occur in the same proportions; e.g. 95% of the atoms in a sample of caesium-137 decay to stable barium-137 through the intermediate metastable form of barium-137m, while the remaining 5% decay by the direct route.

Having now completed our description of the main transformation processes and the emissions they produce, we shall consider the rate at which these processes occur and the means we have for measuring radioactivity.

20.3   Radioactive decay rates

Radioactivity is a random process. We can never predict when a particular atomic nucleus will disintegrate. However, we *are* able to make predictions about the behaviour of large numbers of atoms such as we deal with in practice. (In a similar way, we are not able to predict whether potential parents will conceive a male or a female embryo, but we can say with some confidence that in a group of 100 potential parents, approximately half will have boys and half girls.)

20.3.1   *Activity*

The rate of decay of a radionuclide is known as its **activity**. The activity of a sample is the rate at which the sample undergoes transformations, i.e. the number of transformations per unit time.

The SI unit of activity is the becquerel (Bq), which is defined as an activity of *one* transformation per second. The becquerel represents an incredibly low activity, and in practice the megabecquerel (MBq) or gigabecquerel (GBq) is used, where

$$1 \text{ MBq} = 10^6 \text{ Bq}$$

and

$$1 \text{ GBq} = 10^9 \text{ Bq}$$

One gram of radium has an activity of 3.7×10^{10} transformations per second and this defines the traditional unit of activity, the curie (Ci), which is still used, particularly in the popular news media ($1 \text{ Ci} = 3.7 \times 10^{10} \text{ Bq}$). Table 20.1 shows the wide range of activity levels encountered in a number of different radionuclide applications.

20.3.2   *Decay of activity*

It has been found that for any particular radionuclide, whatever the size of the sample, the same percentage of its atoms is always transformed in the same intervals of time. For example if in a sample containing 20 million atoms, 2000

Table 20.1   Examples of approximate radioactivity levels employed in a range of different applications

Application	Activity (Bq)
Cobalt-60 radiotherapy source	2×10^{14}
Technetium-99m injection for bone scan imaging[a]	5×10^8
Luminous paint containing radium-226 on dials of old aircraft instruments and watches	4×10^5
Americium-241 source in domestic smoke alarms	3.3×10^4
Naturally occurring potassium-40 in the human body	4.2×10^3

[a] Adams (1995).

atoms (i.e. 0.01% of the total) break down per second, then in a smaller sample of the same radionuclide, containing (say) 5 million atoms, 500 atoms would break down per second (because 500 is 0.01% of 5 million). However, as we saw in Section 20.3.1, the number of nuclear transformations occurring per unit time is **activity**. The activity of the first sample is therefore 2000 disintegrations per second (i.e. 2000 Bq), while the activity of the second sample is 500 disintegrations per second (500 Bq). In fact, for a given radionuclide, the activity (A) of a sample depends *only* on the number of atoms that it contains. If the sample contains n atoms, then A is found to be directly proportional to n:

$$A \propto n$$

However, the number of atoms (n) of radionuclide in a sample is always falling because the original atoms are gradually being transformed into different material (the daughter products). Consequently, the activity of a radioactive sample always decreases with time.

Activity tells us the number of transformations occurring per second. It therefore tells us the rate at which the number of atoms of original material is falling. In other words, activity (A) is the *rate of change* of n with respect to time. Using the symbolism of the calculus, we can write this as:

$$A = \frac{dn}{dt}$$

(pronounced 'dee en by dee tee'), but:

$$A \propto n$$

Therefore:

$$\frac{dn}{dt} \propto n$$

and

$$\frac{dn}{dt} = -\lambda n$$

where λ is a constant of proportionality known as the **decay constant**. The minus sign indicates that dn/dt is negative, showing that n is *decreasing* rather than increasing with time.

20.3.2.1   Decay constant

Each radionuclide has a fixed characteristic value of decay constant, indicating how rapidly or slowly it decays. The decay constant of a radionuclide is the number of atoms of radionuclide breaking down per unit time expressed as a fraction of the total number of atoms of the nuclide present. The SI unit of decay constant is *per second* (s^{-1}). In the example quoted in Section 20.3.2 above, the decay constant (λ) can be calculated from the figures used:

$$\lambda = \frac{2000}{20\,000\,000}$$
$$= 10^{-4}\,s^{-1}$$

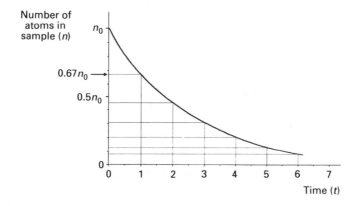

Fig. 20.6   The number (n) of atoms of radionuclide in a sample reducing with time (t). Initially (at time $t = 0$), the number of atoms present is n_0. As each nucleus undergoes radioactive disintegration, the number of atoms of the original radionuclide decreases. After one unit of time has elapsed, the number of atoms has reduced (in the example shown) to 0.67 of its initial value. After two units of time, the number of atoms reduces to 0.67 of its previous value ($0.67 \times 0.67 \approx 0.45$). After three units of time, the number is reduced to 0.67 of this value ($0.67 \times 0.45 \approx 0.30$), and so on. This pattern, which is repeated ad infinitum, is a characteristic feature of an exponential relationship.

20.3.2.2   Exponential decay of activity

The expression $dn/dt = -\lambda n$ can be mathematically converted into an alternative form:

$$n = n_0 e^{-\lambda t}$$

where n_0 is the number of atoms of radionuclide in the original sample (i.e. when $t = 0$) and e is the **exponential constant**. Note the similarities between this expression and those previously encountered in Sections 7.11.2 and 7.11.3 (capacitor charging and discharging) and in Section 17.1.1 (attenuation of X-rays and gamma rays).

It is clear that an **exponential relationship** exists between time (t) and the number of atoms (n) remaining in the sample. Figure 20.6 shows the familiar appearance of the exponential decay curve obtained by plotting n against t.

Of course, it is not feasible to count the number of atoms of radionuclide left in a sample, but it is certainly possible to measure its *activity* by detecting and measuring the rate at which particles and/or gamma-ray photons are emitted from the sample. For example, a Geiger counter (Section 19.2.1.7) could be used for this purpose. Because activity (A) is directly proportional to the number of atoms present, it also decays exponentially with time, and we can therefore write:

$$A = A_0 e^{-\lambda t}$$

where A is the activity after time t, A_0 is the initial activity of the sample (i.e. when $t = 0$), e is the exponential constant and λ is again the decay constant. Figure 20.7 shows the decay activity of a radioactive sample.

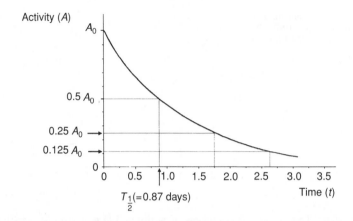

Fig. 20.7   The characteristic exponential decay in the activity of a (fictitious) radionuclide sample. The steepness of the curve depends on the decay constant of the radionuclide. The time axis is scaled in days. Initially, the activity of the sample is A_0. After about 0.87 days its activity has reduced to 0.5 A_0 (half its initial value). This time period is therefore known as the radioactive half-life ($T_{\frac{1}{2}}$) of the radionuclide. After a further 0.87 days, the activity has halved again (to 0.25 A_0), and after three half-lives the activity is down to $0.125 A_0$. In theory, no matter how much time elapses, the activity will never reach zero.

20.3.2.3   Radioactive half-life

Each radionuclide has its own characteristic decay rate, which we can specify either by means of the decay constant or by noting the time taken for the activity of the radionuclide to decrease by 50%. We call this time the **radioactive** or **physical half-life ($T_{\frac{1}{2}}$)**. It is indicated on the graph in Fig. 20.7.

The value of half-life for different radionuclides varies tremendously, from infinitesimally small fractions of a second (e.g. 10^{-9} s) to over a billion years (e.g. 10^{10} years).

Decay constant and half-life are related by the equation:

$$\lambda = \frac{0.693}{T_{\frac{1}{2}}}$$

Table 20.2 shows some of the radionuclides used in medicine, indicating their half-lives and the nature of their emissions.

In medicine, samples with short half-lives are useful for several reasons:

(1)   They are cheaper to manufacture. (They are artificial isotopes.)
(2)   The patients and staff receive less radiation dose because the activity reduces more quickly.
(3)   When the treatment or investigation is over, the residual activity is low.

However, when radioisotopes are used for external beam radiotherapy, long half-lives are required so that the source does not deteriorate too quickly and need replacing too frequently.

Table 20.2   Examples of radionuclides and their medical applications[a]

Radionuclide	Half-life	Decay mode[b]	Gamma-ray photon energy[c] (MeV)	Application
Radium-226	1620 years	α, γ	0.186[d]	Therapy source (needles)
Americium-241	433 years	α, γ	0.043–0.060	Bone densitometry
Caesium-137	30.1 years	β⁻, γ	0.662	Teletherapy source
Cobalt-60	5.27 years	β⁻, γ	1.17 and 1.33	Teletherapy source
Iridium-192	74.0 days	β⁻, ec, γ	0.28–0.61	Therapy source (wires)
Chromium-51	27.7 days	ec	0.32	Blood-volume estimation
Iodine-131	8.06 days	β⁻, γ	0.28–0.64	Thyroid uptake
Xenon-133	5.25 days	β, γ	0.08	Imaging
Gallium-67	3.26 days	ec	0.09–0.30	Imaging
Gold-198	2.70 days	β⁻, γ	0.41	Therapy source (grains)
Technetium-99m	6.02 hours	it	0.141	Imaging

[a] Radionuclides are listed in descending order of their half-lives.
[b] Decay modes include isomeric transition (it) and electron capture (ec) (see Sections 20.2.4 and 20.2.6).
[c] The gamma-ray energies shown are the most dominant energy or range of energies emitted.
[d] Decay of radium-26 is complex and only its immediate gamma-ray emission has been included.

Let us work through two typical problems involving the half-life of a radioisotope.

Worked examples
(1)   A sample of iodine-131 with a half-life of 8 days is to be used for thyroid uptake studies. The delivery of the sample from the supplier takes 16 days. If an activity of 1 MBq is required to carry out the investigation, what should the activity of the sample be when it is despatched from the supplier?
      This problem has deliberately been made straightforward by providing a time period (16 days) which is a whole-number multiple of the half-life (8 days) of the radionuclide involved. In such cases we can arrive at the solution by using an empirical approach based on our understanding of half-life.
      Remember that every 8 days, the activity of iodine-131 reduces by 50%. Then:
      • Eight days before the study, the activity of the sample would have been *twice* its final activity; i.e. $2 \times 1 = 2$ MBq.
      • Sixteen days before the study, the activity would have been *twice* its value at 8 days; i.e. $2 \times 2 = 4$ MBq.
      So 16 days before use, when the sample leaves the supplier, its activity should be 4 MBq.
(2)   Arrangements are made for a patient to have a radionuclide scan on 23 May. The radiopharmaceutical (labelled with technetium-99m) is prepared in advance so that its activity will be 500 MBq at 10.30 AM when the injection is due to be administered. If the minimum activity required to ensure a successful scan is 300 MBq, by how long can the injection be

delayed before its activity falls below this critical level? The half-life of technetium-99m is 6 h.

In this problem, we cannot use the empirical approach of the previous example, because a fall from 500 to 300 MBq is *not* a simple 50% decrease; we are therefore not dealing with whole number multiples of half-life. To arrive at a solution we must resort to a more mathematical approach, using the equation for exponential decay of activity:

$$A = A_0 e^{-\lambda t}$$

where A_0 is the initial activity (500 MBq), A is the activity at time t (300 MBq), e is the exponential constant and λ, the decay constant, can be calculated from the half-life $(T_\frac{1}{2})$, because $\lambda = 0.693/T_\frac{1}{2}$ (Section 20.3.2.3). Thus:

$$\lambda = \frac{0.693}{21\,600} \quad (6\,\text{h} = 21\,600\,\text{s})$$
$$= 3.2 \times 10^{-5}\,\text{s}^{-1}$$

The time t, taken for the activity of the sample to fall from 500 to 300 MBq, is the answer to our problem!

We can now use the exponential equation to calculate the value of t, but the equation must first be rearranged into the form:

$$e^{\lambda t} = \frac{A}{A_0}$$
$$= \frac{300}{500}$$
$$= 0.6$$

Now, by taking logs of both sides of the equation:

$$-\lambda t = \log_e 0.6$$
$$= -0.51 \quad \text{(obtained using the 'ln' function on an}$$
$$\text{electronic calculator)}$$

so that

$$t = \frac{0.51}{3.2 \times 10^{-5}}$$
$$= 1.6 \times 10^4\,\text{s}$$
$$= 4.4\,\text{h}$$

The activity will take just under $4\frac{1}{2}$ h to fall to an unusable level. The injection must therefore be administered to the patient by 3 PM on 23 May for the investigation to be successful.

20.3.3 *Specific activity*

Radioisotopes are rarely available in their pure state. Because the radioactive isotopes of an element are chemically identical to its stable isotopes, it is difficult, if not impossible, to separate the unstable from the stable forms of the element. Depending on how it was produced (see Section 20.4), a radionuclide sample may therefore also contain *stable* nuclides of the same element. Indeed, the radioactive component may form only a small percentage of the sample as a whole. Additionally, both the stable and unstable isotopes of the element are often combined with other non-radioactive elements to form chemical compounds; e.g. technetium-99m is commonly bound to sodium and oxygen to form the compound **sodium pertechnetate**. Consequently, a radionuclide sample contains a greater or smaller amount of non-radioactive carrier material or 'baggage' which adds to its mass without contributing to its activity.

To take account of the inactive part of a radionuclide sample, the **specific activity** of the sample is quoted. Specific activity is defined as the activity per unit mass of the sample. Its SI unit is the becquerel per kilogram ($Bq\ kg^{-1}$). Because radionuclide preparations are often in solution, specific activity is more conveniently expressed in terms of the activity *per unit volume*, e.g. in megabecquerels per millilitre ($MBq\ mL^{-1}$). A knowledge of the specific activity of a preparation enables us to determine what mass (or volume) of the product needs to be used to obtain a specified activity.

Worked example
The specific activity of a solution of sodium pertechnetate is 600 $MBq\ mL^{-1}$. What volume is required to provide an activity of 400 MBq?

$$\text{Specific activity} = \frac{\text{activity}}{\text{volume}}$$

so

$$\text{Volume} = \frac{\text{activity}}{\text{specific activity}}$$
$$= \frac{400}{600}$$
$$= 0.67\ \text{mL}$$

The volume required is therefore 0.67 mL.

20.4   Production of radionuclides

We established in Section 20.1.1.1 that while some radioisotopes (e.g. radium-226) occur naturally, many (e.g. technetium-99m) are manufactured artificially. There are four commercial sources of artificial radionuclides (Ott et al., 1988):

20.4.1   *Nuclear fission in a nuclear reactor*

The spent uranium-fuel rods from a nuclear reactor contain all the elements from zinc ($Z = 30$) to terbium ($Z = 65$), but the fuel rods are highly radioactive and the extraction and purification of individual radionuclides from the rods is difficult. When these problems *can* be overcome, the products obtained have high specific activity. Medically useful radionuclides produced in this way include iodine-131, caesium-137 and molybdenum-99.

20.4.2   *Neutron activation of stable nuclides in a nuclear reactor*

Neutron activation or **neutron capture** occurs when stable nuclides are exposed to neutron bombardment in a nuclear reactor. The previously stable nucleus absorbs or *captures* a neutron and emits a gamma-ray photon. The process is sometimes known as an **n,γ-reaction** (pronounced 'en gamma'). The absorption of a neutron increases by 1 the nucleon number of the nuclide. The specific activity of products obtained by neutron activation is low because many nuclei do not capture a neutron and therefore remain stable. Medically useful radionuclides produced in this way include iron-59 and chromium-51.

20.4.3   *Bombardment with high-energy particles in a particle accelerator*

Particle accelerators such as the **cyclotron** and the **linear accelerator** function by using powerful electromagnetic fields to accelerate charged particles in a circular or linear vacuum tube. Particle energies of up to 100 MeV are used to bombard stable target nuclides, converting them to radionuclides. The manufacturing process is versatile because not only can the target nuclide material be changed, but also the particles with which it is bombarded can be altered. For example, the high-energy accelerated particles can include **deuterons** (^2_1H, the nuclei of **deuterium** or 'heavy hydrogen') and various helium nuclei (^4_2He and ^3_2He). Because the resulting radionuclides nearly always have a different proton number from the target material, they have different chemical properties. They can therefore be chemically separated from the target material and provide a product with very high specific activity. Medically useful radionuclides produced in particle accelerators include oxygen-15, gallium-67, indium-111 and iodine-123.

20.4.4   *Radionuclide generator*

One of the difficulties encountered in the medical applications of radionuclides is the reduction in activity which takes place between the production of the nuclide and its subsequent use. This is particularly true of the short-half-life radionuclides that are used for diagnostic imaging (Section 20.6.1). The solution to the problem is to create the nuclides with a **radionuclide generator**. The principle underlying radionuclide generators is to use a long-half-life parent radionuclide whose daughter product is a radionuclide with a short half-life. The parent radionuclide, prepared by one of the means described above, is shipped to a site close to or inside the centre, where the short-half-life daughter nuclide is required. The radionuclide generator provides a means of chemically separating the daughter product from its parent so that it is available whenever needed. Probably the most common example encountered in radiography is the **technetium-99m generator**. In this device, the parent radionuclide, molybdenum-99 ($T_{\frac{1}{2}} = 2.7$ days), decays by β^- emission into technetium-99m ($T_{\frac{1}{2}} = 6$ h), which is eluted or 'milked' from the generator in the form of a bacteriologically sterile solution of sodium pertechnetate.

20.5   Medical applications of radionuclides

The medical uses of radioactive materials can be divided into two broad categories: *therapeutic* applications (radiotherapy) and *diagnostic* applications. Examples of each of these applications are given below.

20.5.1   Therapeutic applications

In radiotherapy, radionuclides are used as sources of ionising radiation and/or ionising particles to which malignant tissue is particularly sensitive. Exposure of the abnormal tissue to such ionising agents prevents or severely inhibits cell division, thereby arresting or slowing down the growth of malignant disease. The radiotherapy can be administered:

- *Internally*, either by the introduction of **sealed sources** (small wires, needles or capsules) into the tissue, or by the injection or ingestion of **unsealed sources** (usually in solution)
- *Externally*, by **external beam therapy** (**teletherapy**), using powerful gamma-ray emitters such as cobalt-60 or caesium-137

20.5.2   Diagnostic applications

Radionuclides are used in a variety of ways to help diagnose and monitor a patient's disease or injury. Diagnostic investigations can either be undertaken on tissue samples in the laboratory (in vitro studies) or be carried out directly on the living person (in vivo studies).

20.5.2.1   In vitro studies

A sample of the patient's tissue (e.g. blood) is removed and the radionuclide is used, for example, to carry out a **radioimmunoassay** or measurement of the levels of one of its constituents.

20.5.2.2   In vivo studies

The radionuclide is introduced into the living patient (e.g. by injection or inhalation). Examples of in vivo procedures include the following:

- *Physiological studies* in which the function of various organs (e.g. kidney and thyroid) is investigated and measured. A chemical labelled with radionuclide is introduced into the body and its uptake by an organ or system is monitored.
- *Blood volume studies* in which the total blood volume of an individual can be estimated by measuring its diluting effect on a known amount of radionuclide injected into the blood stream.
- *Imaging studies* in which measurement of the spatial distribution in an organ or system, of a previously introduced radionuclide, enables an image of the

organ or system to be created. This process of **radionuclide imaging** is the next topic of study in this chapter.

20.6   Radionuclide imaging

Radionuclide imaging ('isotope scanning') is the technique of producing diagnostic images by analysing the radiation emitted from a patient who has previously been given radioactive medication.

To examine a patient by this method there are four essential requirements:

(1)   **The radiopharmaceutical.** This is a pharmaceutical preparation that can be safely and easily administered to the patient, that will concentrate in the organ or tissues under investigation and that contains a radionuclide emitting a suitable level of gamma radiation.

(2)   **The radiation detection system.** This must be capable of detecting and measuring the level of radiation emerging from the patient.

(3)   **The analysing system.** This must be able to compute the position in the patient of the source of each photon of radiation received by the detectors. This enables a two-dimensional image to be generated, showing the pattern of distribution of the radiopharmaceutical within the patient.

(4)   **The display and recording system.** This presents the image to the operator in an acceptable form and provides a permanent record if required.

Let us examine each of these features in more detail.

20.6.1   *Radiopharmaceuticals*

A vast range of these preparations is available. Many of them, when administered to the patient, participate in the normal (or abnormal) physiology of the body. Depending on their exact chemical nature, they may concentrate in specific organs or tissues. In this respect their behaviour is similar to that of the radiological contrast agents used in excretion urography.

All radiopharmaceuticals include in their molecular structure a radionuclide *label*, which enables their movements within the body to be traced and physiological function to be assessed.

20.6.1.1   Choice of radionuclide label

A number of points must be considered when selecting the radionuclide label:

(1)   The chemical properties of the nuclide must be such that they combine to form a wide range of chemical compounds, each of which must be non-toxic and compatible with the physiology of the patient.

(2)   The **specific activity** of the nuclide (Section 20.3.3) must be high enough to ensure that only small quantities of the preparation need be administered.

(3) The emissions from the nuclide must be of a suitable type, i.e. gamma rays of sufficiently high energy to escape from the patient without undue attenuation, but not so high that the detection of the gamma rays becomes unreliable. There should preferably be no alpha or beta emissions, because these give an unwanted dose to the tissues of the patient.

(4) The nuclide must have a suitable radioactive decay rate. A very short half-life means that the activity reduces so rapidly that too little time is available to carry out any diagnostic imaging. A long half-life increases the radiation hazard to the patient if the nuclide is retained permanently in the body. If the nuclide is excreted quickly, handling of waste from the patient may present problems.

Technetium-99m

The radionuclide **technetium-99m** (^{99m}Tc) is the popular choice for most imaging applications because it satisfies all the criteria listed above (Section 20.6.1.1):

- It is chemically versatile and can be labelled onto a range of compounds, allowing most body organs and systems to be imaged.
- It is conveniently available (from a technetium generator) in a form (sodium pertechnetate) which is of high specific activity and is immediately usable.
- Being metastable, it emits only gamma photons and at an energy (140 keV) which is ideal for imaging purposes.
- Its decay rate ($T_{\frac{1}{2}} = 6$ h) gives the minimum radiation dose to the patient consistent with providing an adequate time to complete the imaging study.

20.6.1.2 Biological and effective half-life

As we saw in Section 20.6.1.1 (above), both the radioactive decay rate of the nuclide and its excretion rate from the body are important factors in determining the radiation dose received by the patient. We must therefore consider two new concepts: **biological half-life** and **effective half-life**.

- *Biological half-life* of a pharmaceutical preparation is the time taken for the quantity of pharmaceutical within the patient to reduce to one-half due to its excretion from body. Biological half-life is a *general* concept which can be applied to any pharmaceutical preparation, whether or not it is radioactive. It depends on the rate of excretion of the pharmaceutical and hence on both its chemical nature and the physiology of the patient.
- *Effective half-life* is the time taken for the activity of a radiopharmaceutical within the patient to reduce to one-half due to both radioactive decay *and* biological excretion. A simple relationship exists between effective half-life, $T_{\frac{1}{2}}$ (effective); biological half-life, $T_{\frac{1}{2}}$ (biological); and radioactive (physical) half-life, $T_{\frac{1}{2}}$ (radioactive):

$$\frac{1}{T_{\frac{1}{2}} \text{ (effective)}} = \frac{1}{T_{\frac{1}{2}} \text{ (biological)}} + \frac{1}{T_{\frac{1}{2}} \text{ (radioactivity)}}$$

Worked example

If $T_{\frac{1}{2}}$ (biological) $= 24$ h and $T_{\frac{1}{2}}$ (radioactive) $= 6$ h, calculate the effective half-life, $T_{\frac{1}{2}}$ (effective):

$$\frac{1}{T_{\frac{1}{2}}\text{ (effective)}} = \frac{1}{24} + \frac{1}{6} = \frac{1}{24} + \frac{4}{24} = \frac{5}{24}$$

Thus:

$$T_{\frac{1}{2}}\text{ (effective)} = \frac{24}{5} = 4.8\text{ h}$$

20.6.2   Radiation detection system

In Section 19.2.4, we discussed the process of scintillation as a method of detecting and measuring ionising radiations. In a scintillation crystal, the absorption of a single photon of X- or gamma rays causes the instantaneous release of a number of visible light photons seen as a faint flash of light within the crystal. The detection of each flash of light makes it possible to *count* the number of photons of ionising radiation absorbed in the crystal. This is the principle of the **scintillation counter** used as a radiation detector in radionuclide imaging equipment.

A scintillation crystal of thallium-activated **sodium iodide** is commonly employed to trap gamma-ray photons and convert them into light pulses. A highly responsive light-sensitive device known as a **photomultiplier tube** (Section 15.4.1) detects the arrival of light photons and converts each flash of light into an electrical pulse.

A lead collimator is attached to the front of the detector so that it only receives gamma-ray photons travelling in a specified direction. The collimator is a lead block through which a large number of holes have been drilled in precisely defined directions. The detector is protected from background radiation by a lead shield forming part of its housing.

20.6.2.1   Gamma camera

The most common design of gamma-ray detector used for imaging purposes is the **gamma camera**.

The gamma camera (Fig. 20.8) employs a large crystal of thallium-activated sodium iodide (e.g. 40-cm diameter) monitored by a hexagonal array of 61 or 75 photomultipliers. Various types of collimators are used. For example, a **parallel-hole collimator** may be used, allowing the crystal to receive gamma rays from a large area of the patient. The sodium iodide crystal is optically coupled to the photomultiplier tubes. This minimises light leakage, which would result in failure to detect some of the light pulses.

20.6.3   Analysing system

The purpose of the analysing system is twofold:

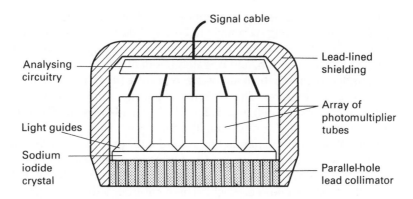

Fig. 20.8 Longitudinal section of the detector head of a gamma camera.

(1) **Position analysis.** The precise position in the scintillation crystal of the source of each light pulse is computed by comparing the signal strengths from each of the photomultiplier tubes. This enables the coordinates of each scintillation to be determined and therefore the location in the patient of the source of the gamma-ray photon which produced the scintillation.

(2) **Signal-strength analysis.** The strength of signal originating from each gamma-ray photon detected is examined with a **pulse height analyser** (Section 19.2.4). This device rejects very *weak* signals, created by low-energy scattered radiation, and very *strong* signals, created by simultaneous scintillations. Consequently, the only signals accepted for onward transmission are those from scintillations triggered *by primary* gamma-ray photons arriving in the patient directly from the radionuclide.

Positional and other signal data are digitised in readiness for computer processing prior to image display and storage.

20.6.4 *Display and recording system*

The signal derived from each tiny volume **(voxel)** of tissue in the gamma camera's field of view indicates whether or not a gamma-ray photon was detected from that location. For each point, therefore, the signal has just *two* possible states: ON (if a gamma photon *was* detected) and OFF (if a gamma photon *was not* detected). This type of signal, having only two states, is known as a **bistable** signal. An imaging computer collects these data, together with the associated positional data, and converts them into a form which can be used to generate an image. The image data, representing the spatial distribution of the gamma-ray photons detected in the patient, can be handled in various ways to give, for example, a real-time television (TV) display or recorded images.

20.6.4.1 **Real-time television display**

When gamma-camera signals are integrated (i.e. added up) over a period of time, a total count (and count rate) can be determined. Because there is a critical minimum count necessary to produce a good-quality image, the count rate determines for how long data have to be acquired (i.e. the scan time) to produce a successful image. If the count rate is sufficiently high, the image may be constructed rapidly enough, and updated frequently enough, for a **dynamic study** to be undertaken, in which a moving, **real-time** (live) image is displayed on the screen of a TV monitor. The TV screen image comprises an array or **matrix** of picture elements (**pixels**), e.g. 512×512 (=262 144 pixels). The gamma-camera image is made up of a much smaller matrix whose size is determined by the number of holes in the parallel-hole collimator (e.g. 6000–30 000 holes). Consequently, *a group* of pixels is used to represent each position in the patient for which data are available. Each pixel has two states: ON (activated, i.e. white) and OFF (deactivated, i.e. black). The computer activates a group of pixels if gamma-ray photons were detected, but not if no photons were detected. To construct a complete image, data are required for *all* the points in the area of patient being investigated.

20.6.4.2   Recorded images

Gamma-camera images can be recorded in several ways (Ball & Price, 1995). Examples include the following:

- **Digital data storage.** The digital output from the gamma camera may be recorded on data-storage media, such as **magnetic** or **optical discs** (CDs and DVDs). Images can then be recalled and manipulated at a later date.
- **Hard-copy storage.** The signals supplying the TV monitor can also be fed to a **laser imager**. This device produces a convenient and permanent *photographic* record of the gamma-camera images on high-resolution film.

20.6.4.3   Image enhancement

The imaging computer which forms part of the gamma-camera system can be used to manipulate or *enhance* the characteristics of the image to obtain maximum information. For example, image artefacts may be removed, or a multi-colour image may be produced.

20.6.5   *Summary*

The combination of gamma camera and digital computer forms an extremely powerful diagnostic tool, which plays an important role in complementing traditional radiological techniques.

In the next chapter we shall consider the *biological* effects of ionising radiation and discuss the measures which may be taken to minimise any hazards.

Chapter 21
Radiation Safety

21.1   Introduction

Ionising radiation damages living tissue. The damage caused may be relatively minor, e.g. simple ionisation of water, or may result in the cell becoming *initiated*, i.e. having the potential to develop into a fatal cancer. However, radiation can be used to treat cancers when applied in a controlled manner. Whether radiation is used diagnostically or therapeutically, it always has the potential to produce cancer.

X-rays and radioactivity were known to be harmful within years of their discovery and there are many examples of early radiation workers suffering serious radiation damage. It is, therefore, essential that safety measures are considered when dealing with radiation.

However, before discussing the regulations controlling the use of radiation in hospitals, we need to consider the origins of radiation exposure and how an exposure to radiation affects human cells.

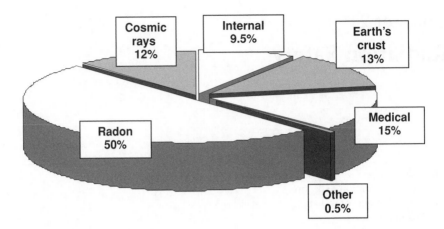

Fig. 21.1   Sources of radiation exposure. (*Source*: HPA, 2005a.)

21.2   Sources of radiation

We live in an environment in which approximately 85% of the radiation dose to the population of the UK arises from natural sources, while the remaining 15% arises from man-made sources (Health Protection Agency (HPA), 2005a). The major sources of radiation are shown in Fig. 21.1.

21.2.1   Natural sources

All individuals are exposed to radiation from naturally occurring sources. The major sources of this exposure are as follows:

- **Radon gas (50%).** Radon gas ($^{222}_{86}$Rn) is a daughter product of the radioactive decay of uranium-238. Uranium-238 occurs naturally and is found particularly in granite. Radon gas diffuses easily through soil, dispersing into the air. However, it can become trapped inside and underneath buildings and can prove to be a hazard. Radon is more likely to be trapped in modern houses that may be double-glazed, draught-proofed and with cavity wall insulation and therefore poorly ventilated. Radon gas emits alpha particles, which when breathed in, result in localised damage to the lungs. As alpha particles are not very penetrating, the only real hazard from inhalation of radon gas is the production of radiation-induced cancer of the lung. It is estimated that in the UK approximately 1000 lung cancer deaths per year are attributable to radon gas (Cancer Research UK, 2004).

  The level of radon gas exposure is dependent on the geology of the area but the south-west of the UK is recognised as an area with high radon levels. Radon gas is responsible for approximately 50% of our total radiation dose from natural sources.
- **Earth's crust and building materials (13%).** This source refers to gamma rays originating from rocks, soil and building materials. The earth's crust contains

many naturally occurring radioisotopes, which become incorporated into building materials such as sand and cement. The radiation dose received from these sources can differ considerably from location to location, depending on local geology, numbers of buildings, roads etc.

- **Cosmic rays (12%).** Cosmic radiation originates from outer space and enters the earth's atmosphere. Some of the radiation is absorbed by the earth's atmosphere, but a significant proportion reaches the surface and contributes to population dose. This means that passengers in high-flying aircraft generally receive greater doses than people on the ground, as there is less atmosphere above them to attenuate the radiation. On a flight from London to New York, the passengers will receive a radiation dose of approximately 0.04 mSv, which equates to the dose received from having two chest radiographs (HPA, 2005a).
- **Internal sources (9.5%).** These are due to our food and drink. Many items of food and drink contain some naturally occurring radioactive material, and therefore we are constantly ingesting sources of radiation into our bodies; e.g. eating 135 g of Brazil nuts results in a radiation exposure of approximately 0.01 mSv (HPA, 2005b). The radioactive isotopes that we eat and drink may be incorporated into our own tissues, which become radioactive, and we ourselves are then contributing to our own radiation dose.

21.2.2 Man-made sources

The main artificial sources of radiation are:

- **Medical exposures (15%).** Medical exposures are by far the major source of man-made radiation, and include X-rays and radionuclides used in diagnosis and treatment. The doses received during radiotherapy are far greater than those used in diagnostic radiography. However, because many more people undergo diagnostic procedures than radiotherapy, the major contribution for medical exposures is from diagnostic sources. It is interesting to note that approximately 97% of the radiation dose from man-made sources comes from medical exposures.
- **Other sources (0.5%).** This group includes radioactive fallout, environmental pollution, some consumer products and occupational exposures. As can be seen in Fig. 21.1, this group of radiation sources makes only a minor contribution to the overall dose received by the population of the UK.

21.3 Biological effects of ionising radiation

In earlier chapters, the production and attenuation of radiation have been discussed. When considering the biological effects of radiation it is important to know what type of radiation is incident on the tissues of the body. Different types of radiations produce greater or lesser degrees of damage to tissue; we therefore use different units to express the degree of biological damage done to the tissues.

21.3.1   Radiation units of measurement

21.3.1.1   Absorbed dose

As we saw in Section 19.1, absorbed dose is the amount of energy transferred from the beam of radiation to the irradiated material (in this case, to the tissues of the body). Energy is measured in joules and the unit of absorbed dose is the gray (Gy); hence:

$$1 \text{ gray} = 1 \text{ joule per kilogram}$$
$$= 1 \text{ J kg}^{-1}$$

Absorbed dose is a measure of the amount of energy deposited but it does not take into account the varying biological damage caused by different types of radiation. Absorbed dose does not, therefore, give an accurate measure of the biological effects of radiation. An adjustment has to be made to the absorbed dose to take into account the type of radiation incident upon the body tissues.

21.3.1.2   Dose equivalent

The unit of dose equivalent is the sievert (Sv). Dose equivalent relates the absorbed dose to the degree of biological damage caused by a particular type of radiation. This is achieved by applying a **quality factor** related to the type of radiation. The quality factor can be considered to be a scaling factor relating absorbed dose to biological effect. Hence:

$$\text{Dose equivalent (Sv)} = \text{absorbed dose} \times \text{quality factor}$$
$$= \text{Gy} \times \text{QF}$$

where the quality factors are as given in Table 21.1.

21.3.1.3   Effective dose

With any exposure to radiation, several types of tissues will lie in the radiation beam. Some tissues are more sensitive to radiation than others, so an adjustment to the dose equivalent is necessary to reflect the relative risk of damage to the various tissues. The unit of effective dose is also the sievert (Sv), as we are still measuring damage to tissue. The adjustment applied to the value of the dose equivalent is called the **tissue weighting factor**, which reflects the relative

Table 21.1   Radiation quality factors

Type of radiation	Quality factor
X-rays and gamma rays	1
Electrons	1
Neutrons	10
Alpha particles	20

Table 21.2 Tissue weighting factors

Tissue	Weighting factor	Tissue	Weighting factor
Gonads	0.2	Lung	0.12
Red bone Marrow	0.12	Oesophagus	0.05
Bladder	0.05	Skin	0.01
Bone surfaces	0.01	Stomach	0.12
Breast	0.05	Thyroid	0.05
Colon	0.12	Others	0.05
Liver	0.05		

Source: ICRP (1990).

sensitivity of the various tissues to provide a more accurate measure of the biological damage caused by the radiation.

Hence:

Effective dose (Sv) = dose equivalent × tissue weighting factor

$$= Sv \times W_T$$

The weighting factors are given in Table 21.2.

The doses received by the different organs can be combined into a single dose of radiation that *if applied to the whole body* would result in the same risk of cancer as the dose to individual organs in the beam.

Example. Consider a chest radiograph in which the following organ dose was recorded:

Lungs 0.20 mSv (weighting factor 0.12)

Then, applying the tissue weighting factor:

Effective dose = 0.20 × 0.12

= 0.024 mSv

This result means that the risk of developing cancer of the lung from receiving an absorbed dose of 0.20 mSv is the same as that if the whole body received 0.024 mSv.

A major advantage of using effective dose is that it allows different imaging modalities to be compared in determining the risk of developing cancer. An effective dose of 0.1 mSv resulting from a chest X-ray has the same risk of developing cancer as that of an effective dose of 0.1 mSv resulting from a radionuclide imaging procedure or 0.1 mSv from a CT scan.

The relationships between the different units used in establishing the biological effects of ionising radiation are summarised in Fig. 21.2.

21.4 Radiobiology

Radiobiology is the study of how tissues behave when exposed to radiation. However, not all cells react in the same way when radiation is incident upon

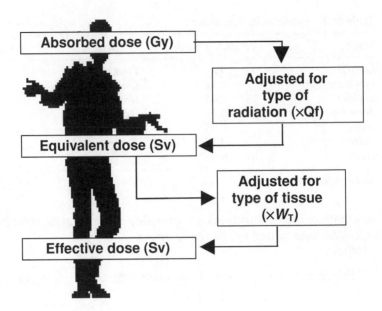

Fig. 21.2   Relationships between units of dose.

them. This difference in reaction to radiation is called **radiosensitivity** and is a statement of how sensitive a particular type of cell is to radiation damage.

21.4.1 *Nature of the hazard*

X-rays and gamma rays are ionising radiations and are therefore capable of removing electrons from atoms. The ionisation of atoms results in the breaking of the covalent bonds of molecules. It is the breaking of these bonds that causes biological damage.

When the tissues of the body are irradiated, the photons of radiation undergo photoelectric and Compton interactions with cells of the tissues. Energy is transferred to the tissues, resulting in the breaking of the chemical bonds between atoms by ionising the atom; e.g.

$$H_2O + photon \rightarrow OH^- + H^+$$

21.4.2 *Nature of the biological damage*

A typical tissue cell has a very complex structure. However, one of the most important components is DNA. The chromosomes within the nucleus are made of DNA and they are responsible, via the activation of genes, for the functioning of the cell. Any radiation damage to the DNA can result in significant biological damage to the cell.

This damage to the DNA can be caused in one of two ways:

- **Direct effect.** Here, the radiation interacts directly with DNA to cause damage.

- **Indirect effect.** Here, the radiation interacts with a molecule of water to produce what are known as free radicals. Free radicals are a group of highly reactive chemicals that can have a damaging effect on the DNA structure. A free radical commonly produced is ionised hydroxyl ($\cdot$OH). As cells consist of approximately 70–80% water, it is not surprising that most of the radiation interactions are of an indirect nature.

Typical effects due to radiation interacting with the cell are:

- Genetic damage (to genes)
- Cell mutation (both physical and physiological)
- Delayed or arrested cell division
- Radiation-induced cancers
- Cell death

The effects detailed above occur in individual cells. However, when a patient is exposed to a beam of radiation or to a radioactive source, it is tissues and systems that are receiving the exposure, rather than a few individual cells. The biological effects of radiation can, therefore, be classified by how radiation interacts with areas of the body and differing tissue types.

21.4.3   Biological effects

The biological effects of radiation can be classified as somatic and genetic effects, which relate to body areas, or as deterministic and stochastic effects, which relate to the type of damage that may be caused.

21.4.3.1   Somatic effects

These effects are the result of irradiation of the body tissues. The major feature of somatic effects is that they are restricted to the individual irradiated; i.e. they are not passed on to future generations. Examples of somatic effects are radiation-induced cancers or radiation cataracts.

21.4.3.2   Genetic effects

Genetic effects are caused by irradiation of the gonads and may be passed on to an individual's offspring. The effects do not appear in the person receiving the exposure but in their descendants as they are caused by damage to the DNA of the sperm or ovum. Examples of genetic effects are leukaemia and mental retardation.

21.4.3.3   Deterministic effects

Deterministic effects are always somatic effects. As the name implies, deterministic effects are determined by the dose received by an individual. The main

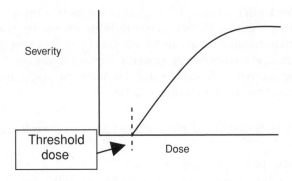

Fig. 21.3   Deterministic effects of radiation.

features of a deterministic effect are:

- There is a **threshold dose** below which the effect will not occur.
- The *severity* of the effect increases with the dose received (Fig. 21.3).

The most common deterministic effects are impaired fertility and cataracts. The threshold dose for cataract formation is approximately 0.5 Gy, with full cataracts being evident at 6.0 Gy.

21.4.3.4   Stochastic effects

Stochastic is a statistical term relating to probability. Stochastic effects can be either somatic or genetic. The main features of stochastic effects are:

- There is no threshold dose. This means that for any exposure there is always a risk of developing cancer. It could, therefore, be said that there is no such thing as a safe dose of radiation.
- The *probability* of an effect occurring increases with the dose received.

The main stochastic effect is cancer. As can be seen from Fig. 21.4, cancer is more likely to develop with increases in radiation dose. Even though the risk may

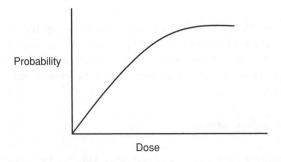

Fig. 21.4   Stochastic effects of radiation.

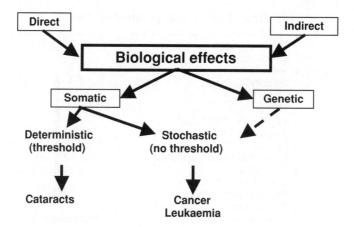

Fig. 21.5   Biological effects of radiation.

be very small at low exposure levels, it is not zero. This relationship between increased dose and the increase in the probability of producing cancer underpins the philosophy of radiation legislation.

Genetic effects, induced in the offspring of an individual, are classed as stochastic because exposure of the testes or ovaries to radiation *may* result in the effect manifesting itself. The greater the level of exposure, the greater the likelihood of the effect occurring.

The biological effects of radiation are summarised in Fig. 21.5.

21.5   Radiosensitivity

Radiosensitivity is a statement of how sensitive a particular type of tissue is to radiation damage. X-rays damage living tissue and the extent of the damage depends on:

- Type of cell irradiated (based on radiosensitivity)
- Volume of tissue irradiated (The greater the volume, the greater the degree of damage.)
- Dose received (The greater the dose, the greater the degree of damage.)

The relative sensitivities of different tissue types are provided in Table 21.3.

Biological effects of irradiation of the tissues may be subclinical or manifest clinically as signs and symptoms suffered by the irradiated individual. The explanation of the biological basis of the relative sensitivity of the various tissues lies outside the scope of this book, but the differing sensitivities of the tissues is reflected in the risk of radiation-induced cancers produced by the various radiological procedures undertaken. These risks will be discussed in the following section.

Table 21.3   Relative radiosensitivity of tissues

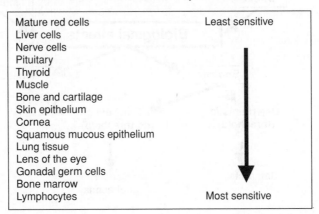

Mature red cells	Least sensitive
Liver cells	
Nerve cells	
Pituitary	
Thyroid	
Muscle	
Bone and cartilage	
Skin epithelium	
Cornea	
Squamous mucous epithelium	
Lung tissue	
Lens of the eye	
Gonadal germ cells	
Bone marrow	
Lymphocytes	Most sensitive

21.6   Principles of radiation protection

The specific aims of radiation protection are to:

- Ensure all exposures are justified
- Prevent deterministic effects by not reaching the necessary threshold dose
- Limit stochastic effects by keeping doses low, as probability increases with dose

The International Commission on Radiological Protection (ICRP) has identified three basic principles of radiation protection:

1. Justification
2. Optimisation
3. Limitation

The principles of justification and optimisation apply to everyone: staff, patients and members of the public. The principle of limitation, however, applies to radiation workers only.

21.6.1   *Justification*

The principle of justification means that no exposure to ionising radiation shall be undertaken unless it results in a net benefit to the individual receiving the exposure. Essentially, this means that unless there is a good reason for a person to receive a dose of radiation, the exposure should not be made. Justification is one of the major elements of radiation legislation in the UK (Her Majesty's Stationery Office (HMSO), 2000, regulation 6).

Justification is the first step in radiation protection as no exposure is justifiable without a valid clinical indication. The best form of radiation protection is not to receive an exposure to radiation at all. In arriving at the decision as to whether an exposure is justified, we make use of the risk–benefit relationship and every exposure must result in a net benefit for the patient.

21.6.1.1   Risk–Benefit relationship

Radiation damages living tissue and when deciding whether an exposure should take place, we have to weigh up the risks to the patient from radiation against the potential benefit of having the exposure.

Radiology involves striking a balance between benefit and risk for the patient, where:

- The benefit is successful diagnosis and treatment.
- The risks are:

    (a)   Radiation-induced cancers in the individual
    (b)   Serious hereditary effects in descendants

Typical risks from common radiological examinations are given in Table 21.4, where it can be seen, for example, that the risk of developing cancer from having a chest X-ray is one in a million. This means that for every million people having the examination, one will develop cancer over the next 15 to 20 years as a result of the radiation exposure.

When applying the principle of justification, the benefit to the patient of having the exposure must outweigh the risks; e.g. the benefit of establishing the extent of a pneumothorax outweighs the tiny risk of inducing cancer; therefore, the procedure is justified.

In applying the risk–benefit relationship to a proposed exposure, a criterion often applied is that the exposure is justified if the result of having the examination will change the clinical management of the patient.

The risk of producing serious hereditary effects in the offspring of the person receiving the exposure stems from radiation damage to the DNA of the chromosomes when the ovaries or testes have been irradiated.

Table 21.4   Risks arising from radiological examinations

Examination	Risk	Risk of serious hereditary effects in first two generations	
		Female	Male
Chest	1 in 1 million	Less than 1 in 1 billion	
Abdomen	1 in 30 000	1 in 170 000	1 in a million
Pelvis	1 in 30 000	1 in 240 000	1 in 60 000
Lumbar spine	1 in 15 000	1 in 65 000	1 in 1 million
IVU	1 in 8000	1 in 160 000	1 in 1 million
Barium meal	1 in 6700	1 in 150 000	1 in 10 million
Barium enema	1 in 3 000	1 in 30 000	1 in 100 000
CT abdomen	1 in 2000	1 in 25 000	1 in 100 000

Data from HPA (2005).

21.6.2   Optimisation

Optimisation is the second principle of radiation protection. Once an exposure has been justified, the exposure should be optimised. This principle is commonly referred to as the ALARA principle, where the dose delivered by the exposure should be as low as reasonably achievable to produce the desired outcome. In diagnostic radiography the desired outcome is very often the production of a diagnostic image. In radiotherapy it has to be ensured that exposure of target volumes is individually planned, taking into account that doses to non-target tissues should be kept as low as reasonably achievable. The desired outcome is an effective treatment of the particular pathology. The principle of optimisation also forms part of UK radiation legislation (HMSO, 2000, regulation 7).

By the application of the ALARA principle, the radiation risk to the individual irradiated is kept to a minimum. There are a number of factors in radiological practice which influence keeping the radiation dose low, e.g.:

- **Choice of equipment.** For example, the fastest imaging systems should be used to produce diagnostic images (including digital systems which are replacing many film-based systems), the use of automatic exposure control, pulsed fluoroscopy, etc. In the UK there is a legal requirement for manufacturers to design dose-reducing features into all new imaging equipment (HMSO, 1999).
- **Implementation of effective quality-assurance programmes.** Such programmes ensure that equipment and staff perform to the highest standards.
- **Assessment of dose.** Effective dose monitoring ensures that the lowest dose compatible with producing the desired outcome is achieved.
- **Implementation and use of Diagnostic Reference Levels (DRLs).** DRLs are dose levels for a typical X-ray examination of a group of patients with standard body sizes and for broadly defined types of equipment. It is expected that these reference levels will not be exceeded for standard procedures. The establishment of DRLs and their review at regular intervals should help ensure optimum dose levels for radiographic practice.
- **Correct choice of technique.** Using technique protocols to establish the number of projections, positioning and exposure criteria for the standard radiological examinations will also help to ensure dose optimisation.

The factors identified are only examples of the wide range of measures to assist in keeping dose levels to a minimum. A full discussion of all the measures available is beyond the scope of this book and the reader is encouraged to refer to other sources to supplement, and to explore more fully, the examples given here.

It is the radiographer's responsibility to ensure that, through good practice, radiation doses are kept as low as reasonably achievable.

21.6.3   Limitation

The purpose of the principles of justification and optimisation is to safeguard the interests of the patient, staff and members of the public. We tend to think only of the patient when applying these principles. However, these principles apply to radiographers too. For example, radiographers have to justify why they are in the X-ray room. (This may be fairly obvious because the patient cannot be examined or treated unless the radiographer is present!). When in the room, the principle of optimisation applies to the radiographer, and all doses have to be as low as reasonably achievable. This involves standing behind radiation barriers when making an exposure to ensure that any primary or secondary (scattered) radiation does not reach the radiographer. The principle of optimisation is also behind the reason for wearing a lead-rubber apron when undertaking fluoro-scopic examinations. The lead-rubber apron ensures that any dose received is as low as reasonably achievable by absorbing scattered radiation that may be directed towards the radiographer.

However, the principle of limitation applies to everyone other than the patient, e.g. radiation workers and members of the public. There are strict limits on the radiation dose that can be received. These limits are based on the findings of the ICRP in establishing the stochastic risk of developing a fatal radiation-induced cancer. For radiation workers, a risk of 1 in 1000 is considered to be not unacceptable. For members of the public the maximum risk recommended is 1 in 100 000, one hundred times less than that for a radiation worker.

Remember that two of the aims of radiation protection are to limit stochastic effects and to prevent deterministic effects. Hence dose limits are imposed in the UK by the Ionising Radiations Regulations 1999 to ensure that the risk of radiation-induced cancer is not at an unacceptable level (see Table 21.5).

Dose limits are established above which continued exposure increases the risk to unacceptable levels. A dose limit *does not* mean that doses above the limit are dangerous and that those below are safe – *all* exposures carry a risk of inducing cancer.

The Ionising Radiations Regulations 1999 also identify dose limits for women of reproductive capacity and those who are pregnant:

- The dose limit for the abdomen of a female radiation worker of reproductive capacity is 13 mSv in any consecutive 3-month interval.
- Once a pregnancy has been confirmed and the employer notified, the dose to the fetus should not exceed 1 mSv during the remainder of the pregnancy.

Table 21.5   Radiation Dose limits

	Radiation worker >18 years	Radiation worker <18 years	Other persons
To limit stochastic effects, the effective dose shall not exceed			
Whole body (mSv)	20	6	1
To prevent deterministic effects, the equivalent dose shall not exceed			
Single organ or tissue (mSv)	500	150	50
Lens of the eye (mSv)	150	45	15
Hands, forearms, feet and ankles (mSv)	500	150	50

Adapted from Schedule 4 of the Ionising Radiations Regulations 1999 (HMSO, 1999).

Having considered the effects of radiation exposure on tissues and the principles of radiation protection, we will now consider how radiation safety is implemented in practice.

21.7   Radiation safety in practice

In the European Union (EU), radiation safety measures are governed by the ICRP. Each member nation interprets the recommendations to produce legislation and codes of practice, which become enshrined within the nation's legal structures. Nations not in the EU have their own arrangements for radiation safety.

21.7.1   UK radiation safety legislation

In the UK, radiation safety legislation forms part of the Health and Safety at Work Act 1974. Within the act are a number of pieces of legislation called statutory instruments. Radiation safety falls under the heading of statutory instruments and currently (2007) consists of the following major pieces of legislation:

- **Ionising Radiations Regulations 1999 (IRR 1999).** These regulations came into force on 13 May 2000. They are concerned with the establishment and maintenance of a safe working environment concerning the use of radiation. These regulations cover, for example, the provision and use of protective equipment, establishment of radiation areas and various aspects of equipment design (HMSO, 1999). These regulations do not specifically relate to patients.
- **Ionising Radiation (Medical Exposure) Regulations 2000 (IR(ME)R 2000).** These regulations came into force on 1 January 2001. These regulations are specifically concerned with keeping the radiation exposure to patients as low as reasonably practicable. The main principles underlying these regulations are justification and optimisation (HMSO, 2000).
- **Ionising Radiation (Medical Exposure) (Amendment) Regulations 2006.** These regulations came into force on 1 November 2006. The purpose of these regulations is to update the IR(ME)R 2000 regulations and also to clarify the terminology and definitions used in the original IR(ME)R 2000 regulations (HMSO, 2006).

Many hospitals and clinics use radioactive materials for the diagnosis and treatment of disease. As sources of radiation, these substances present a radiation hazard and are subject to further legislation:

- **Radioactive Substances Act 1993.** These regulations came into force on 1 January 1993. The act is concerned with the use, storage and disposal of radioactive materials (RSA 1993).

- **Radioactive Substances (Hospitals) Exemption (Amendment) Order 1995.** This legislation came into force on 3 October 1995. The legislation is concerned with the exemption of hospitals from the RSA 1993 regulations for the storage and use of radioactive materials in a hospital (HMSO, 1995).

These regulations supersede all previous legislation.

21.7.2   *Practical application of radiation safety*

The radiation legislation noted above consists of numerous documents that cover all aspects of radiation safety, but do so in a very general manner. The regulations have to be interpreted and implemented within the clinical departments to ensure that safe working practices are in place.

We shall look at the practical application of radiation safety under the following headings:

- Administrative aspects
- Radiation protection measures
- Personnel dose monitoring

21.7.2.1   Administration of radiation safety

The Ionising Radiations Regulations 1999 and the Ionising Radiation (Medical Exposure) Regulations 2000 lay down many of the administrative requirements for establishing and maintaining a safe working environment. These can be considered under a number of headings:

Organisation of radiation protection (IRR 1999)
The employer (e.g. the hospital trust) is ultimately responsible for the management of radiation safety. The employer achieves this through a number of radiation safety experts:

Radiation protection adviser (RPA). The RPA is usually a physicist and is employed to advise the employer on radiation safety and compliance with the regulations. This includes advising on the production of local rules and on the use of new radiation equipment and rooms where ionising radiation is employed.

Radiation protection supervisor (RPS). Every department in which ionising radiation is used must have an RPS, who understands the requirements of the regulations applying to radiation safety. The RPS is responsible for ensuring that radiation safety measures are implemented and radiation safety standards are maintained.

Radiation safety committee. The purpose of this committee is to oversee all radiation safety issues and ensure that the reports and recommendations of the RPA are acted upon.

Designation of areas (IRR 1999)
In order for radiation safety to be applied, we must know *where* the potential hazards are present. This is achieved by designating areas of hazard as either a **controlled area** or a **supervised area**. This designation may not be permanent, e.g. when the X-ray unit is isolated from the mains electricity supply. In this case the unit is incapable of producing X-rays so there are no hazards to be identified.

> **Controlled area.** This is any area where a person is likely to receive an effective dose greater than 6 mSv per year or an equivalent dose greater than three-tenths of any relevant dose limit (IRR 1999) (Table 21.5). In practice, all X-ray rooms are designated as controlled areas. All controlled areas must have the appropriate radiation-hazard warning signs in place at entry points and a means of indicating when an exposure is about to take place. This is usually achieved by an illuminated sign, linked to the exposure circuit and positioned outside the entrance to the X-ray room.
>   Access by staff to controlled areas has to be formalised in a written **system of work**.
> **Supervised area.** This is an area where the radiation risk is not as great as that in a controlled area. It is defined as any area where a person is likely to receive an effective dose greater than 1 mSv per year or an equivalent dose greater than one-tenth of any relevant dose limit (IRR 1999) (Table 21.5).

Designation of classified persons (IRR 1999)
When considering radiation safety, occupationally exposed employees who may be at risk need to be identified. On this basis a **classified person** is a person who is likely to receive an effective dose in excess of 6 mSv per year or an equivalent dose which exceeds three-tenths of any relevant dose limit (IRR 1999) (Table 21.5).

A classified worker must be individually monitored and under medical surveillance by an appointed doctor. When newly designated as a classified worker, a medical examination is carried out to:

- Assess the medical fitness of the employee for the work to be carried out with ionising radiation
- Act as a 'baseline' against which any future changes in health can be assessed

In practice, the majority of radiographers are not designated as classified workers, as they are very unlikely to exceed the stated radiation dose limits.

Local rules (IRR 1999)
All ionising radiation legislation needs to be applied to the particular area in which ionising radiation is used, e.g. a hospital X-ray department. As every imaging department is different in layout, number of rooms, types of equipment and examinations carried out, the regulations have to be applied to meet the local situation. **Local rules**, which are the application of the national regulations to a local area, have to be drawn up.

Local rules have to be written down and appropriate to the radiation risk and nature of the procedures undertaken. The local rules should be read by everyone using radiation and contain, for example,

- Details of designated areas
- Name of the RPS
- System of work for access to controlled areas
- General information on radiation safety

System of work (IRR 1999)
If a non-classified worker is to enter a controlled area, access can be permitted only under a **system of work**. A system of work is a written document which gives details of protocols and procedures to restrict, as far as is reasonably practicable, the exposure to ionising radiation of employees and others. A system of work would include, for example, details of who can enter a controlled area and for what purpose. Radiographers enter controlled areas under a system of work, as generally they are not designated as classified workers.

Duty holders (IRR 2000)
IR(ME)R 2000 identifies four main duty holders:

1. Employer
2. Referrer
3. Practitioner
4. Operator

> **Employer.** The employer takes ultimate responsibility for ensuring that all aspects of radiation safety as detailed in IR(ME)R 2000 are implemented in areas in which ionising radiation is used.
> **Referrer.** This term applies to the individual making the request for a procedure using ionising radiation, i.e. referring the patient. A referrer can be any health care professional, providing that he or she has been adequately trained in accordance with the employer's procedures. Today, it is common in many hospitals to have nurses and physiotherapists referring patients for a radiological examination. This was not possible under previous regulations. A referrer must supply adequate medical data relevant to the examination to allow the justification process to take place (see Section 21.6.1.1). This includes recording the clinical indications for the request and may involve making the patient's notes available to the radiographer.
> **Practitioner.** This person is responsible for justifying and authorising the exposure and plays a key role in reducing unnecessary exposures. The practitioner is usually a radiologist but can also be a radiographer.
> **Operator.** The operator is the person carrying out the practical aspects of a medical exposure, including the selection of equipment and technique to ensure that the principle of ALARA is applied. All radiographers are classed as operators under the requirements of IR(ME)R 2000.

Adequate training (IRR 2000)
IR(ME)R 2000 requires that all practitioners and operators have successfully completed training and possess adequate theoretical knowledge and practical experience in a range of topic areas, relating to the use of ionising radiation in the examination of patients. The training requirements are detailed in Schedule 2 of IR(ME)R 2000. In practice, this means that **adequate training**, as defined in the regulations, requires the practitioner and operator to be either a radiographer or a radiologist.

21.7.2.2   Practical radiation protection measures

In the previous section we considered the rules and regulations concerned with radiation protection. In this section we review some of the practical measures that can be used in the clinical setting to ensure that any radiation doses received by patients, staff and others are kept as low as reasonably achievable. It is beyond the scope of this book to cover all the aspects of radiographic technique where specific protection measures are applied. However, we will consider some general topic areas that can be universally applied.

Use of lead
Many protection measures depend on the use of lead in one form or another. Lead has a high proton number ($Z = 82$) and a high density. At the radiation energies employed in diagnostic radiography the main attenuation process is photoelectric absorption. As the mass attenuation coefficient for the photoelectric process is proportional to Z^3, lead with its high proton number is an effective protective material.

Lead can be used as a radiation barrier in a number of ways:

- **Room construction.** In the X-ray room, lead is sandwiched between layers of wood in the construction of doors, mobile barriers and control cubicle surrounds, etc. Lead can be used in powder form mixed with concrete, plaster or glass to provide an effective radiation barrier in walls or as windows in control cubicles and mobile barriers.
- **Accessory equipment.** Lead is also used in radiographic equipment to provide radiation protection, e.g. lining the X-ray tube and in the construction of lead cones and collimation devices. Gonad shields and flexible lead-rubber sheets provide protection, as do lead-rubber aprons and lead-rubber gloves.

Lead equivalent. As lead can be used in many different ways in the construction of radiation protective materials and devices, we need to be able to compare the effectiveness of these materials as a radiation barrier. This can be done by quoting their lead-equivalent values.

The **lead equivalent** of a material is defined as the thickness of lead that offers the same degree of protection as the stated thickness of material for a given radiation quality. For example, a solid concrete wall 15 cm thick provides the same degree of protection from 100 keV X-rays as 2.4-mm lead. We can say, therefore, that the lead equivalent of 15 cm of concrete is 2.4 mm at 100 keV. Similarly, the lead-rubber aprons used in imaging departments have lead equivalents from 0.25 mm upwards.

Correct radiographic techniques

By using the correct radiographic techniques, the ALARA principle can be applied. Considerations of dose optimisation by radiographic techniques include:

- Strict application of the justification of a particular exposure
- Following imaging protocols set by the imaging department
- Careful collimation of the beam
- Avoiding repeat exposures

This list is by no means exhaustive, and there are many other ways of reducing patient and staff doses. You should explore these issues more fully in other texts to ensure that you are providing the highest standard of care to the patient by complying with the principle of optimisation (ALARA).

Precautions with early pregnancies

Up to this point our discussion of radiation safety has been concerned with patients, staff and members of the public. However, if a woman is pregnant and needs an examination involving ionising radiation, the potential harm to the fetus has to be considered. One way in which the radiation dose to the fetus can be avoided is by using an alternative investigative technique, such as ultrasound, to establish a diagnosis.

For a woman who is not pregnant the ovaries are considered to be the critical organs being irradiated. The radiation dose risk assessment is based on the potential to produce deterministic and stochastic effects in the woman and any children she may have. However, in the pregnant woman, the critical structure is the fetus. Radiation may produce effects in the fetus and consideration of the radiation dose, fetal age and tissue radiosensitivity is important.

IR(ME)R 2000 states that whenever a female of reproductive capacity is to undergo an examination involving the use of ionising radiation in the area of the pelvis, where appropriate, the pregnancy and breastfeeding status of the woman must be established. Radionuclides are excreted from the body in breast milk, as well as by the more traditional physiological pathways, so radioactivity in the breast milk would result in the infant receiving an unnecessary dose of radiation.

There are two main protocols used in establishing whether the examination should be carried out:

- 28-day rule
- 10-day rule

28-day rule. The patient is asked if she is or might be pregnant. If the answer is no then the examination can proceed. Any other answer requires that the first day of the last menstrual period is established. The procedure to be followed is shown in Fig. 21.6.

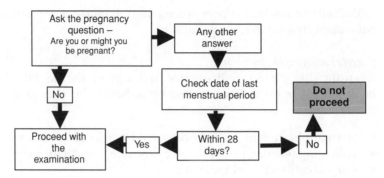

Fig. 21.6   Flow chart for implementation of the 28-day rule.

The 28-day rule is followed for low-dose procedures, which include most routine radiographic investigations where the abdomen or pelvis is irradiated. For examinations where the fetal dose may be in tens of milligray, the 10-day rule should be used.

10-day rule. Any exposure that delivers doses in tens of milligray to the fetus may carry significant risks for the foetus. These examinations include CT of the pelvis and the barium enema. For example, for a barium enema, the risk of the fetus developing a fatal cancer by the age of 15 years is 1 in 5000 (National Radiological Protection Board, 1998). The 10-day rule should therefore be used.

Under the 10-day rule, the examination may proceed only if the woman's menstrual period commenced in the previous ten days. Ten days is used because the chances of a woman being pregnant up to that time are minimal. The procedure is detailed in Fig. 21.7.

21.7.2.3   Personnel monitoring

The Ionising Radiations Regulations 1999 state that staff designated as classified workers must be continuously monitored. Although not required by the regulations, radiographers are also individually monitored. There are two main

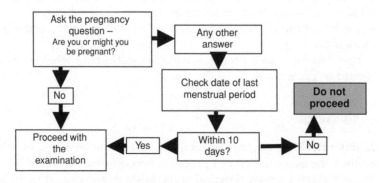

Fig. 21.7   Flow chart for implementation of the 10-day rule.

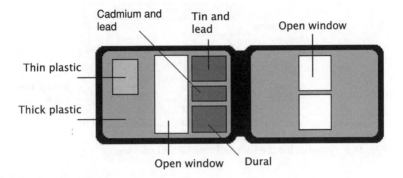

Fig. 21.8 Film badge holder showing the various filters used.

ways in which personnel monitoring is undertaken: film badge dosimetry and thermoluminescent dosimetry.

Film badge dosimetry

For many years, this was the main method of undertaking personnel monitoring. The system is based on the ability of radiation to cause blackening of film. The essential components of the film badge holder are shown in Fig. 21.8.

A small piece of photographic film is used as the radiation detector, similar in size to a periapical dental film. The film has two coatings of emulsion: one fast and one slow. This arrangement allows the film to record a wide range of doses (typically, 0.1–200 mSv). Small doses will be seen on the fast emulsion but high doses would fully blacken this emulsion. For high doses, the fast emulsion is stripped off during the reading process and the high dose is recorded by the slow emulsion. The film badge can therefore measure the small doses that may occur under normal working conditions, and also any high, accidental exposures.

The various filters incorporated into the film badge holder range from no filtration (in the open windows) through to differing thicknesses of plastic and a range of metal filters. The use of these filters allows for an estimation of the radiation energy that has fallen on the monitor. The relative densities on the film behind the various filters allow an estimation of beam quality to be made.

The reading of the film is undertaken by a dose-monitoring service and the results, plus a new piece of film, are supplied for the next monitoring period. The result of the read-out from the film is sent to the RPS of the department.

Thermoluminescent dosimetry

The process of thermoluminescence has been described in Section 19.2.3.1. For personal dosimeters the two detectors are teflon discs impregnated with lithium fluoride. One disc is positioned beneath the open window to monitor skin dose, whilst the other lies under the thick plastic dome and monitors depth dose in the tissues of the body. The teflon discs are fitted into a plastic support which, in turn, is sealed in light-tight wrapping and placed in the holder (Fig. 21.9).

Unlike the film badge dosimeter, a range of filters is not required, because the response of lithium fluoride to radiation is very similar to that of human tissue

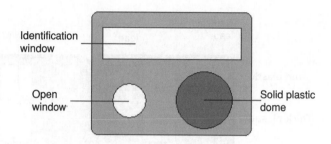

Fig. 21.9   Holder for the thermoluminescent dosimeter.

and it can therefore be considered tissue equivalent. Any dose received and recorded on a thermoluminescent dosimetry (TLD) is therefore a good indicator of tissue dose, regardless of beam quality.

The TLD is returned to the monitoring provider for reading. A major advantage of the TLD over the film badge is that the TLD can be read by a computer and the results are computer generated. Also, the TLD, once heated for the reading process, can be reused.

Both film badge and TLD monitors are classed as retrospective types of monitors, as they record the dose that has been received but have to be read at a later date. Dosimeters are available that monitor in 'real time' the dose falling on them and give an instant read-out on a digital display. Some of the more sophisticated types of real-time monitors also sound an audible alarm to indicate that radiation is being detected.

21.8   Concluding remarks

In this section, we have considered many aspects of radiation safety. However, we strongly recommend that you read this chapter in conjunction with the radiation safety policies and protocols used in your own place of work. Radiation safety is an important responsibility for all radiographers and other workers using ionising radiation and should form a major part of clinical practice. It is only by using radiation in a justified manner that the radiation protection principle of ALARA can be effectively applied.

We have now completed our discussion of those aspects of radiography which involve the use of ionising radiation. In the final two chapters which follow, we explore the physical principles underlying ultrasonography and magnetic resonance imaging.

Chapter 22
Ultrasound

Sound waves
   Frequency
   Speed
   Wavelength
   Attenuation
   The decibel
   Acoustic impedance
   Reflection and refraction
   Doppler effect
Ultrasound
   Pulse–echo principle
   Generation, detection and focusing of ultrasound
Ultrasound image production
   A-scans
   B-scans
   Real-time scanning
   Three- and four-dimensional scanning
   Doppler scanning
Biological effects of ultrasound
Frequently asked questions

22.1 Introduction

Most imaging departments now offer a diagnostic ultrasound scanning service. This is a technique for producing diagnostic images through the use of high-frequency sound waves rather than ionising radiations. One outstanding advantage to be gained is that the risk to the patient is greatly reduced if not eliminated completely. Additionally, it is possible to obtain images of certain anatomical structures which cannot easily be demonstrated by conventional radiography. To understand the physics of ultrasound, we need to firstly study some of the characteristics of sound.

22.1.1 What are sound waves?

It is important to realise that sound waves are *not* a form of electromagnetic radiation. Sound is the process of transferring energy from one place to another by a series of collisions between adjacent molecules in the medium through which the sound is passing. Imagine a row of balls arranged on a snooker table, as shown in Figure 22.1. If we were to strike ball A with our cue, it would impact ball B. This, in turn, would collide with ball C and so on along the entire row.

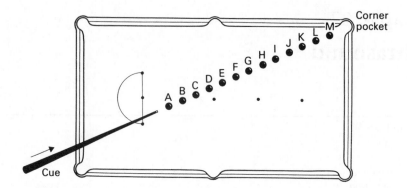

Fig. 22.1 The passage of a disturbance along a row of balls on a snooker table.

Eventually, the last ball (M) would be struck and would (hopefully) drop into the corner pocket.

This illustrates the passage of a single isolated disturbance, but the same logic would apply if ball A was hit repeatedly. The disturbances would pass in sequence along the row of balls. We would see a 'wave' travel along the row. Sound travels through matter in a very similar way as a series of collisions or pressure changes passing through the medium. The disturbances are conveyed more efficiently, and more rapidly, if the individual molecules are closely packed together. The closest molecular packing is found in solid materials; thus, in general, sound waves travel more quickly and with less loss of energy through solids than through liquids or gases.

Sound will not travel at all through a vacuum because there are no molecules present to pass on the disturbances.

22.1.2 Frequency of sound (f)

The rate of repetition of the original disturbances determines the frequency of the sound wave. The human ear is able to detect sounds whose frequencies lie within the range of about 20 Hz up to 20 000 Hz, the **audible frequency** range (1 Hz = one disturbance per second). The note of lowest pitch on a piano has a frequency of about 30 Hz, while 4000 Hz is the highest. Sound frequencies of less than 20 Hz are felt rather than heard, while frequencies above 20 kHz are impossible for us to detect without special equipment. Our ability to hear the higher audible frequencies deteriorates as we get older. Sound of frequency greater than 20 kHz is known as 'ultrasound'. The ultrasound used in diagnostic imaging has a frequency range of 1–15 MHz (1 MHz = 10^6 Hz).

22.1.3 Speed of sound (c)

As we have said, the speed at which sound travels depends on the medium through which it passes. Through air sound travels at 300 m s^{-1}, through water at 1480 m s^{-1} and through iron at about 5000 m s^{-1}. However, these figures are not constant and are affected by prevailing conditions such as temperature

Table 22.1 Speed of sound in different media

Medium	Speed of sound (m s^{-1})
Air	330
Fat	1450
Water	1480
Muscle	1590
Bone	4080

and pressure. However, in all instances sound travels far more slowly than electromagnetic radiation. This explains why we see a flash of lightning before we hear the clap of thunder, even though both are created at the same time.

Table 22.1 gives the values of the speed of sound for various biological tissues and other materials commonly found in the human body.

22.1.4 Wavelength of sound (λ)

The relationship $c = f\lambda$ is as valid for sound waves as it is for electromagnetic waves, but the values of c, f and λ are quite different.

In air, a low-frequency sound, e.g. 20 Hz, has a wavelength of about 16 m, while a sound of 20 kHz has a wavelength of only 16 mm.

Diagnostic ultrasound has its wavelengths in the range 0.02–0.3 mm in air and 0.1–1.5 mm in the body tissues.

22.1.5 Attenuation of sound

As sound is transmitted through a medium it becomes attenuated. Its intensity reduces as its energy is absorbed and dispersed in the medium, and the sound becomes scattered in direction.

The amount by which sound is attenuated depends on a number of factors, e.g.

(1) **The transmitting medium.** A tenuous medium attenuates sound more than a dense medium. (Air is a particularly poor transmitter of sound.)
(2) **The distance travelled.** Sound becomes more attenuated the further it travels.
(3) **The frequency of the sound.** High-frequency sounds are attenuated more than low-frequency sounds, which is why ships' fog horns use low frequencies to give greater range.

N.B. This last point illustrates an important difference between the behaviour of X-rays and sound: the penetration of X-rays increases with frequency, but the penetration of sound waves *reduces* as their frequency increases.

22.1.5.1 The decibel

The fall in sound intensity as sound is attenuated by passage through a medium can be expressed as a fractional change. For example, if the incident intensity is I_0 and the transmitted intensity I_t, then the fractional reduction in intensity is I_t/I_0. In practice, however, it is more convenient to use a *logarithmic* scale to express a fall in intensity. The effect of attenuation may be expressed in **bels** (B), where

$$\text{Attenuation in bels} = \log_{10}(I_t/I_0)$$

but it is more common to use a smaller unit, called the **decibel** (dB), where

$$1 \text{ bel} = 10 \text{ decibel}$$

Therefore, attenuation in decibels $= 10 \log_{10}(I_t/I_0)$.

The decibel scale simplifies the calculation of the combined effect of two (or more) attenuators. The *total* attenuation (expressed in decibels) produced by a combination of different attenuators is given by the arithmetic sum of their individual attenuations (in decibels).

It is important to realise that the decibel scale is a *relative* scale representing a comparison between two quantities (in this case, intensities).

Loudness

The decibel scale is also used to indicate the loudness of sound. In this context, the intensity of sound is compared with a predefined reference value. Table 22.2 shows examples of the loudness of various sounds expressed on the decibel scale. Because of the logarithmic nature of the decibel scale, an incremental change of 10 dB represents a *tenfold* change in sound intensity.

Table 22.2   Loudness of various sounds, expressed on the decibel scale[a]

Sound source	Loudness (dB)
Threshold of hearing	0
Whisper	20
Conversational speech	50
Traffic on busy street	70
Factory noise	80
Thunder	100
Jet aircraft take-off	120
Pain threshold	130
Space rocket launch	140–190

[a] To arrive at these values, the intensity of each sound is compared with the intensity of a standard reference source.
Source: Microsoft (2005).

22.1.6   *Acoustic impedance (z)*

To differentiate between the sound-transmitting properties of different media, the concept of **acoustic impedance** (characteristic impedance) is used. Its value depends on the speed of sound in the medium and the density of the medium:

Acoustic impedance (z) = density (ρ) × speed of sound (c)

or

$$z = \rho c$$

The SI unit of acoustic impedance is the kilogram per square metre per second $(\text{kg m}^{-2}\,\text{s}^{-1})$.

Beams of sound undergo important modifications when they meet a boundary between media of different acoustic impedances.

22.1.7   *Reflection and refraction of sound*

When sound waves meet a boundary or *interface* between two different media, they may suffer sudden changes of direction due to reflections or refractions. Figure 22.2 shows the reflection of sound taking place at an interface. The sound waves bounce off the interface like a ball off a wall.

The angle (i) at which the incident sound wave meets the interface is equal to the angle (r) at which the reflected sound wave leaves; i.e.

Angle of incidence (i) = angle of reflection (r)

If the incident beam is at right angles to the interface $(i = 0)$, the sound will be reflected back on itself, as shown in Fig. 22.3. We shall see later that these special circumstances have a particular significance in ultrasound imaging.

When the two media forming the interface have vastly different values of acoustic impedances, a large fraction of the original sound will be reflected and very little will be transmitted through the interface. For example, this would be

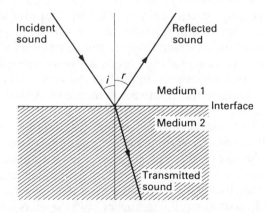

Fig. 22.2   The transmission and reflection of sound at an interface between two media.

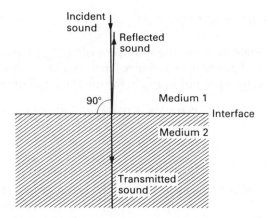

Fig. 22.3   Reflection of sound at 90° to an interface between two media.

the case if the interface were between air and human tissue when over 99% of the sound would be reflected.

Conversely, when the interface is between two very similar media, the reflection would be comparatively weak and most of the sound would be transmitted. Figure 22.2 shows that the transmitted sound wave also suffers a change of direction as it passes through the interface. We say it has been **refracted**. Changes of direction such as this can make it very difficult to determine the true location of the source of a sound wave.

22.1.8   *Doppler effect*

If a sound source is moving towards or away from an observer, the sound appears to undergo a change in frequency. If the source is approaching, the observer perceives the sound frequency to be *higher* than that emitted from the source. Conversely, if the source is receding, the observer perceives the frequency to be *lower* than that of the source.

This phenomenon of apparent frequency change is known as the **Doppler effect**. The change in frequency is called the **Doppler shift**. The magnitude of the Doppler shift depends on the relative speed of approach or recession of the source and the observer. Doppler shift is dramatically demonstrated when an ambulance passes by at high speed while sounding its alarm. The observer experiences the sudden drop in pitch of the siren as the relative motion of the ambulance changes from approach to recession. A similar effect is heard when a low-flying aircraft passes overhead.

Doppler shift can also be experienced if sound is *reflected* from a moving interface. If the interface is moving towards or away from the observer standing alongside the source, the echo appears to have a different frequency from that emitted from the source. If the interface is approaching, the echo is of higher frequency than that of the source. If the interface is receding, the echo is of lower frequency. In both cases, the frequency shift depends on the speed of approach or recession of the interface.

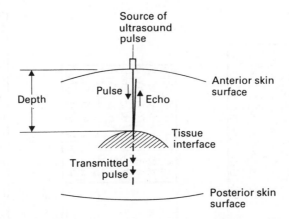

Fig. 22.4 Section through the body showing the echo returning from a tissue interface.

Having discussed some of the general properties of sound we can now concentrate on the special features of ultrasound.

22.2 Pulse–echo principle

The use of ultrasound for diagnostic imaging depends on the so-called **pulse–echo principle**. A short pulse of ultrasound is generated and directed as a narrow beam into the patient's body. Sooner or later the beam will meet an interface between different tissues and reflections will occur. If the interface is orientated correctly (i.e. at 90° to the beam), the reflections will return along the same path as the original pulse and may be detected as an echo (see Fig. 22.4).

The time interval between the generation of the original pulse of ultrasound and the detection of the returning echo, combined with a knowledge of the speed of sound through the tissues, allows an estimate to be made of the total distance travelled by the pulse. The longer the time interval, the greater is the distance travelled because:

Distance travelled = speed of sound × time taken

Halving the total distance travelled gives the depth of the tissue interface (Fig. 22.4). Repeating this process many times in different directions may provide sufficient information about the location of the tissue interfaces to enable a two-dimensional (2D) image to be constructed, showing the relative positions and shapes of the interfaces.

Let us next examine how ultrasound pulses are generated and how the echos are detected.

22.3 Generation of ultrasound

To create a pulse of ultrasound we need to set up mechanical vibrations of the required frequency. We might perhaps imagine that a device such as a loudspeaker

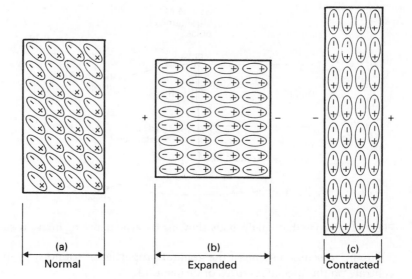

Fig. 22.5 The piezoelectric effect. The diagram shows a crystal whose molecules possess polar properties (see Section 4.4.3). Each polar molecule is represented by an egg-shaped electrical dipole, having a net positive charge at one end and a net negative charge at the other, showing (a) the crystal in its relaxed state; (b) the effect of applying a potential difference across the faces of the crystal, causing the molecules to rotate and the dimensions of the crystal to change, with the transverse dimension being expanded; (c) the effect of reversing the applied potential with the new orientation of the molecules causing the transverse dimension to contract. Note that for the purposes of explanation, the rotation of the molecules has been grossly exaggerated.

could be modified to carry out the task. During its normal operation, the cone or diaphragm of a loudspeaker is forced to vibrate by the rapidly changing magnetic field generated by an alternating electric current. However, if we were to try to force the loudspeaker cone to oscillate at ultrasound frequency, we would fail because the mechanical movements of the system are too sluggish. It has too much inertia.

Instead, we make use of a phenomenon known as the **piezoelectric effect** (see Section 4.4.3). When an electrical potential difference is applied across a crystal of quartz, its polar molecules alter their orientation slightly, causing the thickness of the crystal to change. The crystal expands or contracts according to the polarity of the potential difference applied (see Fig. 22.5). Such crystals possess a *natural frequency* of vibration (known as the **resonant frequency**) whose value depends on the size and shape of the individual crystal. In a similar way church bells each have a natural frequency at which they vibrate when struck. In an ultrasound probe, the piezoelectric crystal is set 'ringing' by the application of a pulse of electricity. The size and shape of the crystal are chosen to provide the crystal with a resonant frequency which corresponds to the frequency of the ultrasound we wish to generate. The crystal's oscillations are made to die away very rapidly, thus producing *a pulse* of ultrasound.

22.4   Detection of ultrasound

As well as creating pulses of ultrasound we need to be able to detect the returning echoes. Luckily, the piezoelectric crystal can also be used as a detector.

If the crystal has mechanical pressure applied to it (i.e. it is 'squeezed') then an electrical potential difference is generated across the crystal. Thus when the echo of a pulse of ultrasound arrives back at the crystal, the crystal is compressed by the pressure wave and a weak electrical signal results. The signal is amplified (magnified) electronically and used to determine the pulse–echo return time.

Because the crystal which generates the ultrasound pulse has also to detect the returning echo, two conditions must be satisfied:

(1)   The crystal must be 'quiet' when the returning echo arrives. It cannot both transmit and receive at the same time. In practice, between 1000 and 10 000 pulses per second may be transmitted from the piezoelectric crystal – the **pulse repetition rate**. Each individual pulse is followed by a short period of quiet, allowing the crystal an opportunity to detect the returning echo.
(2)   The echo should return along the same path as that of the original pulse. If the echo travels in any other direction, it will miss the crystal and only a very weak signal will be detected. From our study of the reflection of sound we know that only when the pulse meets an interface at right angles will this condition be met.

22.5   Focusing an ultrasound beam

An ultrasound beam is better able to resolve fine details of structure in the patient if it is transmitted as a narrow or convergent rather than divergent beam. This requirement for a focused beam may be achieved either by shaping the emitting surface of the piezoelectric crystal or by the use of a **sound lens** through which the beam is transmitted and which produces convergence of the sound by means of refraction. However, even convergent sound beams eventually begin to spread and the focusing effect occurs only over a fairly restricted range (see Fig. 22.6).

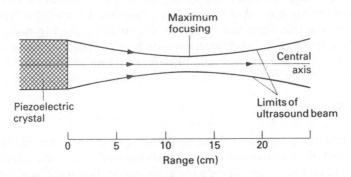

Fig. 22.6   Example of a focused beam of ultrasound.

The higher ultrasound frequencies are more suitable for achieving fine focusing, and thus good resolution, but lack the ability to penetrate deep tissues adequately. The lower frequencies which are more penetrating are not capable of such high resolution of detail. The practical solution is a compromise between adequate penetration and acceptable resolution.

22.6   Producing the image

There are a number of ways in which an image may be constructed from use of the pulse–echo principle described in Section 22.2. The two simplest forms of display are known as the 'A-scan' (or A-mode) and the 'B-scan' (or B-mode).

22.6.1   A-scan

This is the simplest application of the pulse–echo principle. The measure of echo return time from an interface is plotted on the horizontal axis of a graph displayed on the screen of a cathode-ray tube (a primitive TV screen). The vertical axis shows the magnitude of the echo. A value of the speed of sound in tissue is assumed (usually 1540 m s^{-1}) and the horizontal timescale is recalibrated in distance units.

Worked example
What distance would a return time of 0.2 ms signify?

$$\text{Total distance} = \text{speed of sound} \times \text{time}$$
$$= 1540 \times \frac{0.2}{1000}$$
$$= 0.308 \text{ m}$$
$$= 30.8 \text{ cm}$$

However, this is the distance to the interface *and back*. Thus, the depth of the interface must be:

$$\frac{30.8}{2} = 15.4 \text{ cm}$$

Figure 22.7 shows the appearance of an A-scan with several echoes displayed representing a number of interfaces detected. Clearly, this type of image has limited applications but could, for example, be used to make measurements of the distance between interfaces such as the parietal bones of the skull of a fetus. This measurement, the **biparietal diameter**, gives a good indication of fetal maturity and is of great value in the management of pregnancies.

22.6.2   B-scan

In this mode, ultrasound beams pointing in many different directions are employed. Each individual beam records the positions of the interfaces it meets as bright points on the cathode-ray tube screen. Figure 22.8a illustrates four such beams transversing the patient and Fig. 22.8b shows the corresponding screen

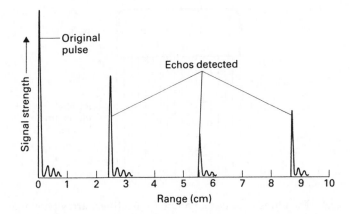

Fig. 22.7 Example of an A-scan showing echos received from interfaces at distances of 2.5, 5.6 and 8.7 cm.

display. In practice, many thousands of points are recorded, giving a screen image of acceptable resolution and continuity of detail. Different echo signal strengths are reproduced as points of differing brightness, giving a so-called **greyscale** image. The image is a 2D representation of a section through the subject.

In the early B-scan equipment a probe containing a *single* piezoelectric crystal was employed. The probe was manipulated by hand with the ultrasound beam directed towards the anatomical features being imaged. In order to build up a complete image of the structure under examination, the beam had to be directed manually at several different angles.

Modern units use multi-element probes. These are probes containing typically 240 individual piezoelectric crystals. In one type of probe, the individual

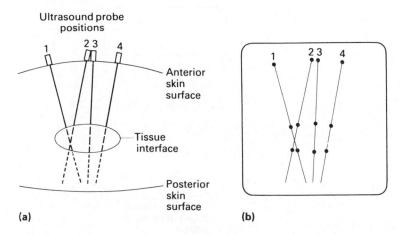

Fig. 22.8 (a) A sample of four ultrasound beams traversing a patient during a B-scan. (b) The cathode-ray tube screen image corresponding to the beam directions shown in (a).

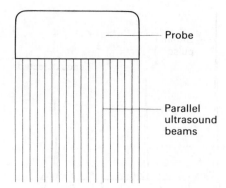

Fig. 22.9 The ultrasound beam pattern from a **linear array** type of multi-element probe.

elements are set parallel to each other in a **linear array** (Fig. 22.9). A second type of multi-element probe, the **sector scanner**, generates an ultrasound beam, which is swept back and forth automatically through an angle of up to 125° (Fig. 22.10). The sweeping action of the beam is produced either by mechanical rotation of the elements inside the probe or by careful phasing of the emission of pulses from the elements.

22.6.3 Real-time scanning

With both sector scanners and linear array probes the image is constructed *instantaneously* on the screen. The image is renewed perhaps 30 times per second, thus updating the position of the structures displayed and demonstrating, *as it*

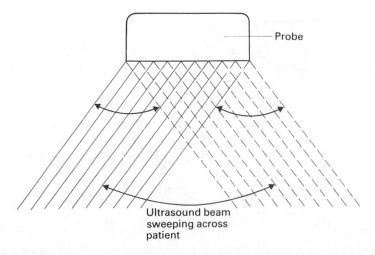

Fig. 22.10 The ultrasound beam pattern from a **sector scanner** type of multi-element probe.

happens, any movement of the anatomical features. This is known as **real-time** scanning.

The B-scan image may be recorded permanently in various ways: by photographing the analogue screen display on film, by capturing an analogue video signal with a videotape recorder or laser imager or by saving the image data in digital format and storing it on an optical disc (e.g. DVD).

22.6.4   Three- and four-dimensional scanning

Conventional ultrasound images are 2D, but if numerous 2D image data are collected sequentially, powerful software can be used to construct a 3D computer model of the structure under study. The model can be rotated on the display screen to improve visualisation of the various tissue planes and anatomical details. The 3D model also permits the creation of images that reproduce the surface contours of a fetus, thus producing a life-like rendering of its appearance.

From 3D images it is possible to move a step further and produce 4D images, the fourth dimension being time. In essence, 4D images are real-time, moving, 3D images. This imaging modality is used, for example, when studying a moving organ, such as the fetal heart, or demonstrating the physical activity of a fetus in the womb. A series of 3D image data are collected by **gated acquisition** over a very short time span. Playing back the resulting images in rapid sequence creates a moving image. Such 4D ultrasound images are often called **dynamic scans**.

22.6.5   Doppler scanning

Modern ultrasound **duplex scanners** can make use of the **Doppler effect** (Section 22.1.8) to detect and measure the movement of anatomical structures within the body, as well as producing B-scan images. One application of Doppler ultrasound is in the investigation of blood flow through arteries and veins or through the heart. The ultrasound beam is detected after being reflected off the cellular components of blood, and the frequency change (**Doppler shift**) is used to determine the rate of flow.

In modern equipment, the Doppler shift information is superimposed as a colour image on top of the normal greyscale B-scan image. Different colours are used to signify different flow rates and directions; e.g. red represents flow towards the transducer, blue flow away from the transducer and yellow turbulent flow. **Doppler colour-flow mapping** is of great value in cardiology and in diagnosing cardiac abnormalities in the human fetus.

22.7   Biological effects of ultrasound

The current position set out in the 2006 revision of the *Clinical Safety Statement for Diagnostic Ultrasound* issued by the European Federation of Societies for Ultrasound in Medicine and Biology (EFSUMB, 2006) is summarised below.

Diagnostic ultrasound has been widely used in clinical medicine for many years, with no proven deleterious effects. However, if used imprudently, diagnostic ultrasound could be capable of producing harmful effects. Ultrasound produces heating, pressure changes and mechanical disturbances in tissue. Diagnostic levels of ultrasound can produce temperature rises that are hazardous to sensitive organs and the embryo or fetus, but no non-thermal biological effects have yet been demonstrated in humans.

In view of the known sensitivity of the embryo and fetus in early pregnancy, and the lack of information on possible subtle biological effects of diagnostic levels of ultrasound on the developing human embryo or fetus, care should be taken to limit the exposure to ultrasound to the minimum commensurate with an acceptable clinical assessment.

Based on scientific evidence of ultrasound-induced biological effects to date, there is no reason to withhold diagnostic scanning during pregnancy, provided it is medically indicated and is used prudently by fully trained operators. This includes routine scanning of pregnant women.

The range of clinical applications and the number of patients undergoing ultrasound examinations are increasing. New techniques with higher acoustic output levels are being introduced. It is therefore essential to maintain vigilance to ensure the continued safe use of ultrasound.

22.8   Frequently asked questions

The detailed operation of ultrasound scanning equipment is beyond the scope of this book, but there are a number of questions that student radiographers often ask, which we shall briefly consider.

22.8.1   *Why is an oil or gel applied to the patients' skin?*

The purpose of these materials is to exclude all the air from between the emitting face of the probe and the patients' skin. The presence of air would cause 99% of the beam to be reflected from the skin surface and thus prevent the passage of ultrasound into the patient. Materials used for this purpose are known as **acoustic coupling agents**.

22.8.2   *What is a transducer?*

A **transducer** is a device which converts energy from one form to another. In diagnostic ultrasound, the probe containing the piezoelectric crystals is often called a transducer because it converts electrical energy into sound and vice versa. (An X-ray tube is also a transducer, although the term is rarely used in this context.)

22.8.3   *What piezoelectric materials do ultrasound scanners employ?*

Quartz is a naturally occurring piezoelectric crystal. However, modern ultrasound scanners generally use more efficient synthetic materials, such as **lead zirconate titanate**, better known as **PZT**.

Chapter 23

Magnetic Resonance Imaging

Basic principles of magnetic resonance imaging
  Precession
  Resonance
  Relaxation
  T_1 and T_2 recovery
  Pulse sequences
MRI equipment
  Magnet
  Gradient coils
  RF coils
  Computer

Introduction

The principle of **nuclear magnetic resonance** spectroscopy has been used for many years to interrogate small samples. In the last 30 years, advances in technology have permitted the development of **magnetic resonance imaging** (MRI) equipment for clinical applications. The subject is a complex one and the purpose of this section is to give the reader a brief introduction to the fundamental principles underpinning MRI and the equipment required to perform MRI.

23.1 Basic principles of MRI

We stated in Section 8.2 that magnetism results from the movement of electric charge. Charged particles inside atoms may exhibit two types of movement, e.g. electrons spinning on their own axes as well as orbiting the nucleus. The particles in the nucleus also spin on their own axes. In nuclei which contain an odd number of nucleons, this spin gives rise to a net magnetic effect or **magnetic moment** and the nucleus resembles a **magnetic dipole** (see Section 8.4). The magnetic moment of the nucleus can be depicted as vector, in which the arrowhead indicates the direction of the magnetic moment and the length of the arrow represents its magnitude (Fig. 23.1). Those nuclei possessing a magnetic moment will interact with an external magnetic field. Table 23.1 shows examples of isotopes whose atomic nuclei exhibit a magnetic moment.

For a number of reasons, $^{1}_{1}\text{H}$, the most common isotope of hydrogen, is the material currently chosen for MRI. Its nuclei contain only a single proton. Hydrogen is chosen because:

- Hydrogen is found in great abundance in body tissues (approximately 10% of body mass).

Table 23.1 Examples of isotopes whose nuclei exhibit a magnetic moment[a]

Isotope	Proton number	Nucleon number
Hydrogen-1	1	1
Carbon-13	6	13
Nitrogen-15	7	15
Oxygen-17	8	17
Fluorine-19	9	19
Sodium-23	11	23
Phosphorus-31	15	31

[a] Note that they all possess odd nucleon numbers. Of the isotopes listed, hydrogen-1 is by far the most abundant in body tissues.

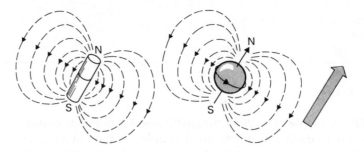

Fig. 23.1 Magnetic field around a bar magnet (left), spinning proton (middle) and corresponding vector diagram (right).

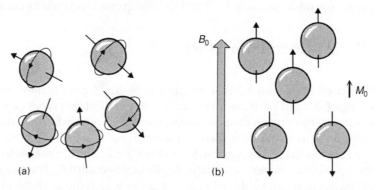

Fig. 23.2 (a) Random orientation of dipoles; (b) dipoles aligned under the influence of the external magnetic field B_0.

- The single proton in the hydrogen nucleus results in a stronger magnetic moment than other elements in the body.

Consequently, hydrogen produces an MR signal 1000 times greater than that from any of the other elements in the body.

   The magnetic moments of spinning protons are orientated randomly (Fig. 23.2a). However, under the influence of a strong external magnetic field, the magnetic moments tend to align themselves with the field. While high-energy protons tend to align themselves *antiparallel* to the applied field (B_0), low-energy protons tend to align *parallel* because they do not have sufficient energy to oppose the applied field (Fig. 23.2b). This results in a small net magnetisation (M_0) in the tissue in the same direction as B_0, known as the longitudinal or Z-axis.

23.1.1 Precession

Although we have said that the spinning protons align themselves with the applied magnetic field, this is not the complete story. In fact, the protons 'wobble' or **precess** around the direction of the applied field (Fig. 23.3a), an effect often compared with the precession of a spinning top. The *frequency* of precession (the number of 'wobbles' per second) depends on the strength (B_0) of the applied magnetic field. Increasing the field strength results in a higher precession frequency (Fig. 23.3b).

For a given strength of applied field, the protons of different elements precess at different frequencies. The frequency of precession (ω), sometimes known as the **Larmor frequency**, is directly proportional to the applied field strength (B_0):

$$\omega \propto B_0$$

so

$$\omega = B_0 \lambda$$

where λ is the constant of proportionality, known as the **gyromagnetic ratio**.

For example, if the applied field strength is 1 T, the frequency of precession for hydrogen is 42.57 MHz, while in a 0.5-T field it is 21.28 MHz. The nuclei of other elements have different values of gyromagnetic ratio, allowing each element

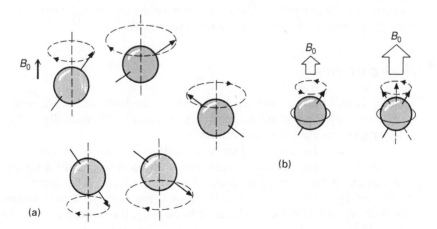

Fig. 23.3 (a) Precession around the longitudinal axis; (b) effect on precessional frequency of increasing the applied field strength.

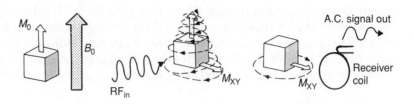

Fig. 23.4   The 90° flip angle following the application of an RF pulse (middle) and detection of the net transverse magnetisation (M_{XY}) as an a.c. signal (right).

to be imaged separately from the others. Unfortunately, the net magnetisation effect on tissue of aligning its hydrogen nuclei is so small compared with the strength of the applied magnetic field that we are unable to measure the effect directly in any useful way.

23.1.2 Resonance

If the precessing hydrogen protons are subjected to a pulse of radio frequency (**RF**) electromagnetic radiation at right angles to the direction of the applied field and at precisely the precessional frequency, the nuclei will absorb energy and their axes of precession can be flipped through an angle of 90°. This matching or tuning of the radio frequency to the precessional frequency is known as **resonance**, and the RF pulse of radiation is known as a **90°RF pulse**. The magnitude of the angle depends on the amplitude and duration of the RF pulse.

Resonance not only results in a change in direction of the net magnetisation from the longitudinal axis to the transverse axis, but also causes the nuclei to precess *in phase* with each other. A radio **receiver coil** situated in the transverse plane and tuned to the precessional frequency will detect this net magnetisation as a voltage (signal). The magnitude of the signal is dependent on the net magnetisation in the transverse plane (see Fig. 23.4).

23.1.3 Relaxation

After the RF pulse is switched off, the net magnetisation (M_0) will again be influenced by the applied magnetic field (B_0) and will gradually realign with it. This process is known as **relaxation**.

As a result of relaxation there is a gradual increase in magnetisation in the longitudinal plane, known as **recovery**, and a corresponding decrease in magnetisation in the transverse plane, known as **decay**. The decrease in signal recorded by the receiver coil in the transverse plane is known as **free induction decay** and its value can be used to measure the proton density of a sample (Fig. 23.5).

During relaxation, two separate events occur, which contribute to the reduction in net transverse magnetisation (M_{XY}).

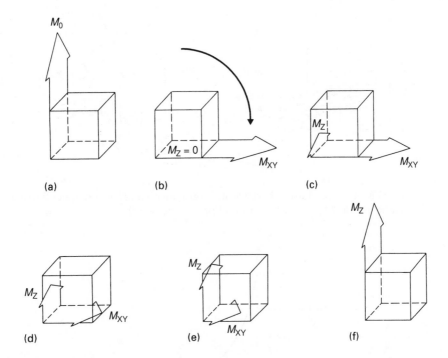

Fig. 23.5 Net transverse magnetisation immediately before (a) and after (b) the application of an RF pulse, where M_0 (longitudinal magnetisation) is zero and M_{XY} (transverse magnetisation) is at a maximum; (c)–(f) show the decay of M_{XY} and regrowth of M_Z over time (spin–lattice relaxation – T_1 recovery).

23.1.4 T_1 recovery

The rate at which recovery to the longitudinal plane occurs is known as **spin–lattice relaxation** (T_1). Recovery follows an exponential pattern, and T_1 is defined as the **time constant** for this relationship, being the time taken for the recovery of 63.2% of the net magnetisation to the longitudinal axis (see also Section 7.11.2.1). Different tissues have different T_1 recovery rates. Fat has a very short T_1 time (about 200 ms), whereas cerebrospinal fluid has a long T_1 recovery time (about 2500 ms). These differences are used to display tissue as a greyscale image.

23.1.5 T_2 recovery

We stated earlier that one of the effects of the RF pulse was to make the protons precess in phase. During relaxation, the decay occurs in the net transverse magnetisation as a result of loss of phase coherence (Fig. 23.6). This is known as **spin–spin relaxation**, and T_2 is the time constant for this decay, being the time taken for the net transverse magnetisation to decay to 36.8% of its original value (Fig 23.7). T_2 decay occurs as nuclei interact magnetically with neighbouring nuclei. Because it takes place much more rapidly than T_1 recovery, T_2 is shorter than T_1.

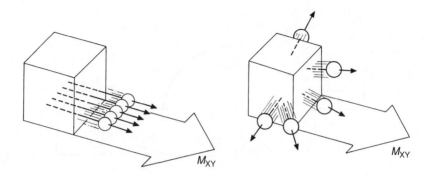

Fig. 23.6   Loss of phase coherence and consequential reduction in net transverse magnetisation M_{XY} (spin–spin relaxation – T_2 recovery).

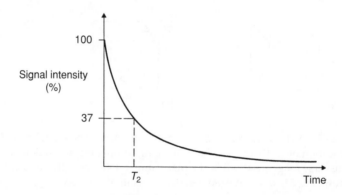

Fig. 23.7 T_2 decay curve.

23.1.6   *Pulse sequences*

An MRI examination will comprise a combination of RF pulses, signal acquisition and recovery times, which are beyond the scope of this text. However, two terms which the reader may encounter are:

(1)   **Repetition time (TR)** – which is the time between sequential applications of the RF pulse
(2)   **Echo time (TE)** – which is the time interval between the application of the RF pulse and the moment when peak signal is detected in the receiving coil (see Fig. 23.8)

By altering the pulse sequence parameters, different weighting can be selected to produce either a predominantly T_1-weighted image or a T_2-weighted image. For example, a TR of 500 ms and a TE of 20 ms will produce a T_1-weighted image, but a TR of 2000 ms and a TE of 80 ms will produce a T_2-weighted image.

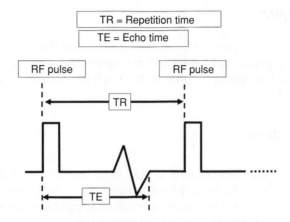

Fig. 23.8 Repetition time (TR) and echo time (TE) in relation to the sequence of RF pulses.

Further study will reveal other sequences such as **saturation recovery**, **inversion recovery** and, more recently, **MAST** and **STIR**!

23.2   Equipment requirements

23.2.1   *Magnet*

A powerful magnet is needed to produce a static uniform external magnetic field. Magnets may be **electromagnets** or **permanent magnets**. Electromagnets are normally **superconductive** (requiring the use of cryogenic materials). Magnetic field strengths range from 0.5 to 3.0 T, up to 30 000 times more powerful than the earth's magnetic field.

23.2.2   *Gradient coils*

Gradient coils are located inside the bore of the magnet to provide linear variations in the field strength along three mutually perpendicular (X, Y and Z) axes. These provide a means of obtaining the spatial resolution necessary to enable different slices to be selected.

23.2.3   *RF coils*

RF coils are used to transmit the RF signal and receive the MR signal from the selected slice (i.e. transceiver coils). Small dedicated **body coils** (e.g. head, neck, knee, shoulder and breast) are normally used to receive the signal, as they can be positioned close to the part under examination to detect weak signals.

23.2.4   Computer

A powerful computer is used to store the raw data and construct the image through a process of **projection reconstruction** similar to that used in computerised tomography. **Spin-warp** or **phase-encoded** methods may also be employed.

23.3   Conclusion

There is clearly much more to MRI than we have been able to include here. However, the basic principles described above will equip the reader to delve further into some of the many specialised texts (e.g. Westbrook et al., 2005) and recent journal articles available on the subject.

Appendix
Maths Help File

The purpose of this *Maths Help File* is to provide additional detail on, and explanation of, the mathematical techniques employed in the main text. This will act as a reminder to readers whose mathematical knowledge is a little rusty and hopefully, will provide welcome clarification for readers to whom *any* maths presents difficulty. The explanations are numbered to facilitate quick reference from the main text. For guidance on how to use this section, see p. xi.

Mathematical index notation and powers of 10

In the imaging sciences, we often have to deal with very large and very small numbers; e.g. X-rays travel at a speed of 300 000 000 m s^{-1}; an electron carries an electric charge of 0.00000000000000000016 C; X-rays have a wavelength of about 0.00000000001 m and a frequency of about 30 000 000 000 000 000 000 cycles per second.

To handle such numbers we use a 'shorthand' method which requires an understanding of the concept of indices or powers of numbers, especially powers of the number 10. For example, for numbers greater than 1:

- 10 can be written 10^1
- 100 10^2
- 1000 10^3
- 10 000 10^4
- 10 000 000 10^7, etc.

Notice that in each case the index is *equal* to the number of noughts in the original number. Using this notation we can write:

- The speed of X-rays as 3×10^8 metres per second
- The frequency of X-rays as 3×10^{19} cycles per second
- A number such as 1 500 000 as either 15×10^5 or 1.5×10^6

For numbers smaller than 1, we can write:

- 1/10 (=0.1) as 10^{-1}
- 1/100 (=0.01) as 10^{-2}
- 1/1000 (=0.001) as 10^{-3}
- 1/10 000 (=0.0001) as 10^{-4}
- 1/10 000 000 (=0.0000001) as 10^{-7}, etc.

Notice that in these cases the index is negative and its value is *one more* than the number of noughts to the right of the decimal point. Using this notation we can write:

- The charge on an electron as 1.6×10^{-19} C
- The wavelength of X-rays as 1×10^{-11} m, or just 10^{-11} m

Multiplication using powers of 10

Multiplication is achieved simply by adding the indices:

- $10^2 \times 10^3 = 10^{2+3} = 10^5$ (because $100 \times 1000 = 100\,000 = 10^5$)
- $10^2 \times 10^{-5} = 10^{2+(-5)} = 10^{-3}$ (because $100 \times 0.00001 = 100/100\,000 = 1/1000 = 10^3$)
- $10^{-12} \times 10^{-2} = 10^{-12+(-2)} = 10^{-14}$ (because $1/1\,000\,000\,000\,000 \times 1/100 = 1/100\,000\,000\,000\,000 = 10^{-14}$)
- $3.5 \times 10^8 \times 2 \times 10^{-5} = 3.5 \times 2 \times 10^{8+(-5)} = 7 \times 10^3$

Division using powers of 10

Division is achieved simply by subtracting the indices:

- $10^3 \div 10^2 = 10^{3-2} = 10^1$ (10) (because $1000 \div 100 = 10$)
- $10^5 \div 10^{-2} = 10^{5-(-2)} = 10^7$ (because $100\,000 \div 0.01 = 100\,000 \div 1/100 = 10\,000\,000$)
- $10^{-5} \div 10^{-2} = 10^{-5-(-2)} = 10^{-3}$ (because $0.00001 \div 0.01 = 1/100\,000 \div 1/100 = 1/100\,000 \div 100 = 1/1000$)
- $10^{-5} \div 10^7 = 10^{-5-7} = 10^{-12}$ (because $0.00001 \div 10\,000\,000 = 1/100\,000 \div 10\,000\,000 = 1/1\,000\,000\,000\,000$)
- $6.4 \times 10^6 \div 3.2 \times 10^{-2} = 2 \times 10^8$ (because $6\,400\,000 \div 0.032 = 6\,400\,000 \div 3.2/100 = (6\,400\,000 \div 3.2) \times 100 = 200\,000\,000$)

Squares and cubes, square roots and cube roots, etc.

To square a number expressed in powers of 10, simply double the index:

- $(10^6)^2$ $=10^{6\times2}$ $=10^{12}$
- $(2.5 \times 10^5)^2$ $=2.5^2 \times 10^{5\times2}$ $=6.25 \times 10^{10}$
- $(10^{-3})^2$ $=10^{-3\times2}$ $=10^{-6}$

To cube a number, multiply the index by 3:

- $(10^2)^3$ $=10^{2\times3}$ $=10^6$, etc.

To take a square root, divide the index by 2:

- $\sqrt{(10^{14})}$ $=10^{14/2}$ $=10^7$
- $\sqrt{(10^{-6})}$ $=10^{-6/2}$ $=10^{-3}$
- $\sqrt{(9 \times 10^6)}$ $=\sqrt{9} \times \sqrt{(10^6)}$ $=3 \times 10^3$

To take a cube root, divide the index by 3.

Miscellaneous points

1.3.1

- Any number raised to the power zero equals 1:

    e.g. $10^0 = 1$, $27^0 = 1$, $y^0 = 1$, etc.

- Fractional indices represent roots of numbers:

    e.g. $10^{1/2}$ (or $10^{0.5}$) $= \sqrt{10}$ (the square root of 10)
    $10^{1/3}$ (or $10^{0.33}$) $= \sqrt[3]{10}$ (the cube root of 10)

- Note also that:

    $10^{3/4}$ (or $10^{0.75}$) $= \sqrt[4]{(10^3)}$ (the fourth root of 10 cubed)

Logarithms

1.4

The logarithm of a to the base b is the power to which b must be raised to equal a. Therefore, the logarithm of a to the base b is c ($\log_b a = c$) if $b^c = a$; e.g. the logarithm of 2 to the base 10 is 0.3 ($\log_{10} 2 = 0.3$) because $10^{0.3} = 2$. Other examples of logarithms to the base 10 are given in Table A.1.

Logarithms expressed to the base 10 are known as **common logarithms**. In mathematics, it is also common to encounter logarithms expressed to the base e, where e is the exponential constant and is approximately equal to 2.718. Logarithms to the base e are known as **natural** or **Napierian logarithms**.

Note that it is not possible to express the quantity zero as a logarithm except in the form minus infinity ($-\infty$), i.e. $\log_{10} 0 = -\infty$ and $\log_e 0 = -\infty$. Consequently, it is not possible to plot the value zero on a graph which uses a logarithmic scale.

Table A.1   Examples of the approximate values of logarithms to the base 10

Number	Log_{10} value (approx.)
1	0
2	0.30
3	0.48
4	0.60
5	0.70
6	0.78
7	0.85
8	0.90
9	0.95
10	1
20	1.30
0.1	-1
0.2	$-1 + 0.30$[a]

[a] Note that logarithmic quantities such as $-1 + 0.30$ are usually written in the form $\bar{1}.30$ and pronounced 'bar one, point three zero'.

1.5 Reciprocals and negative powers

Note that:

- 10^{-2} is the same as $1/10^2$.
- $1/10^{-2}$ is the same as 10^2.

This notation is frequently used in the abbreviations for units of measurement (see Section 1.2.3.1). For example, it is more correct to abbreviate:

- The unit of speed (metres per second) as m s^{-1} than as m/s
- The unit of acceleration (metres per second squared) as m s^{-2} than as m/s^2
- The unit of electric field strength (volts per metre) as V m^{-1} than as V/m

2 Significant figures

The measurement of physical quantities is always an inexact science. It is not possible to measure *any* quantity with absolute accuracy (see also Section 4.5.3). Consequently, when a quantity is expressed in figures, there is a limit to the accuracy implied. For example, we have quoted the value of gravitational acceleration (g) as 9.81 m s^{-2}. This implies that its value could be 9.806 or 9.812, or indeed *any* value between (say) 9.8050 and 9.8149: we have rounded the value to three significant figures, implying that although its value is closer to 9.81 than it is to 9.82 or to 9.80, its value is not *precisely* 9.81 m s^{-2}. When calculations are made involving such approximations, we must remember that the result can be no more accurate than the accuracy of the *least accurate* of the individual values employed in the calculation.

In the calculation of work done (Section 1.3.4.1), the values of mass (50 kg) and distance (25 cm) are quoted to two significant figures. It is not sensible, therefore, to quote the results of our calculation with any greater accuracy than two significant figures; i.e. the final answer should be expressed as 120 J rather than 123 J. In general, the accuracy of the results of a computation should always reflect the accuracy of the individual measurements on which the computation was based. To quote with any greater accuracy is scientifically dishonest, since it misleads the reader!

3 Manipulating an equation (Section 1.3.4.2)

The original form of the equation is:

$$\mathrm{KE} = \frac{1}{2}mv^2$$

but we wish to rearrange the formula to enable us to calculate the value of v. First, interchange the left and right sides of the equation, bringing v to the left-hand side (LHS) of the equation:

$$\frac{1}{2}mv^2 = \mathrm{KE}$$

Now eliminate the $\frac{1}{2}$ factor by multiplying both sides of the equation by 2:

$$2 \times \frac{1}{2}mv^2 = 2 \times KE$$

so

$$mv^2 = 2KE \quad \left(\text{because } 2 \times \tfrac{1}{2} = 1\right)$$

Now eliminate the m factor by dividing both sides of the equation by m:

$$\frac{mv^2}{m} = \frac{2KE}{m}$$

so

$$v^2 = \frac{2KE}{m} \quad \text{(because the } m \text{ factors cancel on the LHS)}$$

The value of v can now be obtained by taking the square root of both sides of the equation:

$$\sqrt{v^2} = \sqrt{(2KE/m)}$$

so

$$v = \sqrt{(2KE/m)} \quad \text{(because the square root of } v^2 \text{ is } v)$$

The general principle involved throughout the manipulation of formulae or equations is always to carry out exactly the same operation on both sides of the equation.

The use of Δ (delta) (Section 2.3.2)

The Greek letter Δ (delta) is frequently used in science to indicate 'a change in' whatever quantity follows it. The Greek letter θ (theta) here represents temperature, so $\Delta\theta$ (delta theta) means change in temperature. A positive value for $\Delta\theta$ represents a *rise* in temperature, while a negative value represents a *fall* in temperature.

Manipulation of formulae (Section 2.3.4)

First, we interchange the left and right sides of the equation:

$$mc\,\Delta\theta = Q$$

Then divide both sides of the equation by the factor mc:

$$\frac{mc\,\Delta\theta}{mc} = \frac{Q}{mc}$$

so

$$\Delta\theta = \frac{Q}{mc} \quad \text{(because the factors } mc \text{ cancel on the LHS)}$$

The general principle involved throughout the manipulation of formulae or equations is always to carry out exactly the same operation on both sides of the equation.

6 Calculus notation (Section 2.4.1)

It is common to represent rates of change by expressions derived from the branch of mathematics called the **calculus**. In the present case, the rate of flow of energy is treated as a rate of change of energy with time and is written in the form:

$$\text{Rate of energy flow} = \frac{dQ}{dt} \quad \text{(pronounced 'dee queue by dee tee')}$$

where dQ ('dee queue') means change of energy and dt ('dee tee') means the change of time (i.e. interval of time) in which the change of energy occurred. In many respects, the use of d to represent the change in a variable is similar to the use of the Greek Δ (delta) that we encountered in Section 2.3.2.

7 Constants of proportionality (e.g. Sections 2.4.1.1, 3.3.4 and 14.3.5.2)

In mathematics, a *proportional* relationship can always be transformed into an equation by the introduction of a factor known as a constant of proportionality. For example, a proportional relationship between two quantities a and b which may be expressed in the form:

$$a \propto b$$

can be transformed into an equation by introducing a constant c, giving:

$$a = b \times c$$

The value of c depends on the precise nature of the quantities a and b. In Section 2.4.1.1, the proportional relationships between dQ/dt and the factors on which it depends can be combined directly into a single equation in which the constant of proportionality (e.g. k or σ) is also one of the factors; e.g.

$$\frac{dQ}{dt} = \frac{k A(\theta_1 - \theta_2)}{l} \quad \text{(for thermal conduction)}$$

and

$$\frac{dQ}{dt} = \sigma AT^4 \quad \text{(for thermal radiation)}$$

Similarly, in Section 3.3.4, the relationship determining the force between two electric charges includes a constant of proportionality (k):

$$F = \frac{kq_1q_2}{d^2}$$

Calculus notation (Section 3.3.3)

The expression dq/dt is a further example of the use of the symbolism employed in the branch of mathematics known as the **calculus**. It merely means the rate of change of electrical charge (q) with respect to time (t) – in other words, the rate of flow of charge.

The value of pi (π) (Section 2.4.1.1)

The mathematical constant **pi** (π) is defined as the ratio of the length of the circumference of a circle to its diameter. Because its value cannot be expressed precisely either as a fraction or as a decimal number, pi is known as an **irrational number**. Expressed decimally, the first eight digits of pi are 3.1415926.... In Section 2.4.1.1, we have used 3.14 as an approximation for pi, correct to three significant figures.

Calculus notation (Sections 5.2.6 and 9.4)

As we saw in Chapter 2, the **calculus** notation is often employed to denote rates of change. Here, changes in potential (V) with respect to distance (x), flux linkage (N) with respect to time (t), and current (I) with respect to time (t) can be written in the form dV/dx, dN/dt and dI/dt, respectively.

Manipulation of formulae (Sections 6.2.1.1)

First, multiply both sides of the equation by the factor V:

$$VC = \frac{VQ}{V}$$

so

$$VC = Q \quad \text{(because the factor } V \text{ cancels on the RHS of the equation)}$$

Then divide both sides of the equation by the factor C:

$$\frac{VC}{C} = \frac{Q}{C}$$

so

$$V = \frac{Q}{C} \quad \text{(because the factor } C \text{ cancels on the LHS of the equation)}$$

Remember, the general principle involved throughout the manipulation of formulae or equations is always to carry out exactly the same operation on both sides of the equation.

12 The value of the exponential constant (*e*) (Section 7.11.2.1)

The value of the mathematical **exponential constant** (*e*) cannot be expressed precisely either as a fraction or as a decimal number. Like pi (π), it is an **irrational number**. On a typical eight-digit electronic calculator, the value of *e* is given as 2.7182818. In the worked examples which follow Section 7.11.2.2, we have used 2.72 as an approximation for *e*, correct to three significant figures.

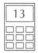

13 Manipulation of exponential formulae (Section 7.11.2.2, worked example 4)

The task is to isolate the factor *t* from the exponential equation:

$$I = I_0 e^{-t/T}$$

First, interchange the LHS and RHS of the equation to bring *t* to the left side:

$$I_0 e^{-t/T} = I$$

Next, eliminate I_0 from the LHS by dividing both sides by I_0:

$$e^{-t/T} = \frac{I}{I_0}$$

However, $e^{-t/T}$ is the reciprocal of $e^{t/T}$; in other words, $e^{-t/T} = 1/e^{t/T}$. So,

$$\frac{1}{e^{t/T}} = \frac{I}{I_0}$$

Inverting both sides gives:

$$e^{t/T} = \frac{I_0}{I}$$

Now take the natural logarithmic value of both sides (i.e. the log to the base *e*):

$$\log_e e^{t/T} = \log_e \frac{I_0}{I}$$

so

$$\frac{t}{T} = \log_e \frac{I_0}{I} \quad \text{(By definition, the log }_e e^a = a.)$$

Multiply both sides by *T* to eliminate *T* from the LHS:

$$\frac{T \times t}{T} = T \log_e \frac{I_0}{I}$$

so

$$t = T \log_e (I_0/I) \quad \text{(The factor } T \text{ cancels on the LHS.)}$$

Remember once again that the general principle involved throughout the manipulation of formulae or equations is always to carry out exactly the same operation on both sides of the equation.

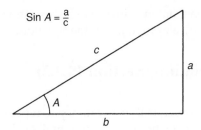

Fig. A.1 The sine of an angle. In the right-angled triangle shown, the sine of angle *A* is the ratio of the length (*a*) of the side opposite *A* to the length (*c*) of the hypotenuse: $\sin A = a/c$.

Sine of an angle and sine waves (Sections 10.2.1.1 and 14.3.1)

A sine is a mathematical function derived from the branch of mathematics known as trigonometry. It is one way of expressing the magnitude of an angle. In a right-angled triangle, such as that shown in Fig. A.l, the sine of the angle *A* is the ratio of the length (*a*) of the side of the triangle, which is *opposite* to the angle *A*, to the length (*c*) of the *hypotenuse* of the triangle:

$$\sin A = \frac{a}{c}$$

The sine of an angle of zero degrees is *zero* ($\sin 0° = 0$). As the angle is increased in size, the sine value also increases up to a maximum of 1 when the angle is 90° ($\sin 90° = 1$). Increasing the angle beyond 90° results in the sine of the angle decreasing through *zero* for an angle of 180° ($\sin 180° = 0$) to a negative maximum of −1 for an angle of 270° ($\sin 270° = -1$). Continuing the angle through a full circle (360°) brings the sine value back to zero ($\sin 360° = 0$). Further increases in the angle repeat the cycle of change in the value of the sine of the angle.

If a graph is plotted of the value of the sine of an angle against the value of the angle, this cyclic nature of sine values is clearly demonstrated (Fig. A.2). The characteristic wave-like pattern of the graph is known as a **sine wave**. Many

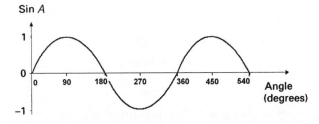

Fig. A.2 The characteristic shape of a sine wave. The graph shows how the value of the sine of an angle changes with the value of the angle itself. The pattern is repeated every 360° for both positive and negative angles.

natural wave phenomena, such as electromagnetic waves, can be modelled mathematically by employing the sine function.

 ## Calculus notation (Section 14.3.3)

As we have seen previously, it is common to represent rates of change by expressions derived from the branch of mathematics called the **calculus**. In the present case, the rate of flow of energy is treated as a rate of change of energy with time and is written in the form:

$$\text{Rate of energy flow} = \frac{dE}{dt} \quad \text{(pronounced 'dee ee by dee tee')}$$

where dE ('dee ee') means change of energy and dt ('dee tee') means the change of time (i.e. interval of time) in which the change of energy occurred.

 ## Logarithmic straight-line graphs (Sections 17.1.1 and 19.3.3.1)

The general equation describing a straight line is of the form:

$$y = mx + c$$

where y is the quantity plotted on the vertical axis, x is the quantity plotted on the horizontal axis, m is a constant which determines the angle of slope of the line and c is a constant which determines the point at which the line intersects the x and y axes.

For the straight-line graph shown in Fig. 17.5, the quantity plotted on the vertical axis is the logarithmic value of the dosimeter reading Q, while the quantity plotted on the horizontal axis is the attenuator thickness x. The general equation $y = mx + c$ therefore becomes:

$$\log Q = mx + c$$

This can be rewritten in the form:

$$Q = e^{mx+c} \quad \text{(because by definition, if } \log_e a = b, \text{ then } a = e^b)$$

but

$$e^{mx+c} = e^{mx} \times e^c \quad \text{(Adding indices is equivalent to multiplying the quantities.)}$$

so

$$Q = e^{mx} \times \text{constant} \quad \text{(The quantity } e^c \text{ is a constant.)}$$

and

$$Q \propto e^{mx} \quad (e^c \text{ is a constant of proportionality.)}$$

Remember that m determines the slope of the straight line. If the line slopes downwards to the right, as in Fig. 17.5, m has a *negative* value. In the context of beam attenuation, m is given the value $-\mu$, so:

$$Q \propto e^{-\mu x}$$

Manipulation of exponential formulae (Section 17.1.2.1)

From the relationship $I = I_0 e^{-\mu x}$, we wish to separate out the factor μ. The first step is to isolate the term $e^{-\mu x}$ (by dividing both sides of the equation by I_0) and place it on the LHS of the equation:

$$e^{-\mu x} = I/I_0$$

Then take logarithms of both sides of the equation:

$$-\mu x = \log_e I/I_0 \quad \text{(because by definition, } \log_e e^a = a\text{)}$$

Now divide both sides by $-x$:

$$\mu = \frac{-1}{x} \log_e I/I_0$$

Remember once again that the general principle involved throughout the manipulation of formulae or equations is always to carry out exactly the same operation on both sides of the equation.

'Correction' of the negative sign (Section 17.1.2.1)

The fraction I/I_0 is always less than 1 because the transmitted intensity is always less than the incident intensity. This gives a negative value for $\log_e I/I_0$ because the log of *any* number less than 1 is negative. Consequently, when this negative value is multiplied by the term $-1/x$, the result is always a positive value for μ.

Decay constant (λ) and half-life ($T_{\frac{1}{2}}$) (Section 20.3.2.3)

It is a straightforward matter to deduce the relationship $\lambda = 0.693/T_{\frac{1}{2}}$ from the general equation:

$$A = A_0 e^{-\lambda t}$$

First, isolate the term $e^{-\lambda t}$ and bring it to the LHS of the equation:

$$e^{-\lambda t} = A/A_0 \quad \text{(by dividing both sides of the equation by } A_0\text{)}$$

Next, take logarithms of both sides of the equation:

$$-\lambda t = \log_e A/A_0 \quad \text{(By definition, } \log_e e^a = a.\text{)}$$

Now isolate the decay constant λ on the LHS of the equation by dividing both sides by $-t$:

$$\lambda = \frac{-1}{t} \log_e A/A_0$$

However, when the time period (t) is equal to the half-life ($T_{\frac{1}{2}}$), by definition, the ratio $A/A_0 = \frac{1}{2} = 0.5$, so that

$$\lambda = \frac{-1}{T_{\frac{1}{2}}} \log_e 0.5$$

and

$$\lambda = \frac{-1}{T_{\frac{1}{2}}} \times -0.693$$

(because $\log_e 0.5 = 0.693$ from the 'ln' function on a calculator)

Therefore

$$\lambda = \frac{0.693}{T_{\frac{1}{2}}}$$

Derivation of $n = n_0 e^{-\lambda t}$ (Section 20.3.2.2)

Readers familiar with the **integral calculus** may wish to examine how the expression $n = n_0 e^{-\lambda t}$ is derived from the expression $dn/dt = -\lambda n$.

First, rearrange the expression by dividing both sides by n and multiplying both sides by dt:

$$\frac{dn}{n} = -1 dt$$

Now, integrate both sides:

$$\int \frac{dn}{n} = \int -1 dt$$

$$\log_e n = -\lambda t + \text{constant}$$

However, when $t = 0$, $n = n_0$; therefore, the constant $= \log_e n_0$, so that

$$\log_e n = -\lambda t + \log_e n_0$$

$$\log_e n - \log_e n_0 = -\lambda t \quad \text{(subtracting } \log_e n_0 \text{ from both sides)}$$
$$\text{of the equation)}$$

$$\log_e (n/n_0) = -\lambda t \quad \text{(because } \log a - \log b = \log a/b)$$

so

$$n/n_0 = e^{-\lambda t} \quad \text{(because if } \log_e a = b, \text{ then } a = e^b)$$

and

$$n = n_0 e^{-\lambda t} \quad \text{(multiplying both sides of the equation by } n_0)$$

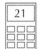

Manipulation of formulae (Section 20.3.2.3, worked example 2)

We wish to manipulate the expression $A = A_0 e^{-\lambda t}$ to bring the term $e^{-\lambda t}$ to the LHS of the equation.

First, interchange the LHS and RHS of the equation:

$$A_0 e^{-\lambda t} = A$$

Then divide both sides by A_0.

$$e^{-\lambda t} = A/A_0 \quad (A_0 \text{ cancels on the LHS of the equation.})$$

Remember once again that the general principle involved throughout the manipulation of formulae or equations is always to carry out exactly the same operation on both sides of the equation.

References and Bibliography

Adams T. J. (1995) *A comparative study of plain radiography and radionuclide imaging of the carpal bones following injury*. HDCR thesis, College of Radiographers.

Aird E. G. A. (1988) *Basic Physics for Medical Imaging*. Heinemann Medical Books, Oxford.

Arnold M. (1994) Through the magnifying glass: the curious world of quantum physics. *Radiography Today*, **60**, 15–18.

Ball J. & Price T. (1995) *Chesneys' Radiographic Imaging*. Blackwell Science, Oxford.

Blackwell R. (1988) Safety of diagnostic ultrasound. In *Practical Ultrasound* (ed. R. A. Lerski). IRL Press, Oxford.

Breithaupt J. (1995) *Understanding Physics for Advanced Level*. Stanley Thornes, Cheltenham.

Cancer Research UK (2004) *Radon gas in ordinary homes increases lung cancer risk, particularly for smokers*. Cancer Research UK Press Release, 21 December 2004, accessed 2 October 2007 from http://info.cancerresearchuk.org/news/archive/pressreleases/2004/december/62528.

Carter P. H. (ed.) (1994) *Chesneys' Equipment for Student Radiographers*. Blackwell Science, Oxford.

Cayless M. A. & Marsden A. M. (eds.) (1997) *Lamps and Lighting*. Edward Arnold, London.

Close F. (1992) The quark structure of matter. In *The New Physics* (ed. P. Davies). Cambridge University Press, Cambridge.

Cutnell J. D. & Johnson K. W. (2007) *Physics*. John Wiley, New York.

Darton M. & Clark J. O. E. (1994) *The Dent Dictionary of Measurement*. Dent, London.

Davison M. (1982) X-ray computed tomography. In *Scientific Basis of Medical Imaging* (ed. P. N. T. Wells). Churchill Livingstone, Edinburgh.

Dinman B. D. (1980) The reality and acceptance of risk. *Journal of the American Medical Association*, **244**, 1226.

Duffin W. J. (1990) *Electricity and Magnetism*. McGraw-Hill, Berkshire.

Epp E. R. & Weiss H. (1966) Experimental study of the photon energy spectrum of primary diagnostic X-rays. *Physics in Medicine and Biology*, **11**, 235.

European Federation of Societies for Ultrasound Medicine and Biology (EFSUMB) (2006) *Clinical Safety Statement for Diagnostic Ultrasound – 2006 Revision*, accessed 24 June 2007 from http://www.efsumb.org/ (home page).

Evans G. (1991) *An evaluation of high kilovoltage chest radiography*. HDCR thesis, College of Radiographers.

Fullick P. (1994) *Physics*. Heinemann Advanced Science, London.

Graham D. T., Cloke P. J. & Vosper, M. (2007) *Principles of Radiological Physics*. Churchill Livingstone, Edinburgh.

Hale J. & Thomas J. W. (1985) Radiation risks for patients having X-rays. *Nurse Practitioner*, **10**, 12.

Hall E. J. (1990) *Radiobiology for the Radiologist*. Lippincott, Philadelphia.

Halliday D., Resnick R. & Walker J. (2001) *Fundamentals of Physics*. John Wiley, New York.

Hawking S. W. & Mlodinow L. (2005) *A Briefer History of Time*. Bantam Books, London.

Hay G. A. (1982) Traditional X-ray imaging. In *Scientific Basis of Medical Imaging* (ed. P. N. T. Wells). Churchill Livingstone, Edinburgh.

Health Protection Agency (2005a) *Essex HPU Factsheet on Air Quality – Radiation*. HPA website, accessed 2 October 2007 from http://www.hpa.org.uk/essex/factsheets/radiatn.htm.

Health Protection Agency (2005b) HPA website, accessed 2 October 2007 from http://www.hpa.org.uk/radiation/.

Her Majesty's Stationery Office (1974) *Health and Safety at Work etc Act 1974*. HMSO, London. Online at Health and Safety Executive website, accessed 2 October 2007 from http://www.hse.gov.uk/legislation/hswa.pdf.

Her Majesty's Stationery Office (1993) *Radioactive Substances Act 1993*. HMSO, London. Online at Office of Public Sector Information website, accessed 2 October 2007 from http://www.opsi.gov.uk/acts/acts1993/Ukpga_19930012_en_1.htm.

Her Majesty's Stationery Office (1995) *The Radioactive Substances (Hospitals) Exemption (Amendment) Order 1995*. Statutory Instrument 1995 No. 2395. HMSO, London.

Her Majesty's Stationery Office (1999) *The Ionising Radiations Regulations 1999*. Statutory Instruments 1999 No. 3232. HMSO, London.

Her Majesty's Stationery Office (2000) *The Ionising Radiation (Medical Exposure) Regulations 2000*. Statutory Instruments 2000 No. 1059. HMSO, London.

Her Majesty's Stationery Office (2006) *The Ionising Radiation (Medical Exposure) (Amendment) Regulations 2006*. Statutory Instruments No. 2523. HMSO, London.

Hey T. & Walters P. (2003) *The New Quantum Universe*. Cambridge University Press, Cambridge.

Horder A. (1971) *The Manual of Photography, Formerly the Ilford Manual of Photography*. Chilton Book Co., Philadelphia.

Hutchings R. (1990) *Physics*. Macmillan, London.

IEC (2001) *Safety of laser products Part 1: Equipment classification and requirements: IEC 60825-1*. International Electrotechnical Commission, Geneva.

International Commission on Radiological Protection (1990) Recommendations of the International Commission on Radiological Protection 1990. *Annals of the ICRP*, **21**(1–3). ICRP Publication 60.

Jackson F. I. (1964) The air-gap technique; and an improvement by anteroposterior positioning for chest roentgenography. *American Journal of Radiology*, **42**, 688–691.

Jaundrell-Thompson F. & Ashworth W. J. (1970) *X-ray Physics and Equipment*. Blackwell Scientific Publications, Oxford.

Jenkins F. A. & White H. E. (2001) *Fundamentals of Optics*. McGraw-Hill, New York.

Kaye G. W. C. & Laby T. H. (1995) *Tables of Physical and Chemical Constants*. Longman, New York. Online at the National Physical Laboratory website, accessed 24 June 2007 from http://www.kayelaby.npl.co.uk/.

Kraus J. D. & Marhefka R. J. (2002) *Antennas For All Applications*. McGraw-Hill, New York.

Kreel L. (1979) *Medical Imaging CT U/S IS NMR – A Basic Course*. HM+M, Aylesbury.

Lawrence D. J. (1977) Kodak X-omatic and Lanex screens and Kodak films for medical radiography. *Medical Radiography and Photography*, **53**, 2.

Microsoft (2005) *Encarta Reference Library – Premium 2005*. DVD-ROM. Microsoft Corporation, USA.

Minchin S. L. (1996) *An audit of pregnancy checking procedures prior to X-ray examination*. BSc thesis, University of Wales College of Medicine.

Moore P. & Hunt G. (1997) *The Atlas of the Solar System*. Chancellor Press, London.

Muncaster R. (1993) *A-Level Physics*. Stanley Thornes, Cheltenham.

National Physical Laboratory (NPL) (2007) *The Avogadro Project*. National Physical Laboratory, accessed 24 June 2007 from http://www.npl.co.uk/mass/avogadro.html.

National Radiological Protection Board (1998) *Diagnostic Medical Exposures. Advice on exposure to ionising radiation during pregnancy*. NRPB, HMSO, London.

Nelkon M. & Parker P. (1995) *Advanced Level Physics*. Heinemann, Oxford.

Oborne D. J. (1995) *Ergonomics at Work*. John Wiley, New York.

Oshorn A. G., Hendrick R. E. & Kanal E. (1992) *Introduction to Magnetic Resonance Imaging – A Basic Primer*. Nycomed, Oslo, Norway.

Ott R. J., Flower M. A., Babich J. W. & Marsden P. K. (1988) The physics of radioisotope imaging. In *The Physics of Medical Imaging* (ed. S. Webb). Institute of Physics Publishing, Bristol.

Ramsey L. J. (1970) Origin of British X-ray film sizes. *Radiography*, **36**, 191.

Ridgway A. & Thumm W. (1973) *The Physics of Medical Imaging*. Addison-Wesley, Reading, MA.

Siel (undated) *Siel X-ray Quality Assurance Products* (Product catalogue). Siel Imaging Equipment Ltd., Aldermaston.

Stather J. (1994) Visual display units – report of an advisory group on non-ionising radiation (Chairman Sir Richard Doll). *NRPB Radiological Protection Bulletin*, **154**, 6–10.

Sternheim M. M. & Kane J. W. (1991) *General Physics*. John Wiley, New York.

Thorpe J. S. (1949) Electron focusing in a demountable X-ray tube. *Journal of Scientific Instruments*, **26**, 203.

Watson J. (1988) *Optoelectronics, Tutorial Guides in Electronic Engineering*, Vol. 14. Van Nostrand Reinhold, London.

Wegener O. H. (1992) *Whole Body Computed Tomography*. Blackwell Science, Oxford.

Westbrook C. (1999) *Handbook of MRI Technique*. Blackwell Publishing, Oxford.

Westbrook C., Kaut Roth C. & Talbot, J. (2005) *MRI in Practice*. Blackwell Publishing, Oxford.

Wilson F. A. (1993) *An Introduction to Satellite Communications*. Babani, London.

Wilson J. & Hawkes J. F. B. (1987) *Lasers – Principles and Applications*. Prentice Hall, Hemel Hempstead.

Workman A. & Cowen A. R. (1994) Tutorial on the image quality characteristics of radiographic screen-film systems and their measurement. Medical Devices Directorate Evaluation Report, MDD/94/34. HMSO, London.

Young H. D. & Freedman R. A. (1996) *University Physics*. Wesley Publishing, Reading, MA.

Index